GOOD AND BAD FOOD SCIENCE

Separating the wheat from the chaff

Good and Bad Food Science

Separating the wheat from the chaff

Leo Goeyens

ASP

Boekverzorging: theSWitch
Coverontwerp: Stephanie Jacobs

© 2019 Academic and Scientific Publishers nv
Keizerslaan 34 B
1000 Brussels
Tel. +32 (0) 2 289 26 56
Fax +32 (0) 2 289 26 59
info@aspeditions.be
www.aspeditions.be

ISBN 978 90 5718 878 7
NUR 913
Legal deposit D/2019/11.161/028

Content

Preface

Préface

I would first like to say that I have never before read a book such as this: richly documented with clarity and precision and in question and answer format. The book is like no other and could also have been entitled "Looking for Front Runners in the Field of Sustainability".

Building on his PhD in Chemistry and teaching qualifications in higher education and drawing on his experience in the field, author Leo Goeyens has collaborated either as main contributor or in a coordinating capacity on roughly 100 publications published in prestigious scientific journals including "Science of the Total Environment" and "Food Additives & Contaminants" and others published by Kluwer Academic Publisher.

In partnership with Luc Pussemier – international expert in sanitary and environmental risk assessment – two books were produced: "AgricultureS et Enjeux de

D'emblée j'affirme n'avoir jamais lu un ouvrage pareil, abondamment documenté avec clarté et précision, sous forme de questions et réponses. Il ne ressemble à aucun autre livre et pourrait s'intituler : « Looking for Front Runners in the field of sustainability ».

L'auteur Leo Goeyens, fort de son doctorat en chimie et de son agrégation de l'enseignement supérieur, associés tous les deux à son expérience sur le terrain, a collaboré soit comme principal auteur soit comme coordonnateur à une centaine de publications parues dans des revues scientifiques prestigieuses comme : « Science of the Total Environment », « Food Additives & Contaminants », ou encore celles produites par « Kluwer Academic Publisher ».

En partenariat avec Luc Pussemier, expert international en évaluation des risques sanitaires et environnementaux, il a écrit deux livres : « AgricultureS et Enjeux de

Société" and "Landbouwsystemen en Maatschappelijke Uitdagingen", both published by Presses Universitaires de Liège.

As soon as you start reading you realise that the author belongs to the world of analytical chemistry and scientific research.

Not only is Leo Goeyens an entertaining story-teller – his account of the extinction of hamsters in Europe is quite revealing in this respect — but he is also a teacher determined to objectively inform his readers about the impact of chemistry on the health of living beings, on the state of our environment and on the potential for the sustainable development of society.

Leo Goeyens reminds us that chemistry is at the crossroads of technosciences, those nano-bio-info-cogno-sciences and technologies, inextricably linked, paradigms of transhumanism, the scientific, intellectual and cultural movement in rapid development aimed at improving living conditions in the world.

But Leo Goeyens also produces many concrete examples (maize monocultures, glyphosate in Roundup, endocrine-disrupting Biphenol A) to show that alongside pure

Sociétés » ainsi que « Landbouwsystemen en Maatschappelijke Uitdagingen », parus aux Presses universitaires de Liège.

Dès les premières pages du présent ouvrage on devine que leur auteur appartient au monde de la chimie analytique et de la recherche scientifique.

Outre ses qualités narratives (lire l'extinction des hamsters en Europe) le livre contient de nombreux éléments pédagogiques décrits dans l'intention d'informer objectivement de l'impact de la chimie sur la santé des êtres vivants, sur l'état de notre environnement et sur le développement durable potentiel pour notre société.

Leo Goeyens rappelle que la chimie se trouve au carrefour des technosciences, ces nano-bio-info-cogno sciences et techniques, sœurs jumelles, paradigmes du transhumanisme, mouvement scientifique intellectuel et culturel en développement rapide destiné à l'amélioration des conditions de vie dans le monde.

Mais voilà que l'auteur nous dévoile par de multiples exemples concrets (p.ex. les monocultures de maïs, le glyphosate dans le Roundup, le Biphénol A perturbateur

science – a factor of progress developed in industrial and university laboratories — there is also a fake science akin to fraud, developed by experts working to further private vested interests to the detriment of the general interest, which is to preserve the Common Good.

These deviant experts stand in the way of the beneficial effects revealed by fundamental and applied science. These effects include, e.g., the antioxidant and antibacterial properties of cinnamon, vitamin A enriched bananas, astaxanthin — a pigment of the carotenoids family used in biodegradable packaging etc.

We follow the author when he denounces the ruthlessness of scientific counterfeiters who take no account of the risk associated with mixing a basic molecule, which may as such be inoffensive, with surfactant additives to arrive at a finished product that could turn out to be a dangerous "cocktail". By way of example, the author describes how the glyphosate molecule was mixed with other ingredients to produce the herbicide Roundup whose use is harmful to human health.

endocrinien, …) qu'à côté de cette science pure, moteur de progrès créé dans des laboratoires industriels et universitaires, se développe une fausse science assimilable à une imposture, pratiquée par des experts à la solde d'intérêts particuliers au détriment de l'intérêt général soucieux du Bien Commun.

Ces experts déviants font obstacle à la progression des effets bénéfiques due à la science fondamentale et appliquée développée par la méthode scientifique (p.ex. la cannelle au rôle antioxydant et antibactérien, la banane enrichie en vitamine A, l'astaxanthine, pigment de la famille des caroténoïdes utilisé dans les emballages biodégradables, …).

Nous suivons l'auteur lorsqu'il montre avec lucidité que ces faussaires de la science négligent la prise en compte de la dangerosité du mélange d'une molécule de base qui peut être inoffensive avec des additifs surfactants ajoutés pour aboutir au produit fini à mettre sur le marché. Il s'agit de l'effet cocktail. Leo Goeyens cite l'exemple de la molécule de glyphosate qui par mélange avec des ingrédients essentiels donne l'herbicide « Roundup » dont l'usage affecte dangereusement la santé.

Leo Goeyens is inspired by the ethical standards of the famous mathematician and philosopher James Clifford – standards which all research workers should observe. In his essay, The Ethics of Belief, which he presented to the Metaphysical Society in 1876, Clifford was revealed as an early advocate of what today is known as the Precautionary Principle.

Clifford argued that it is wrong always, everywhere, and for anyone to believe anything on insufficient evidence. In the face of gradual encroachment by non-scientific science to the detriment of academic integrity, it has become more urgent than ever to reiterate the need to investigate the evidence.

Researchers have an intellectual and moral duty to analyse all the available evidence to eliminate any doubt and to use their free and sovereign judgement.

Here, it is worth recalling how freedom of speech was defined by the Mathematician Henri Poincarré in an address at the Université Libre de Bruxelles: "Thought must never submit, neither to a dogma, nor to a party, nor to a passion, nor to an interest, nor to a preconceived idea, nor

L'auteur dans cette problématique s'inspire de l'éthique de la croyance qui doit être propre aux chercheurs, proposée en 1876 par James Clifford, célèbre mathématicien et philosophe. Dans son exposé à la Metaphysical Society, intitulé « The Ethics of Belief » Clifford se pose en précurseur du fameux Principe de Précaution.

Selon cette éthique on a tort, partout et toujours, qui que l'on soit, de croire sur la base d'éléments de preuve insuffisants. Enquêter sur ces preuves est un impératif qu'il demeure urgent de rappeler, devant l'emprise progressive d'une science non scientifique au détriment de l'intégrité académique.

Le chercheur a le devoir d'enquêter sur la validité des preuves considérées afin d'éliminer les doutes, de se servir de son entendement, libre et souverain.

Il convient ici de se rappeler la définition de la liberté de pensée énoncée par le mathématicien Henri Poincaré à l'Université Libre de Bruxelles : « La pensée ne doit jamais se soumettre, ni à un dogme, ni à un parti, ni à une passion, ni à un intérêt, ni à une idée préconçue,

to whatever it may be, save to the facts themselves, because, for thought, submission would mean ceasing to be."

International institutions like ECODA (European Confederation of Directors' Associations) should constitute an ethics-based core common to all business enterprises operating in the life sciences sector that are committed to preserving diversity as a real source of wealth. This core of enterprises would defend the values and set the moral standards that all enterprises and researchers are expected to observe.

To conclude, this is a must-read book for all those among us who are eager to remain in good health and are anxious to contribute to building a sustainable future for the planet.

ni à quoi que ce soit, si ce n'est aux faits eux-mêmes, parce que pour elle se soumettre ce serait cesser d'être. »

Il en résulte qu'il est souhaitable que les institutions internationales telle qu'ECODA (European Confederation of Directors Associations) constituent un noyau éthique, commun à toutes les entreprises du secteur du vivant, sans en altérer la diversité, source de richesses. Ce noyau rappellerait les valeurs à respecter et servirait de norme aux règles morales attendues dans le comportement des entreprises et des chercheurs concernés.

En guise de conclusion, c'est un livre à lire par tout citoyen soucieux de posséder une bonne santé et de vivre durablement dans un environnement amical et chaleureux.

Honorary Professor Eng.
Pierre Klees
February 2019

Professeur honoraire Ir.
Pierre Klees
Février 2019

THIS BOOK IS ABOUT CHEMISTRY, BUT IT IS NOT A CHEMISTRY BOOK

Food contains vital as well as life-threatening components

The Oxford living dictionary defines chemistry as *the branch of science concerned with the substances of which matter is composed, the investigation of their properties and reactions, and the use of such reactions to form new substances*[1]. A rather simple definition, I would say, and one that focuses on the complexity of chemical sciences. Every single material, even our own bodies, is made up of chemicals. And chemistry is involved in everything we do: from washing our hands and cleaning our homes to launching a space shuttle, from manufacturing clothes and furniture to growing and cooking food.

Food chemistry affects body chemistry

Food science deals with the three major components of food: carbohydrates, lipids and proteins. Carbohydrates are sugars and starches; they are the chemical fuels needed for our body cells to function. Lipids (fats and oils) are essential building elements of cell membranes and they are needed to lubricate and cushion organs within the body. Proteins are complex molecules composed of some 100 to 500 and more amino acids that are chained together and folded into three-dimensional shapes necessary for the structure and function of every cell. Our bodies can synthesize some of these. However, eight of them, the essential amino acids, must be taken in as part of our food. Food chemistry is also concerned with the inorganic components of food such

---

1   Available online at: https://en.oxforddictionaries.com/definition/chemistry.

as water and minerals as well as with essential micronutrients of which only (extremely) small quantities are required – the different vitamins and enzymes, for example.

Food chemists improve the quality, safety, processing, storage and taste of our food. They test products to supply information used for the nutrition labels or to determine to what extent packaging and storage affect the safety and quality of the food. Flavourists work with chemicals to change the taste of food. They also study and develop other ways of improving sensory appeal, e.g. by enhancing colour, odour or texture. Food chemists are also involved in the fine-tuning of techniques and methods to identify and quantify food contaminants to be able to protect us from contaminations, harmful practices or (deliberate) adulterations.

Complexity is the common thread throughout food chemistry. The chemistry that takes place in our tea cup constitutes a very apt illustration of this fact: it shows that our foods and drinks can contain both healthy chemicals as well as poison.

There is much more to tea than just a great brew

From a chemistry point of view, tea is the ultimate mystery and challenge to food and analytical chemists. Tea leaves are packed with different compounds, the main ones being polyphenols, which can be up to ~40 % of the dry weight of the leaf. There are also amino acids, enzymes, methylxanthines such as caffeine, minerals and vitamins and more than 700 aroma compounds in trace amounts. Moreover, after fermentation of freshly plucked green tea leaves only ~30 % of the original green leaf constituents remain chemically unchanged, whereas the remaining ~70 % have been chemically altered to give reaction products of unknown structure, referred to as thearubigins[2] [Drynan et al. 2010; Kuhnert et al. 2013]. In black tea there are ~30.000 molecules – yes, thirty thousand – formed during fermentation or oxidation and only a handful have

---

2   They are polymeric catechins (phenolic compounds) that are formed during the enzymatic oxidation (called fermentation in the tea trade) of tea leaves. In contrast to theaflavins, thearubigins contain polysaccharides and proteins in the polymer [Izawa et al. 2010].

been well studied. Fermentation is often used to describe the process of making tea, but it is essentially an oxidation process: the polyphenols[3] are exposed to oxygen and oxidase enzymes, which convert the polyphenols into theaflavins[2] and thearubigins. This oxidation process can be manipulated and controlled to change the chemical composition and therefore also the appearance, aroma, flavour and taste, which results in different types of tea with different chemical components.

In the traditional production method the tea leaves are spread out in warm air and allowed to wither until they are soft enough to roll without the surface of the leaf splitting. Rolling is sometimes done by hand, but machines that lightly crush the leaf are normally used. The rolled lumps of leaf are then left in cool, humid atmospheric conditions for up to four hours to absorb oxygen. The chemical change in the leaf turns them from green to a coppery red colour.

The final stage requires the leaf to be oxidised or fermented. The main difference between tea types is largely based on the level of oxidation. Black teas, for instance, are fully oxidised. The leaves are left to oxidise in a temperature and humidity controlled room, turning completely brown before being dried. Because of this process, black tea has fewer green catechin polyphenols than other tea types, but contains up to 20 % thearubigins and ~2 % theaflavins, which are formed during oxidation. Green teas, on the other hand, are not oxidised, because heat is applied – through steaming or pan firing – very soon after harvesting. As a result the green catechins are not oxidised and the colour of the leaf is preserved. Yellow and white teas are also subject to very little oxidation. Green, white and yellow teas contain higher levels of polyphenols than black tea, their percentage being similar to that of the fresh tea leaves.

Huge chemical variety, huge chemical complexity!

---

3   The most potent polyphenol in tea is epigallocatechin gallate, which belongs to a group of flavonoid phytochemicals called catechins; the polyphenols in tea seem to operate in a variety of ways. They may help halt the damage that free radicals do to cells [Berkeley Wellness, University of California].

Kitchens are tea labs

One of the most prized and amazing characteristics of tea is the huge array of natural flavours and aromas that can be obtained from the single tea leaf. A tea can be flavoured through the addition of inclusions, by being coated in extracts, or by being scented. Often different methods are combined. Inclusions are blossoms, pieces of dried fruit, herbs or spices that are added to the tea leaves. Essential oils are flavouring agents extracted from the leaves, fruits, blossoms, roots or other parts of a plant. They carry the distinctive scents or flavours that are specific for the plant. Natural flavouring agents are obtained from natural substances with the aid of chemical separation techniques, whereas artificial flavours are created by altering the chemical structure of a naturally occurring molecule to obtain a different, more intense, or less expensive flavour. The latter molecules do not exist in nature.

The final chemical reactions happen in the kitchen. Soaking time and temperature impact the compounds in our cup. When hot water is added to tea, the phenolics are extracted into the aqueous phase along with other tea chemicals. Caffeine is extracted first, followed by the phenolics. At very high temperatures, some highly bitter and astringent phenolics are also extracted. So, if you prefer a less bitter brew, a lower temperature is highly recommended. Moreover, black tea had higher antioxidants in a short hot water infusion, but when steeped for a longer time antioxidant activity was significantly reduced. White tea, on the other hand, was found to have more antioxidants the longer it was brewed [Weerawatanakorn et al. 2015].

In the United Kingdom, many people add milk to their tea. The proteins in milk are thought to form complexes with the tea polyphenols. Ryan & Petit [2010] found that black tea is a valuable source of antioxidants and that the reducing effect of milk on the total antioxidant capacity may be related to the fat content of the milk. The addition of whole, semi-skimmed, and skimmed bovine milk to a tea infusion decreased the total antioxidant capacity of all the tea brands. Skimmed milk decreased the total antioxidant capacity of the tea infusion significantly more than either whole milk or semi-skimmed milk.

Tea is the most frequently consumed beverage worldwide apart from water. All three most popular types of tea, green, black, and oolong (semi-fermented), are manufactured from the leaves of the plant *Camellia sinensis*. Tea possesses significant antioxidative, anti-inflammatory, anti-microbial, anticarcinogenic, antihypertensive, neuroprotective, cholesterol-lowering, and thermogenic properties. Several research investigations, epidemiological studies as well as meta-analyses, suggest that tea and its bioactive polyphenolic constituents have numerous beneficial effects on health, including the prevention of many diseases such as cancer, diabetes, arthritis, cardiovascular disease, stroke, genital warts, and obesity. Controversies regarding the benefits and risks of tea consumption still exist, but the limitless health-promoting benefits of tea seem to outclass the few reported toxic effects. A review by Hayat et al. [2015] highlights both the beneficial effects and the risks associated with tea consumption.

Protecting humans from the harmfulness of contaminated foods has become a daunting task

The term *chemical contamination* refers to the presence of chemicals where they should not be and/or to concentrations of chemicals that are considered unsafe. The origins of chemical contaminants are very diverse: soil, air, water, environment, disinfection by-products, personal care products, packaging materials, agrochemicals, etc. Chemical contaminations affect all mass-produced consumer goods. Even our drinking water and foods are not immune from the attacks of chemical contaminants. Sometimes they occur in disturbingly high concentrations. Food contamination, whether accidental or intentional, brings in its wake serious human health and safety implications [Rather et al. 2017].

Food contamination has long been recorded in history. For example, there is speculation that Ancient Romans suffered chronic to severe lead poisoning due to the ubiquity of lead in lined pots in which acidic foodstuffs were boiled. Today, the growth in agribusiness and globalisation have caused food contamination to spread all over the planet [Carvalho 2017]. Tirado et al. [2010] emphasize the urgent need for intersectoral and international cooperation to better understand the rapidly and severely changing food safety situation.

Chemical contaminants can be present in foods mainly as a result of the use of agrochemicals such as residues of pesticides and veterinary drugs, contamination from environmental sources (water, air and soil pollution), cross-contamination or contaminant formation during food processing, migration from food contact and packaging materials, occurrence of natural toxins and use of unapproved food additives and adulterants [Mastovska 2013]. Environmental contaminants are impurities that are either introduced by humans or occurring naturally. Metal contamination of soils is of particular concern, e.g. cadmium can accumulate in some vegetable crops, and rice grown on soils rich in arsenic is often contaminated with highly toxic, inorganic arsenic species. Both cadmium and arsenic are human carcinogens. Examples of organic environmental contaminants that enter the food chain are polychlorinated biphenyls, dioxins, persistent chlorinated pesticides, brominated flame retardants, polyfluorinated compounds, polycyclic aromatic hydrocarbons, perchlorate, pharmaceutical and personal care products as well as haloacetic acids and other water disinfection by-products [Thompson & Darwish 2019]. Food processing contaminants include the undesirable compounds which are formed in the food during baking, roasting, canning, heating, fermentation, or hydrolysis. Food processing practices give rise to a plethora of chemical compounds whose toxicological effects are still largely unknown [Rasinger et al. 2018]. The direct contact with food packaging materials can lead to chemical contamination due to the migration of some harmful substances into foods. Although Europe has a fairly good legislation in place, there is still a need for updating and improvement [Grob 2017A & B]. Finally, the use of unapproved or erroneous additives is cause for serious concern and requires properly adapted approaches [Weiner 2016].

Nasty chemicals lurking in our cup

Our daily cup of tea has many positive associations: tea is lauded for its antioxidants, the molecules that prevent free radical cell damage. However, recent research has uncovered a connection of a less pleasant kind, i.e. the possibility of pesticides and even carcinogenic chemicals in tea. Independent lab testing by CBC News Canada has found that many tea brands contain pesticides in concentrations exceeding the levels tolerated in Canada. CBC's research found multiple chemicals in eight out of 10 popular brands of green and black tea. Half the teas had pesticide amounts in excess of the allowable limits and eight out of the 10 brands tested contained several different pesticides, with one brand containing residues of 22 different pesticides. In a way, this is not as much of a revelation as one may think. In 2012, Greenpeace found that every one of 18 tea samples from nine Chinese tea manufacturers contained a mixture of at least three different kinds of pesticides[4]. In total, as many as 29 different pesticides were detected. Six of the samples contained more than 10 different kinds of pesticides. Pesticides banned in China for use on tea plants and tea leaves were found in 12 samples from eight different tea companies. Indian tea hardly performed better. About 94 % of 49 Indian tea brands tested by Greenpeace in 2014 contained pesticide residues and 59 % contained at least one pesticide above the maximum residue level (MRL) set by the EU. In 2018, the European Food Safety Authority (EFSA) published a comprehensive report of the 2016 testing of pesticide residues in food in the European Union (EU). Although pesticide levels exceeding the MRL amounted to only 3.9 % in total, for some products, including tea, the levels were much higher. Of the tea samples tested, ~36 % contained no detectable pesticides at all, while ~24 % contained pesticide residue levels exceeding the EU MRL [EFSA 2018].

---

4   This information is available online at: http://www.greenpeace.org/eastasia/Global/ eastasia/publications/reports/food-agriculture/2012/Pesticide%20Hidden%20 Ingredient%20Report%20Final.pdf

The scientific literature is much more cautious. El-Aty et al. [2018] conclude that most contaminants leached into tea brew are not detected or are detected at a level lower than the regulatory limits. This means that levels as such do not pose a public health hazard. However, the traditional practice of overboiling tea leaves should be discouraged as this may increase the risk of more transfer of contaminants from the tea to the brew. Clearly, allowing tea to steep for >3 minutes is not advisable. Moreover, it is recommended that a cup of tea should be consumed at 60-70 C. Heavy metals in tea leaves do not normally constitute a problem for health although their concentrations are sometimes on the high side. Enhanced concentrations may occur in mature leaves; much depends on the soil on which the tea plants grow.

At first sight it seems as though the situation is not as bad as feared. However, concerns remain with regard to the occurrence of high numbers of wanted and unwanted chemical substances in a cup of tea. Chemistry is a science concerned with the investigation of reactions of substances. And since we have not yet identified all 30,000 tea components, we do not know all the reaction products and we have no knowledge of their chemical and toxicological properties.

No one can claim that these components are harmless; no one has thoroughly studied the effects of the cocktail (more about this in the chapters on analysis and control techniques). And there is the rub!

The point of this book is not to turn you into chemists

This book is a collection of case studies, ingenious developments that amazed me and left me with a feeling of admiration or shame and anger. In chemistry there is good and bad news, and there is a great deal of uncertainty.

There is no going back on the development that chemistry has undergone. What then is now the best course of action? There is no simple answer to this question. There is no single miracle solution that can instantly cure all ills. But opportunities are available and new opportunities will continue to emerge. A sound, rational approach is our best tool to keep making progress. Why not think differently about chemistry and particularly about food chemistry, and ask ourselves how willing we are to gamble with our own and other people's health?

This collection of case studies does not attempt to force decisions. It does not fix preferences for one or other approach. It is merely a collection of suggestions from which you, dear readers, can choose freely. It is quite simply a collection of striking ideas upon which you are invited to reflect and which maybe will help you decide on the best course of action for us all.

We should however cease to be merely spectators, allowing things to happen outside our own volition. When it comes to mapping out a plan to combat the growing pandemic of diseases caused by chemical pollutants, contaminant cocktails are still not receiving due attention. The myopic approach that is currently being adopted fails to take stock of the strong scientific evidence.

We should be careful not to miss the opportunity of reducing physical suffering and brain disorders. It is the people who have it in them to cure society of its ills, and not the other way around.

Bibliography

Carvalho [2017]. Pesticides, environment, and food safety, *Food and Energy Security* 6, 2, 48-60

Drynan et al. [2010]. The chemistry of low molecular weight black tea polyphenols, *Natural product reports* 27, 3, 417-462

EFSA [2018]. The 2016 European Union report on pesticide residue s in food, *EFSA Journal* 16, 7, 5348, pp. 139

El-Aty et al. [2018]. Residues and contaminants in tea and tea infusions: a review, *Food Additives & Contaminants: Part A* 31, 11, 1794-1804

Grob [2017A]. Listing approved substances and materials for food contact in Europe: ideas for a better use and further evolvement of the present system. A contribution for discussion, *Journal of Consumer Protection and Food Safety* 12, 3, 271-281

Grob [2017B]. The European system for the control of the safety of foodcontact materials needs restructuring: a review and outlook for discussion, *Food Additives & Contaminants: Part A* 34, 9, 1643-1659

Hayat et al. [2015]. Tea and its consumption: benefits and risks, *Critical reviews in food science and nutrition* 55, 7, 939-954

Izawa et al. [2010]. 4.16 - Human–Environment Interactions – Taste, in *Comprehensive Natural Products II - Chemistry and Biology, Volume 4,* 631-671

Kuhnert et al. [2013]. What is under the hump? Mass spectrometry based analysis of complex mixtures in processed food – lessons from the characterisation of black tea thearubigins, coffee melanoidines and caramel, *Food & function* 4, 8, 1130-1147

Mastovska [2013]. Modern Analysis of Chemical Contaminants in Food, *Food Safety Magazine*, February/March, available online at: http://www.foodsafetymagazine.com/magazine-archive1/februarymarch-2013/modern-analysis-of-chemicalcontaminants-in-food/

Rasinger et al. [2018]. Identification and evaluation of potentially mutagenic and carcinogenic food contaminants, *EFSA Journal* 16, S1, e16085, pp. 9

Rather et al. [2017]. The Sources of Chemical Contaminants in Food and Their Health Implicationsm, *Frontiers in pharmacology* 8, 830, pp. 8

Tirado et al. [2010]. Climate change and food safety: A review, *Food Research International* 43, 7, 1745-1765

Thompson & Darwish [2019]. Environmental Chemical Contaminants in Food: Review of a Global Problem, *Journal of Toxicology*, Article ID 2345283, pp. 14

Weerawatanakorn et al. [2015]. Chemistry and health beneficial effects of oolong tea and theasinensins, *Food Science and Human Wellness* 4, 4, 133-146

Weiner [2016]. Parameters and pitfalls to consider in the conduct of food additive research, Carrageenan as a case study, *Food and Chemical Toxicology* 87, 31-44

LOOKING FOR FRONT-RUNNERS IN THE FIELD OF SUSTAINABILITY

A load of corn!

Well, maybe not all of it is corn. But there's an awful lot of it hiding in our food. A lot more than we ever suspected. We think our supermarkets offer huge varieties of food. Yet, much of that food comes from one single crop [Pollan 2006]. And it all starts with … corn.

Maize (*Zea mays*), also known as corn, is believed to have originated from a wild grass

The history of modern day maize or corn [http://learn.genetics.utah.edu/content/selection/corn/] begins at the dawn of human agriculture some 10,000 years ago, when ancient farmers were living in small groups and shifting their settlements with the seasons. By accurately selecting the kernels before planting they managed to domesticize maize in what is now Mexico. Apparently, they had realized that selecting could produce significant and interesting differences. Some plants grew larger than others, some kernels tasted better or were easier to grind. So, they saved kernels from plants with desirable characteristics and planted them for the following season's harvest. Today, we call this approach selective breeding or artificial selection. Maize cobs became larger over time, with more rows of kernels, eventually taking on the form of the corn we know today. It is clear however that the domestication process must have occurred in many stages over a considerable length of time.

The biological origin of maize has been a long-running mystery. We now know that the wild ancestor of corn was a grass, called teosinte. Teosinte doesn't look much like maize. But at the DNA level teosinte and corn are surprisingly alike. They have the same number of chromosomes and a remarkably similar arrangement of genes. Also, teosinte can crossbreed with modern maize varieties to form maize-teosinte hybrids, and they can go on to reproduce naturally. One of the first scientists to investigate and fully understand the close relationship between teosinte and maize was George Beadle (1903-1989). In the 1930s, he worked on Mendelian asynapsis in corn[5] and was awarded a PhD degree for his work [Beadle 1930] in 1931. In 1935, George Beadle visited Paris for six months to work with Professor Boris Ephrussi (1901-1979) at the Institut de Biologie physico-chimique. Together they initiated the study of the development of eye pigment in *Drosophila*, which later led to investigations on the biochemistry of the genetics of the fungus *Neurospora* for which Beadle and Edward Lawrie Tatum (1909-1975) were awarded the 1958 Nobel Prize for Physiology or Medicine.

The earliest events in maize domestication involved little variation in single genes with huge effects. This suggests that modern varieties descend from one single ancestor. Small changes with dramatic effects explain the sudden appearance of maize in the archaeological record; they show us that evolution does not always involve gradual change over time. Furthermore, the more recent changes in the evolution of modern maize involve high numbers of genes and generate small effects. These minor changes include: (1) types and amounts of starch production, (2) ability to grow in different climates and types of soil, (3) length and number of kernel rows, (4) kernel size, shape, and colour, and (5) resistance to pests. The latter examples tie in with the traditional view of evolution as a gradual change over time. Over thousands of years, selective breeding generated the broad diversity of corn varieties that are grown around the world today.

Maize as well as other cereal grains are the fruits of cultivated grasses. They provide humans with more nourishment than any other food class and nearly half their total caloric requirement. The consumption of these cereals varies from one region to another. Wheat is the preferred cereal

---

5   Asynaptic plants are characterized by a failure of the usual pairing of homologous chromosomes during meiosis. Such plants display a high degree of male and female sterility.

in Central Asia, the Middle East, South and North America, and Europe. Rice is the major cereal in Asia, while maize is preferred in Southern and Eastern Africa, Central America, and Mexico. There are about a dozen cereal crops used for food, but only wheat, rice, and maize are highly important human food sources, accounting for ~94 % of all cereal consumption. Maize contains approximately 72 % starch, 10 % protein, and 4 % fat, supplying an energy density of 365 Kcal per 100 g [Ranum et al. 2014].

The above seems to indicate that Europeans hardly eat any corn. Nothing however could be further from the truth!

Corn is what feeds the cattle that becomes the meat you eat

Current industrial farming practices [Pussemier & Goeyens 2017] often rely heavily on grains. Livestock producers often use corn and soy as a basic ingredient for their animal feed, because these protein-rich grains help animals achieve market weight faster, and because corn and soy are cheaper than other feed options. Corn feeds chickens, ducks, turkeys and other poultry. Corn feeds millions of pigs housed in commercial pigsties as well as countless non-carnivorous fish raised in fish farms. Corn-fed chickens lay the eggs you eat for breakfast. And corn primarily feeds the beef cattle as well as the dairy cows that produce the milk, butter, cheese, yogurt and ice creams.

But that is not the end of it. Take any bag of crisps; candy bar or sweet biscuit; cheese spread; canned soup; salad dressing, mayonnaise or ketchup; frozen junk food or boxed dinner, such as TV dinners, pizzas and macaroni with cheese; coffee creamer; jam or jelly, and you will see the list of ingredients includes such substances as maltodextrin, monosodium glutamate, ascorbic acid, lecithin, mono-, di-, and triglycerides, fructose-glucose syrup. And guess what? These chemicals are predominantly derived from corn, and if you wash them down with a soft drink or juice, you are drinking corn with your corn. Since the 1980s, many soft drinks and most of the fruit juices sold in supermarkets are sweetened with high-fructose corn syrup, an unhealthy ingredient that is added to most of the prepared foods and drinks.

Though fast food outlets appear to offer a vast range of products, their food and drinks have more in common than we are led to believe. According to an earlier study, the multiplicity of choice conceals the fact that the overwhelming majority of takeaway food items is actually based on one single source: corn.

Corn – whether black, brown, white or yellow – is a shooting star in the food firmament. Whether for better or for worse is hard to say. I believe that the obvious lack of some nutrients, such as vitamin B12 and vitamin C, and the poor levels of calcium, folate, and iron have adverse health effects for all living beings, people as well as other animals, living on a corn-rich diet. I also believe that the prevalence of monocultures and intensive livestock breeding cast a worrying shadow over the future of our food. In order to meet the high demand for grain of industrial food animal operations, many smaller farms have been replaced by large corn and soy monocultures, which rely on an elevated input of fertilisers and pesticides. This is very bad news for the environment, and the detrimental effects are often completely unexpected. The next chapter illustrates how an unbalanced diet can turn hamster (*Cricetus cricetus*) mothers into cannibals.

Are we sure corn is the predominant source

So we are. As sure as we can be! I returned to my huge collection of scientific papers and books and discovered convincing evidence for the overwhelming presence of corn provided by the analysis of stable isotope ratios of food samples. Some ten years ago, Jahren & Kraft [2008] from the University of Hawaii discovered the omnipresence of corn by chemically analysing a variety of foods from America's top chains. I could not help being intrigued: the authors of the paper used the same technology as I did many years ago when researching oceanic nitrogen fluxes for my PhD thesis.

Stable isotope ratio determinations are a surprisingly reliable way of tracing the origins of foods. Like all plants, corn gets its energy through photosynthesis, but it uses a metabolic pathway that differs slightly from other major crop plants like rice, wheat or potatoes. The difference is reflected in the plant's ratio of two carbon isotopes – the common carbon-12 and rare carbon-13. Corn has a signature ratio that sets it apart from other crops and by association, the meat of animals that consume the plant also stands out in the same tell-tale way. The results clearly showed that most of the cattle that ended up in the burgers were fed exclusively on corn. Of 162 samples of beef collected by Jahren & Kraft [2008], only 12 (less than 10 %) came from animals that were potentially fed on other sources, like grass or grains. And there were no significant exceptions for chickens: they had all had nothing but corn.

The same scientists also measured the levels of stable nitrogen isotopes in both chicken and beef burgers. The high levels they found of the rare nitrogen-15 isotope[6] indicated that the animals were given corn that had been grown using nitrogen-based fertilisers and that they had been reared in very confined spaces. The fertilization required for corn production results in nitrogen-15 enriched corn seed and silage compared with natural vegetation. Moreover, beef produced in confinement was enriched in nitrogen-15 compared with animals raised outdoors.

Interesting results, but do they really matter?

One could argue that consumers have a right to know where their food comes from. Obviously, most of our food can be traced back to corn monocultures and intensive livestock farming, which even today is regarded as the best way to prevent food shortages. There are however two sides to every coin. On the negative side, there is the greater reliance on monoculture cropping, decreased farmer interest in preserving biodiversity on their land, poor water management and improper fertilizer and pesticide application practices that cause pronounced greenhouse gas emissions. It is imperative that this situation should change and that the change should occur as soon as possible! There is simply no alternative to ecological agriculture. This may sound very

---

6   Natural nitrogen consists of two stable isotopes: nitrogen-14, which makes up the vast majority (~99.63 %) of naturally occurring nitrogen, and nitrogen-15, the concentration of which is ~0.37 %.

final, but it has become virtually impossible to deny that there is only one possible future for agricultural practice: sustainability. Sustainability refers to ecology; it can assume several forms. Fortunately, ecological agriculture is on the rise in many regions. The variety of organisms that are found makes our fields more attractive. The care that many farmers spend on their crops and their livestock farming reflect the respect they show for the environment and for animal welfare [Pussemier & Goeyens 2017].

For the consumer, maize has one serious limitation. While it contains the vitamin B3 or niacin, it is in a bound form that is not readily available to the body. Additionally, it is low in tryptophan, a niacin precursor. Niacin can only be released from the bound form at high pH. The ancient Aztec and Mayan civilizations developed a process, called nixtamalization, which involved soaking the whole maize in a lime[7] solution, followed by grinding to produce a paste, called masa, from which tortillas are made [Caballero-Briones et al. 2000]. This process has two benefits: it converts the hard maize kernels into a more digestible form and releases the bound niacin. Without this process there would have been much higher incidences of pellagra[8] due to niacin deficiency. In Europe, North America, and Africa, where the nixtamalization process was not used, pellagra became a problem in some areas. Eventually, the cereal fortification through niacin addition into maize meal was a real success story in the 1940s. It contributed to the elimination of pellagra as a major health problem in the South Eastern United States.

Eating a balanced diet does not have to be difficult at all. Ultimately, it is as simple as eating more fruit, vegetables, starchy, fibre-rich foods and fresh products, and fewer fatty, sugary, salty and processed foods. That also includes corn. Our diet should not be restricted to corn and corn derivatives alone.

---

7   Lime is a white or greyish-white, odourless, lumpy, very slightly water-soluble solid, calcium oxide, which when combined with water forms calcium hydroxide.

8   Pellagra is a complex disease characterised by diarrhoea, dermatitis and dementia. If left untreated, death is the usual outcome. It occurs as a result of tryptophan and vitamin B3 deficiency.

Bibliography

Beadle [1930]. *Genetical and Cytological Studies of Mendelian Asynapsis in Zea mays*, PhD thesis, Cornell University

Caballero-Briones et al. 2000]. Recent advances on the understanding of the *nixtamalization* process, *Superficies y Vacío* 10, 20-24

Jahren & Kraft [2008]. Carbon and nitrogen stable isotopes in fast food: Signatures of corn and confinement, *Proceedings of the National Academy of Sciences* 105, 46, 17855-17860

Pollan [2006]. *The Omnivore's Dilemma: A Natural History of Four Meals*, Bloomsbury, pp. 450

Pussemier & Goeyens [2017]. *AgricultureS et Enjeux de Société*, Presses Universitaires de Liège, Agronomie – Gembloux, pp. 112

Ranum et al. [2014]. Global maize production, utilization, and consumption, *Annals of the New York Academy of Sciences* 1312, 105-112

Corn turns hamster mothers into cannibals

It is hard to deny that cereal monocultures generate huge losses in biodiversity. The endless sweep of cultivated land as far as the eye can see. No trees or hedges to separate the plots. The total lack of natural vegetation where once insects, reptiles, birds and small mammals used to find shelter. No other shades of colour than those imposed by the seasons: brownish-grey during winter, plain green during spring, ephemeral yellow at harvest time, and depressingly brown during autumn. Even though we know that these vast, uniform cultures lead to a depletion of natural and wild flora and fauna, we still know very little about a number of the disturbances that have unexpectedly caused the eradication of the native fauna including the small, hibernating European hamster (*Cricetus cricetus*).

The European hamster population has been reduced to ~450 individuals

Today, ecological investigations are being conducted to determine the extent to which current agricultural systems influence animal life. Researchers from the University of Strasbourg in France (Tissier et al. 2016 & 2017) for example have for the first time studied the combined role of climate changes and agricultural practices in the alarming decline of the European hamster.

The hamster, once a common rodent on agricultural land, is now on the verge of extinction in France. Despite earlier measures aimed at protecting the hamster, populations are still in sharp decline. The threat of extinction is particularly high in the western part of its distribution area (The Netherlands, France, Germany and Belgium). The European hamster population, still very abundant in French Alsace as late as the 1960s, has been reduced to some 450 individuals today. What is the way of life of this small rodent? Why is its habitat collapsing? What are the challenges that need to be addressed to preserve large Alsatian hamster populations?

The main reason generally put forward for the population decline remains the destruction of the hamster's habitat by the propagation of industrial and inappropriate crops, corn in particular, intensive (and excessive) urbanization causing fragmentation of Cricetus habitats, and increasing winter rainfall [Tissier et al. 2016]. Generally, cereal monocultures are associated with the increased application of (toxic) pesticides and the mechanization of agricultural practice. At first glance, this sounds like a plausible explanation for what can only be described as a very serious and extremely alarming situation.

But there may be more than meets the eye. Apparently, the entire situation has spiralled out of control. Witness this striking title in the scientific literature: *Diets derived from maize monoculture cause maternal infanticides in the endangered European hamster due to vitamine B3 deficiency.* A diet of corn turns hamster mothers into deranged cannibals that devour their offspring [Tissier et al. 2017]. The authors explain how nutritional deficiencies caused by maize monoculture could affect farmland animal fitness and reproduction. They argue that maize overabundance in the diet of farmland animals could be particularly detrimental to the fitness of hamsters. Hamsters also face many other threats, and so there is an urgent need to restore a culture diversity in the agricultural plant schedules to ensure that farmland animals have access to a more diversified and better balanced, animal and vegetable diet.

Hamsters used to find their nourishment in a variety of grains, roots and insects

Earlier investigations examined the impact of pesticide exposures and mechanised ploughing, which can destroy the hamsters' underground caves, especially during hibernation, but the possible link with what they eat has remained largely unexplored.

No more grains, no roots, no insects and no worms! Many Western European hamsters now live in an ocean of corn that hardly provides the rodents with a well-balanced diet. The findings, reported by Tissier et al. [2016], point to industrial scale monocultures as the culprit. The unbalanced diet leaves the animals starving, as the French team discovered. A first set of laboratory experiments with caged wild specimens compared wheat and corn-based diets, with side dishes of clover or worms. Though there was virtually no difference in the number of pups born, when it came to survival rates, the difference was dramatic. About 80 % of the pups born of mothers feasting on wheat-and-clover or wheat-and-worms were weaned. However, only ~5 % of the baby hamsters whose mothers ate corn instead of wheat made it that far.

Corn lacks several micronutrients such as calcium, tryptophan, lysine, riboflavin, and especially vitamin B3. And no animal knows the nixtamalization technique. Vitamin B3 is also known as niacin and nicotinic acid. It is one of the essential human nutrients. Pharmaceutical and supplemental niacin are primarily used to treat hypercholesterolemia[9] and pellagra[10]. Insufficient niacin in the diet is known to cause nausea, skin and mouth lesions, anaemia, headaches, and tiredness in humans [Wikipedia]. An unbalanced corn-based diet has been associated with high rates of homicide, suicide and cannibalism in humans [Ernandes et al. 1996; Ernandes 2002] and may cause pellagra, the disease that

---

9   Hypercholesterolemia refers to levels of cholesterol in the blood that are higher than normal.

10 Pellagra is a disease caused by low levels of vitamin B3 or niacin. It is marked by dementia, diarrhoea, and dermatitis. If left untreated, pellagra can be fatal.

decimated millions of people in North America and Europe between the mid-18th and the mid-20th century [Hegyi et al. 2004].

Even more disturbing is how the pups perished

Hamster mothers stored their living pups with their hoards of maize before eating them. Tissier et al. [2017] reported that the high propensity of corn caused abnormal maternal behaviour, infanticide and siblicide, associated with diarrhoea and skin problems in the pups. The symptoms obviously resemble those observed in humans affected by pellagra [Hegyi et al. 2004] as well as the symptoms of canine black tongue disease.

In an additional set of experiments, the hamsters were offered corn-based diets, one of them with vitamin B3 added. Sure enough, the vitamin B3-enriched diet eliminated the horrific symptoms and prevented the hamster mothers from eating their offspring. The dire consequences of the vitamin B3-deficient corn diet, the scientists concluded, stemmed not from reduced maternal hormones, but rather from a change in the nervous system that induced the same dementia-like behaviour previously diagnosed in humans.

Monoculture in agriculture really is bad news for biodiversity

Given the intensification of maize monoculture across the globe – inherently associated with a reduction in diversity and abundance of other plants, micro-organisms as well as soil fauna – the overabundance of corn compared with other food plants in the diet of farmland animals will be detrimental to the fitness and survival of the latter.

May it not be the same for humans, who intentionally or not, turn their backs on well-balanced and varied diets? The results of the aforementioned studies do not bode well for human health, just as canaries were used to warn coal miners of the presence of toxic gases [Burrell & Seibert, 1914]. Animals serve as sentinels, because of their greater susceptibility, their environmental exposure or their shorter life-span.

Healthy eating means eating the foods that give us the nutrients we need to maintain our health, feel good, and have plenty of energy. These nutrients include proteins, carbohydrates, fat, water, vitamins, and minerals. Evidently, this means eating a wide variety of foods in the right proportions, and consuming the right amount of food and drinks. Fruit and vegetables are vital sources of vitamins and minerals; nutritionists and dieticians recommend they should make up just over one third of the food we eat every day.

Why biodiversity matters

The air we breathe, the water we drink and the food we eat, all rely on biodiversity[11]. Biodiversity is a highly complex and vital feature we should long have been more aware of. I returned to what Prof. Paul R. Ehrlich published ~30 years ago and once more appreciated the still valid conclusions of his highly relevant papers. Ehrlich is the Bing Professor of Population Studies at the Department of Biology of Stanford University and the President of Stanford's Center for Conservation Biology. He believes that discussions tend to focus all too often on the threat faced by prominent endangered species and on deliberate overexploitation by humans seen as the major cause of the threat. Although Ehrlich [1988] is convinced that the concern about direct risks is legitimate, he also draws our attention to these other more obscure and unpleasant truths listed below:

- *The primary cause of the decay of organic diversity is not direct human exploitation or malevolence, but the habitat destruction that inevitably results from the expansion of human populations and human activities.*

---

11 The term biological diversity was first used by wildlife scientist and conservationist, Raymond F. Dasmann (1919-2002). In "A Different Kind of Country" he notes the prevailing global trend toward uniformity and makes a counter-plea for diversity. The term was widely adopted only after more than a decade, when in the 1980s it came into common usage in science as well as in environmental policy. In his book, Dasmann points to the dangers of monocultures and the values of biological diversity as related to stability and adaptability.

- *Many of the less cuddly, less spectacular organisms that Homo sapiens is wiping out are more important to the human future than are most of the publicized endangered species. People need plants and insects more than they need leopards and whales (which is not to denigrate the value of the latter two).*
- *Other organisms have provided humanity with the very basis of civilization in the form of crops, domestic animals, a wide variety of industrial products, and many important medicines. Nonetheless, the most important anthropocentric reason for preserving diversity is the role that microorganisms, plants, and animals play in providing free ecosystem services, without which society in its present form could not persist [Ehrlich & Ehrlich 1981; Holdren & Ehrlich 1974].*
- *The loss of genetically distinct populations within species is, at the moment, at least as important a problem as the loss of entire species. Once a species is reduced to a remnant, its ability to benefit humanity ordinarily declines greatly, and its total extinction in the relatively near future becomes much more likely. By the time an organism is recognized as endangered, it is often too late to save it.*
- *Extrapolation of current trends in the reduction of diversity implies a denouement for civilization within the next 100 years comparable to a nuclear winter.*
- *Arresting the loss of diversity will be extremely difficult. The traditional "just set aside a preserve" approach is almost certain to be inadequate because of factors such as runaway human population growth, acid rains, and climate change induced by human beings. A quasi-religious transformation leading to the appreciation of diversity for its own sake, apart from the obvious direct benefits to humanity, may be required to save other organisms and ourselves.*

Reversing the dramatic decline in (bio)diversity is an essential goal for sustainable development. Biodiversity may be defined as the collection of animal and vegetal species and the environment in which they live. It refers not just to species, but also to ecosystems and differences in genes within a single species. Biologists simply define biodiversity as the "totality of genes, species and ecosystems of a region". Everywhere on the planet, species live together and depend on one another. Every living thing including man is involved in these complex networks of interdependent relationships, which are called ecosystems [http://ec.europa.eu/environment/nature/biodiversity/].

Yet, three predominant aspects are pertinent [Daily 2005]. The first is that ecosystems and their inherent biodiversity are capital assets. Ecosystem capital supplies society with plenty of vital benefits, or "services". Healthy ecosystems clean the water, purify the air, maintain and fertilize the soil, regulate the climate, recycle the indispensable nutrients and provide us with food. They provide raw materials and resources for medicines and many other purposes. They underpin all civilisations and sustain our economies. We could not live without these ecosystem services: it is that simple. The services are what we call our natural capital. Second, traditional approaches to conservation alone are doomed to fail. Natural reserve networks are unlikely to protect more than a tiny fraction of the Earth's biodiversity and ecosystem services over the long run. Third: this means that a new approach to conservation is required – one that makes conservation economically attractive. This of course is an obvious challenge for the 21st century.

Biodiversity is the key indicator of the health of the ecosystem. Even if certain species are affected by pollution, climate change, or human activities, the ecosystem as a whole may adapt and survive. However, the extinction of a species may have unforeseen impacts, sometimes escalating into the destruction of entire ecosystems. The current planetary scale shifts, which characterize the Anthropocene[12] era, pose major though still imperfectly understood threats to humanity and to life in general [Haines et al. 2018].

---

12 The period of time during which human activities had an environmental impact on the Earth regarded as constituting a distinct geological age.

What can we, as individuals, do to help slow the loss of biodiversity

The European diversity is unique, but the loss of biodiversity has accelerated to an unprecedented level. In Europe ~42 % of European mammals are endangered, together with ~15 % of birds and ~45 % of butterflies and reptiles. On 2nd February 2016, the European Parliament adopted a Resolution on the mid-term review of the EU Biodiversity Strategy to 2020. This strategy must finally put a stop to the loss of biodiversity and ecosystem services in the EU and help stop global biodiversity loss by 2020. [http://eur-lex.europa.eu/legal-content/EN/TXT/?uri=CELEX:52015DC0478]. Unfortunately, one is forced to admit that the target to halt biodiversity loss by 2010 has not been met.

What can we, as individuals, do to halt this long-term decline? One of our greatest immediate challenges is to minimize the impacts of new infrastructure development, especially in hotspots of biodiversity in the developing world. Large infrastructure projects are potentially damaging for two reasons. First, some projects have massive direct effects on entire ecosystems. Second, the development of infrastructure frequently catalyzes many other threats and thereby triggers rapid escalation of total pressure on biodiversity [Johnson et al. 2017].

Moreover, there are lots of "small" things we can do to help ease the pressure on biodiversity loss. Pollinators are the key to reproduction for most flowering plants which are essential to the survival of many species on our planet. We should help them [EFSA 2018]. Why not restore the habitats in our gardens and in our communities? National Wildlife Federation [https://www.nwf.org/] has a programme to help us attract wildlife, whether on city balconies or large farms.

Arguably, the action that will have the biggest positive impact on the environment is the reduction of our consumption. Since the consumption of resources is a root cause of biodiversity loss, we should consume less and in particular, be more mindful about what we consume. We need to leverage our purchasing power to help protect biodiversity by consuming products that do not harm the environment [Pussemier & Goeyens 2017]. Why does the food industry have such power as to placate its critics?

Why is there unrestrained consumption of (processed) meat products that are full of antibiotics and hormones that threaten public health, destroy nature, and exacerbate at an astonishing rate the very serious climatic crisis that is undeniably under way?

The more we reduce our demand for new food as well as non-food resources, the less destruction of natural habitat there will be as part of the process to free those resources or the energy required to make those products. And the less waste will end up in incinerators, landfills, and … on the pavements of our cities, the edges of motorways, in watercourses and seas. Hopefully, consumers will no longer litter the streets. Hopefully, industry will increasingly treat waste as a raw material. And hopefully, decision makers will seriously and financially encourage the research we still need to continue to innovate.

To change our habits is one of the true freedoms left to us [Nicolino 2009]!

Bibliography

Allan et al. [2015], Land use intensification alters ecosystem multifunctionality via loss of biodiversity and changes to functional composition, *Ecology Letters* 18, 834-843

Burrell & Seibert [1914]. Experiments with Small Animals and Carbon Monoxide, *Industrial & Engineering Chemistry* 6, 3, 241-244

Daily [2005]. Why biodiversity matters, in Babbit & Sarukhán (Eds.), *Conserving biodiversity,* Washington DC, The Aspen Institute, 15-23

Diaz et al. [2006]. Biodiversity Loss Threatens Human Well-Being, *PLoS Biology* 4, 8, 1300-1305

EFSA [2018]. *Terms of reference for an EU Bee Partnership*, technical report, pp. 18

Ehrlich [1988]. The loss of diversity, in Wilson (ed.), *Biodiversity*, National Academy Press, Washington, DC, 21-27

Ehrlich & Ehrlich [1981]. *Extinction: The Causes and Consequences of the Disappearance of Species*, Random House, New York, pp. 305

Ernandes et al. [1996]. Maize based diets and possible neurobehavioural after-effects among some populations in the world, *Human Evolution* 11, 1, 67-77

Ernandes et al. [2002]. Aztec Cannibalism and Maize consumption: The serotonin deficiency link, *The Mankind Quarterly* 43, 1, 3-40

Foley et al. [2005]. Global Consequences of Land Use, *Science* 309, 570-574

Haines et al. [2018]. Planetary Health Watch: integrated monitoring in the Anthropocene epoch, *The Lancet Planetary Health* 2, 4, e141-e143

Hegyi et al. [2004]. Pellagra: Dermatitis, dementia, and diarrhoea, *International journal of dermatology* 43, 1, 1-5

Holdren & Ehrlich [1974]. Human population and the global environment, *American Scientific* 62, 282-292

Johnson et al. [2017]. Biodiversity losses and conservation responses in the Anthropocene, *Science* 356, 6335, 270-275

Nicolino [2009]. *Bidoche – l'industrie de la viande menace le monde*, Babel, pp. 380

Pussemier & Goeyens [2017]. *Agricultures et Enjeux de Société*, Presses Universitaires de Liège, Agronomie – Gembloux, pp. 112

Tissier et al. [2016]. How maize monoculture and increasing winter rainfall have brought the hibernating European hamster to the verge of extinction, *Scientific Reports*, Article number 25531

Tissier et al. [2017]. Diets derived from maize monoculture cause maternal infanticides in the endangered European hamster due to vitamin B3 deficiency, *Proceedings of the Royal Society B* 284, 2016-2168

Glyphosate has become the world's most widely used weed killer, which could well be serious cause for concern

On 27th November 2017, the EU member states agreed on a five-year renewal period for the controversial herbicide glyphosate, the principal component of Monsanto's Roundup. The decision was taken by EU member state experts, with 18 votes in favour, 9 against and 1 abstention. Heated discussions and many disapproving as well as positive comments in newspapers and magazines had preceded the vote.

Glyphosate, the active ingredient in Monsanto's flagship herbicide Roundup: a contaminant?

Glyphosate may have contaminated the honey production because bees forage on agricultural genetically modified organisms (GMO) such as corn and soybeans, which are sprayed with the weed killer during the growing season. Glyphosate has been a highly controversial substance since March 2015. The International Agency for Research on Cancer (IARC) classified the herbicide glyphosate and the insecticides malathion and diazinon as probably carcinogenic to humans (Group 2A) – the second worst rating possible[13].

---

13 This category is used when there is limited evidence of carcinogenicity in humans and sufficient evidence of carcinogenicity in experimental animals. In some cases, an agent (mixture) may be classified in this category when there is inadequate evidence of carcinogenicity in humans and sufficient evidence of carcinogenicity

For glyphosate, some evidence of carcinogenicity in humans for non-Hodgkin lymphoma (NHL) is based on several exposure studies, mostly agricultural, since the beginning of the 21st Century [Alexander et al. 2007, and references herein]. Dewayne Johnson was the first of hundreds of cancer patients to see his case against agrochemical giant Monsanto go to trial. The former gardener and father of two children was diagnosed with incurable non-Hodgkin's lymphoma in 2014. He had used Monsanto's products Roundup and Ranger Pro in large quantities during the course of his work and was awarded ~290 million dollars' compensation. The jury found Monsanto had acted with malice and oppression, because they knew that what they were doing was wrong and had acted with reckless disregard for human life. Monsanto has denied a link between the active ingredient in Roundup, glyphosate, and cancer, claiming that hundreds of studies have established that the weed killer is safe. Johnson's attorney, Timothy Litzenburg, said he represents more than 2,000 non-Hodgkin's lymphoma sufferers, who used Roundup extensively. In a sharp turn of events, another San Francisco judge slashed Dewayne Johnson's 250 million dollars' punitive award reducing it to 39 million dollars. No doubt we have not heard the last of this yet.

In addition, there is compelling evidence that glyphosate can cause cancer in laboratory animals [IARC Monograph 112; Guyton et al. 2015]. Not all the IARC-report references were well received, however. For example, Séralini et al. [2012] published a controversial study in *Food and Chemical Toxicology*, but the paper was eventually retracted by the editor and later republished in *Environmental Sciences Europe* [Séralini et al. 2014]. The authors evaluated both the effects of feeding laboratory rats with transgenic corn and the effects of exposure to the increasingly common herbicide Roundup, and concluded that pathologies cannot be excluded. They observed severe hepatic and renal disturbances. Moreover, Séralini et al. [2014] questioned the earlier conclusions of a Monsanto team [Hammond et al. 2004], claiming that the initial indicators of organ

---

in experimental animals and strong evidence that the carcinogenesis is mediated by a mechanism that also operates in humans. Exceptionally, an agent, mixture or exposure circumstance may be classified in this category solely on the basis of limited evidence of carcinogenicity in humans [http://ec.europa.eu/health].

toxicity were not "biologically meaningful". But the Séralini et al. study suffers from enormous gaps in the number of animals studied and from incorrect statistical interpretation. Even though some studies are liable to create controversy, there is every reason to believe that, in spite of their weaknesses and shortcomings, such studies will achieve the strategic goal set by their authors, i.e. to blow the whistle on abuses.

Monsanto was accused of ecocide and crimes against humanity, and was denounced for marketing toxic products that killed people. The "advisory" opinion of the court, under the chairmanship of Françoise Tulkens, former judge of the European Court of Human Rights, was delivered on 18th April, 2017 in The Hague, The Netherlands. The document does not however constitute condemnation in the legal sense of the term since it is not "legally binding". In a certain sense, the "opinion tribunal" leadership rehashed typical myths about the modern food system using Monsanto as a symbolic scapegoat.

Hundreds of internal documents and emails were unsealed by Judge Vince Chhabria, who was presiding over litigation brought by people who claim to have developed NHL as a result of exposure to glyphosate. It would seem that Monsanto has influenced and falsified scientific studies for many years. The documents and internal emails produced in 2015 reveal that Monsanto executives have developed a strategy for working with academic and independent scientists in order to convey the company's message that glyphosate does not increase the risk of cancer. Moreover, the Monsanto documents suggest that company officials "ghost wrote" portions of scientific papers to be submitted to peer-reviewed scientific journals [Cornwall 2017]. One of the emails reveals that the company itself secretly wrote a study, even though it was published in the peer-reviewed journal *Regulatory Toxicology and Pharmacology* under the authorship of "independent" scientists [Williams et al. 2000].

Approval for Roundup in both the European Union and the United States has been Monsanto's priority target. The company's strategy sounds very familiar. Big Tobacco served as a showcase. Industry became a subtle device capable of infiltrating culture and science, of subverting medicine and corrupting *en masse*. "Doubt is our product", the famous quote of the tobacco industry, demonstrates and says much about their controversial approach [Proctor 2006]. Industry has clearly understood that debating the science is much easier and more efficient than debating the policy [Michaels 2008].

Williams et al. [2000] concluded that: ... *under present and expected conditions of use, Roundup herbicide does not pose health risks to humans...* Today, almost 20 years later, this conclusion seems to me highly implausible. Several recent articles on the link between glyphosate and kidney disease, autism, rheumatoid arthritis and pulmonary problems are now available [Jayasumana et al. 2014, 2015; Beecham et al. 2016; Sealy et al. 2016; Parks et al. 2017; Hoppin et al. 2017]. Even though link and causality, as also hazard and risk[14], are very different concepts, great care is highly recommended. This theme has been taken up by the EU. Humans and the environment are exposed to a cocktail of chemicals from many different sources. The combined exposure to multiple chemicals can lead to health as well as environmental effects, even if single substances in the mixture do not exceed safe levels. Unfortunately, the assessment and management of mixtures is only partly covered by the current legislation. The Joint Research Center (JRC) recently started performing research on new strategies to assess the combination effects of chemicals [JRC 2018].

The European Food Safety Authority reached fundamentally different conclusions

The assessment of the European Food Safety Authority (EFSA) focused only on the active substance and considered the weight of evidence of all available information. In contrast to the IARC evaluation, the EU peer review experts, with one exception, concluded that glyphosate is unlikely to pose a carcinogenic hazard to humans and that the evidence does not

---

14 Hazard is a potential source of harm or adverse health effect on a person or persons; it is the likelihood that a person may be harmed or suffers adverse health effects if exposed to a hazard.

support classification with regard to its carcinogenic potential [EFSA 2015].

And again, several references quoted in the report have given rise to a great deal of uneasiness. In their review paper, Kier & Kirkland [2013] concluded that the lack of genotoxic hazard potential, evidenced by core gene mutation and chromosomal effect studies, and coupled with the very low human and environmental species systemic exposure potential, indicates that glyphosate and typical glyphosate-based formulations present negligible genotoxicity risk. Both Larry Kier and David Kirkland, however, were paid consultants of the Glyphosate Task Force for the preparation of their review, and Larry Kier was a former employee of Monsanto Company. Employment by a business or research institute whose funding was significantly derived from commercial sources could possibly have created a conflict of interest [Robinson et al. 2013].

EFSA's mission is to provide independent scientific advice to risk managers of the European Commission and Member States and to communicate to all interested parties and to the public at large on risks in the food and feed chain. European Member States must act in such a way as to meet their commitments, even if independent scientific advice is extremely expensive.

The EFSA peer review expert group also concluded that the toxicity of glyphosate needs to be redefined [https://www. efsa.europa.eu/sites/default/files/corporate_publications/files/ efsaexplainsglyphosate151112en_1.pdf]. Pending the completion of gap-filling research, an acute reference dose (ARfD) of 0.5 mg per kg body weight[15] and an acceptable daily intake of 0.5 mg per kg body weight per day were proposed. Moreover, EFSA advocated that the toxicity of each pesticide formulation and its genotoxic potential in particular should be further considered and addressed by Member State authorities while they re-assess uses of glyphosate-based formulations in their own territories.

---

15 The ARfD of a chemical is the estimated amount of a substance in food or drinking water expressed on a body weight basis that can be ingested over a short period of time, usually during one meal or one day, without appreciable health risk to the consumer on the basis of all known facts at the time of evaluation.

Carcinogenic or not? This was a textbook example of the paradoxical situation that affected Europe in 2015/2016. Pending a conclusion by the European Chemicals Agency (ECHA), Europe provisionally authorized glyphosate under certain conditions.

After a great deal of procrastination, the European Chemicals Agency finally reached a conclusion

For ECHA there were no grounds for classifying the controversial herbicide, glyphosate, as a carcinogen, as a mutagen or as a toxic substance for reproduction. ECHA's Committee for Risk Assessment agreed to maintain its current harmonised classification of glyphosate as a substance causing serious eye damage and being toxic to aquatic life with long-lasting effects, and concluded that the available scientific evidence did not meet the criteria to classify glyphosate as a carcinogen, as a mutagen or as toxic for reproduction [https://echa.europa.eu].

As for EFSA, the ECHA classification is based solely on the hazardous properties of the pure substance glyphosate [EFSA 2015] and does not take into consideration the likelihood of exposure to the substance and consequently, does not address the risks of exposure.

What chemical substance are we dealing with?

Glyphosate – its correct International Union of Pure and Applied Chemistry designation is N-(phosphonomethyl)glycine – is the predominant agricultural chemical in the history of the world [Duke & Powles 2008]. The US Geological Survey estimates that in 2011 ~110 million kg of glyphosate were applied in the US for agricultural purposes [Baker & Stone 2013]. Glyphosate is mainly used as active substance in herbicides or weed killers to prevent unwanted plant growth; it is applied to the leaves of the plants, especially the annual broadleaf weeds and grasses that compete with the crops. Its great success was due to its systemic and non-selective action against plant organisms, but also and mainly to increased cultivation of genetically modified soybeans and corn with resistance to glyphosate.

Glyphosate was discovered to be an herbicide by Monsanto chemist John E. Franz in 1970. In 1974 the company began to market the substance under the trade name Roundup [Franz et al. 1997]. Normally, glyphosate is used in agriculture and horticulture to combat weeds before sowing. However, when GMO with resistance to glyphosate are grown, glyphosate is also used after sowing to destroy the weeds that grow among the crops.

The proposed minimum purity of the active substance as manufactured by the members of the European Glyphosate Task Force varies between 950 and 983 g per kg. In other words, every kg of glyphosate is "contaminated" with 17 to 50 g of other chemicals, some of them relevant and others not. N-nitroso-glyphosate and formaldehyde are considered relevant impurities [EFSA 2015]. Depending on the commercial formula, the easily accessible Safety Data Sheets commonly mention that 3 to 4 ingredients – a glyphosate salt, tallow alkylamine ethoxylate, pelargonic and related fatty acids, and bis (2-hydroxyalkyl) cocoalkylamine – as well as some unnamed ingredients, determined not to be hazardous, are dissolved in water. Polyoxyethylene tallow amine (POEA) has been used as a surfactant additive in glyphosate formulations since Monsanto introduced the Roundup brand of herbicide. It was found in current agricultural and household glyphosate formulations from several manufacturers [Tush et al. 2013] and POEA as well as glyphosate and its main metabolite, aminomethylphosphonic acid, were detected in agricultural soils of most of the American states [Tush & Meyer 2016], in surface and ground water, and in sediments [Battaglin et al. 2014]. Although we know that the toxicity of glyphosate formulations to non-target organisms has been attributed to POEA, or to the mixture of POEA and glyphosate more so than to glyphosate alone [Moore et al. 2012], there are far too few studies on the occurrence, fate, and transport pathways of POEA in the environment [Tush et al. 2018].

Are evaluations fundamentally different? Or not?

The crown jewel of Monsanto is a blend of glyphosate with several other co-formulants and few unavoidable impurities and reaction products.

Roundup is simply a very complex mixture. It was perceived as truly ecological and not very toxic for a considerable amount of time. In 2015, IARC classified glyphosate in Group 2A. Later, EFSA and ECHA concluded that the substance was not cancerogenous. Or how to create confusion in Europe! These discrepancies however can be explained. On the one hand, the different agencies did not rely on the same studies and did not apply the same evaluation methods, but above all they did not carry out their investigations on the same products.

The IARC report looked at both the active substance glyphosate as well as the glyphosate-based formulations. The EFSA and ECHA assessments, on the other hand, considered glyphosate only. IARC and EU adopted different approaches. It is the distinction between the effects of one single active substance and those of complex biocide formulations (mixtures of several chemicals) that explains how EFSA and IARC arrived at different conclusions. For the EFSA and ECHA studies, focussing exclusively on glyphosate was more relevant than investigating on formulated products containing several constituents (as well as their impurities and reaction products). This approach had been specifically recommended, since the different components could not be clearly identified.

We know for a fact, however, that humans are chronically exposed to multiple exogenous substances, including environmental pollutants, drugs and dietary components, and we suspect that many among these compounds impact human health and that their combination in complex mixtures could significantly exacerbate their individual harmful effects. Delfosse et al. [2015], for example, clearly demonstrates that a pharmaceutical oestrogen and a persistent organochlorine pesticide, both of them exhibiting low efficacy when studied separately, cooperatively bind to the pregnane X receptor, leading to synergistic activation[16]. Why then focus on the effects of the pure chemical rather than assess biocide formulations? Many scientists have already convincingly evidenced that the effects of mixtures differ from the sums of their individual effects

---

16 When the combined power of a group of things when they are working together is greater than the total power achieved by each working separately [Cambridge Dictionary]; e.g. team work at its best results in a synergy that can be very productive.

[Pape-Lindstrom & Lydy 1997; Laetz et al. 2002; Gore et al. 2015; Delfosse et al. 2015; Krepker et al. 2017]. Today, the "cocktail of contaminants" remains a broadly misunderstood and insufficiently researched concept with a strong social resonance. Now is the time to invest in studies on the cocktail effects of various pollutants.

This is extremely important, because although some studies suggest that certain glyphosate-based formulations may be genotoxic[17], others that look solely at the active substance glyphosate do not show this effect. It is therefore likely that the genotoxic effects observed in glyphosate-based formulations are caused by exposure to several constituent blends of obligatory ingredients and their inherent impurities. It also happens that the genotoxic effect of a mixture exceeds the sum of the individual effects since the different compounds work in synergy. That is why we must be honest enough to recognize that glyphosate-based formulations display higher toxicity than that of the active ingredient alone.

In its assessment, EFSA [2015] suggests that the toxicity of each pesticide formulation and in particular its genotoxic potential should be further investigated and addressed by Member State authorities as they re-assess uses of glyphosate-based formulations in their own territories. This is a pressing matter! So-called "inert" ingredients can increase the ability of pesticide formulations to affect significant toxicologic end points, including developmental neurotoxicity, genotoxicity, and disruption of hormone functions [Cox & Surgan 2006].

One should never forget that herbicides, pesticides, fungicides and ... biocides simply mean chemicals intended to destroy, to kill. The worst news is that pesticides often create pests. The message of Paul Ehrlich [1968] is undeniable: ... *Careless overuse of DDT has promoted to "pest" category many species of mites, little insect-like relatives of spiders. The insects which ate the mites were killed by the DDT and the mites were resistant to DDT. There you have it – instant pests, and more profits for the agricultural chemical industry in fighting these Frankensteins of their own*

---

17 In genetics, genotoxicity describes the property of chemical agents that damages the genetic information within a cell causing mutations [Wikipedia].

creation. What is more, some of the more potent miticides the chemists have developed with which to do battle seem to be powerful carcinogens...

Should we expect unrestrained use of glyphosate in the coming years?

As long as it has not been clearly demonstrated that the product is harmless, large-scale use of glyphosate should be banned by virtue of the precautionary principle that should always be applied by public authorities when managing public health risks. The precautionary principle is relevant in those specific circumstances where risk managers have reason to believe that there are reasonable grounds to be concerned that an unacceptable level of risk to health exists, even though the supporting information and data may not be sufficiently complete to enable a comprehensive risk assessment to carried out.

In Europe, technical matters which should be science-based such authorizing marketing for chemicals or genetically engineered crop plants soon take on a political dimension. Even after the European safety agencies have given a provisional go-ahead, the final decision will still depend on approval by qualified majority of the 28 members states. This usually triggers off aggressive lobbying, demagoguery and domestically focused political calculations with insufficient consideration for the scientific advice. Who, then, is speaking the truth? And why not listen to what the Persian poet Jalal al-Din Rumi (1207-1273) had to say about truth: *"The truth was a mirror in the hands of God. It fell, and broke into pieces. Everybody took a piece of it, and they looked at it and thought they had the truth"*.

Science moves rapidly and increases our knowledge. New approaches, accounting for chemical similarity and overlaying multiple data sources, will play a role in future risk assessments [Guha et al. 2016]. Moreover, it has now been recognized that testing for glyphosate in urine can help determine the level of exposure to glyphosate as well as the nature of related risks and ensure that optimal treatment plans for patients are put in place [Shaw & Pratt-Hyatt 2017].

Premature conclusions must be avoided, however, especially since additional analyses are still required by the European Member States [EFSA 2015]. We must always privilege doubt and a constructive critical mind, permanent questioning, and intellectual (and cultural) commitment at everyone's service [Bannel 2013]. And everybody should bear in mind that the responsibility of national health departments is to protect and promote health, and to prevent diseases and injuries.

The last word has not yet been spoken

New data reports in the scientific literature are published in rapid succession. Whether or not by coincidence, I seldom see these reports in the social media. But, then, if they hardly ever appear, they are likely to go unnoticed – reports such as those referenced below:

Gill et al. [2018] have traced the toxicological effects of glyphosate from lower invertebrates to higher vertebrates. Effects have been observed in earthworms, arthropods, molluscs, echinoderms, fish, reptiles, amphibians and birds. Toxicological effects like genotoxicity, cytotoxicity, nuclear aberration, hormonal disruption, chromosomal aberrations and DNA damage have also been observed in higher vertebrates. It is the entire animal realm that is under threat, including man!

The concentration of glyphosate in beer varies from below the limit of detection up to 150 µg per kg, and significantly higher contents of glyphosate were observed when the label did not mention the country of production and when the beer was sold in local supermarkets [Jansons et al. 2018]. If there is glyphosate in the beer, then it is also in the beer drinkers!

The results obtained by Sritana et al. [2018] explain, at least partly, how glyphosate acts on the oestrogen signalling pathway and induces proliferation of cholangiocarcinoma[18] cells. Denying these data would be unacceptable. Cancer is such a painful disease both for cancer sufferers and those who surround them. But there is more: we should not be blind

---

18 Cholangiocarcinoma is a group of cancers that begin in the bile ducts.

to the fact that chemical cocktails could be hormone disruptors, may cause allergies or intolerances, and trigger many other and different illnesses. Making people ill can never be an option. Maybe the chances of this happening are very small – they should be non-existent!

Bibliography

Alexander et al. [2007]. The non-Hodgkin lymphomas: A review of the epidemiologic literature, *International Journal of Cancer* 120, 1-39

Baker & Stone [2013]. Preliminary estimates of annual agricultural pesticide use for counties of the conterminous United States 2010-11, *U.S. Geological Survey Open-file Report* 2013-1295

Bannel [2013]. *Les nouvelles voies de l'éthique*, Éditions Télètes, pp. 132

Battaglin et al. [2014]. Glyphosate and its degradation product AMPA occur frequently and widely in U.S. soils, surface water, groundwater, and precipitation, *Journal of the American Water Resources Association* 50, 275-290

Beecham & Seneff [2016]. Is there a link between autism and glyphosate-formulated herbicides? *Journal of Autism* 3, article 1

Cornwall [2017]. Update: After quick review, medical school says no evidence Monsanto ghostwrote professor's paper, *Science Daily Newsletter*, March 23

Cox & Surgan [2006]. Unidentified Inert Ingredients in Pesticides: Implications for Human and Environmental Health, *Environmental Health Perspectives* 114, 1803-1806

Delfosse et al. [2015]. Synergistic activation of human pregnane X receptor by binary cocktails of pharmaceutical and environmental compounds, *Nature Communications* DOI: 10.1038/ncomms9089

Duke & Powles [2008]. Glyphosate: a once-in-a-century herbicide, *Pest Management Science* 64, 319-325

EFSA [2015]. Conclusion on the peer review of the pesticide risk assessment of the active substance glyphosate, *EFSA Journal* 13, 11, 4302, pp. 107

Ehrlich [1968]. *The Population Bomb*, Ballantine Books pp. 201

Franz et al. [1997]. Glyphosate: a Unique Global Herbicide, *ACS Monograph No. 189*, American Chemical Society, Washington, DC, US

Gill et al. [2018]. Glyphosate toxicity for animals, *Environmental Chemistry Letters*, 1-26

Gore et al. [2015]. EDC-2: The Endocrine Society's Second Scientific Statement on Endocrine-Disrupting Chemicals, *Endocrine reviews* 36, 6, E1-E150

Guha et al. [2016]. Prioritizing Chemicals for Risk Assessment Using Chemoinformatics: Examples from the IARC Monographs on Pesticides, *Environmental Health Perspectives* 124, 1823-1829

Guyton et al. [2015]. Carcinogenicity of tetrachlorvinphos, parathion, malathion, diazinon, and glyphosate, *Lancet Oncology* 16, 5, 490-491

Hammond et al. [2004]. Results of a 13 week safety assurance study with rats fed grain from glyphosate tolerant corn, *Food and Chemical Toxicology* 42, 1003-1014

Hoppin et al. [2017]. Pesticides are Associated with Allergic and Non-Allergic Wheeze among Male Farmers, *Environmental Health Perspectives* 125, 535-543

Jansons et al. [2018]. Occurrence of glyphosate in beer from the Latvian market, *Food Additives and Contaminants Part A* 35, 9, 1767-1775

Jayasumana et al. [2014]. Glyphosate, Hard Water and Nephrotoxic Metals: Are They the Culprits Behind the Epidemic of Chronic Kidney Disease of Unknown Etiology in Sri Lanka? *International Journal of Environmental Research and Public Health* 11, 2125-2147

Jayasumana et al. [2015]. Drinking well water and occupational exposure to Herbicides is associated with chronic kidney disease, in Padavi-Sripura, Sri Lanka, *Environmental Health* 14, 1, pp. 10

JRC [2018]. *Something from nothing? Ensuring the safety of chemical mixtures,* pp. 2

Kier & Kirkland [2013]. Review of genotoxicity studies of glyphosate and glyphosate-based formulations, *Critical Reviews in Toxicology* 43, 4, 283-315

Krepker et al. [2017]. Active food packaging films with synergistic antimicrobial activity, *Food Control* 76, 117-126

Laetz et al. [2002]. The Synergistic Toxicity of Pesticide Mixtures: Implications for Risk Assessment and the Conservation of Endangered Pacific Salmon, *Environmental Health Perspect* 117, 348-353

Michaels [2008]. *Doubt is their product*, Oxford University Press, pp. 372

Moore et al. [2012]. Relative toxicity of the components of the original formulation of roundup, *Ecotoxicology and Environmental Safety* 78, 128-133.

Pape-Lindstrom & Lydy [1997]. Synergistic toxicity of atrazine and organophosphate insecticides contravenes the response addition method, *Environmental Toxicology and Chemistry* 16, 11, 2415-2420

Parks et al. [2017]. Rheumatoid Arthritis in Agricultural Health Study Spouses: Associations with Pesticides and Other Farm Exposures, *Environmental Health Perspectives* 124, 1728-1734

Proctor [2006]. "Everyone knew but no one had proof": tobacco industry use of medical history expertise in US courts, 1990–2002, *Tobacco Control* 15 (Suppl IV), iv117-iv125

Robinson et al. [2013]. Conflicts of interest at the European Food Safety Authority erode public confidence, *Journal of epidemiology and community health* 0, 1-4

Sealy et al. [2016]. Environmental factors in the development of autism spectrum disorders, *Environment International* 88, 288-298

Séralini et al. [2012]. Long term toxicity of a Roundup herbicide and a Roundup-tolerant genetically modified maize, *Food and Chemical Toxicology* 50, 4221-4231 (retracted)

Séralini et al. [2014]. Republished study: long-term toxicity of a Roundup herbicide and a Roundup-tolerant genetically modified maize, *Environmental Sciences Europe* 26, 14, pp. 17

Shaw & Pratt-Hyatt [2017]. The importance of testing for glyphosate: the world's most widely used herbicide, http://www.immh.org/article-source/2017/2/2/the-importance-of-testing-for-glyphosate-the-worlds-most-widely-used-herbicide

Sritana et al. [2018]. Glyphosate induces growth of estrogen receptor alpha positive cholangiocarcinoma cells via non-genomic estrogen receptor/ERK1/2 signaling pathway, Food and Chemical Toxicology 118, 595-607

Tush et al. [2013]. Characterization of polyoxyethylene tallow amine surfactants in technical mixtures and glyphosate formulations using ultra-high performance liquid chromatography and triple quadrupole mass spectrometry, *Journal of Chromatography* A 1319, 80-87

Tush & Meyer [2016]. Polyoxyethylene tallow amine, a glyphosate formulation adjuvant: soil adsorption characteristics, degradation profile, and occurrence on selected soils from agricultural fields in Iowa, Illinois, Indiana, Kansas, Mississippi, and Missouri, *Environmental Science and Technology* 50, 5781-5789

Tush et al. [2018]. Dissipation of polyoxyethylene tallow amine (POEA) and glyphosate in an agricultural field and their co-occurrence on streambed sediments, *Science of the Total Environment* 636, 212-219

Williams et al. [2000]. Safety Evaluation and Risk Assessment of the Herbicide Roundup and Its Active Ingredient, Glyphosate, for Humans, *Regulatory Toxicology and Pharmacology* 31, 2, 117-165

Shouldn't we say "yes" to genetically edited food crops?

Golden rice: a conflict between strictly ecological and humanitarian positions

According to the World Health Organization, vitamin A deficiency (VAD) is a leading cause of childhood blindness in the developing world. Moreover, VAD weakens the immune system, thereby increasing vulnerability to illnesses such as measles, respiratory infections and diarrhea, frequently leading to death. The deficiency affects more than 140 million pre-school children in 118 nations, and more than 7 million pregnant women. The United Nations Children's Fund (UNICEF) estimates that 1.15 million child deaths are precipitated by VAD each year. Witcher et al. [2001] emphasize that 1 million of the estimated 1.5 million blind children in the world live in Asia. *Each year there are half a million new cases, 70 per cent of which are due to vitamin A deficiency,* the authors wrote. They estimate that every minute a child goes blind somewhere in the world. And, worst of all, the study points out that a majority of them die before their first birthday.

Rice, a major staple food, is usually milled to remove the oil-rich aleurone[19] layer that turns rancid when stored, especially in tropical areas. The remaining edible endosperm[20] lacks several essential nutrients,

---

19 Protein stored as granules in the cells of plant seeds.

20 The endosperm is a nutritive tissue found in the seeds of nearly all the flowering plants after fertilization; it is normally formed in the process of double fertilization, and contains mainly starch in addition to some oil and protein [Maximum Yield].

more particularly provitamin A. Unbalanced rice consumption (without vitamin A rich foods, such as carrots, green leafy vegetables, and chicken or mutton liver, for example) promotes VAD, more particularly in the highly populated areas of Asia, Africa, and Latin America [Ye et al. 2000].

In the 1990s, the Golden Rice prototype was developed by two European scientists, Ingo Potrykus and Peter Beyer. Golden Rice is conventional rice that has been genetically engineered to have high levels of beta-carotene, the precursor to vitamin A [Ye et al. 2000]. Beta-carotene is found in a variety of fruits and vegetables, but rice, which makes up to ~80 % of the daily diet in Asia, contains only very small amounts of beta-carotene. Potrykus and Beyer's rice was greeted with great enthusiasm. The first prototype however did not contain high enough levels of beta-carotene to be an effective source of vitamin A. Subsequently, Paine et al. [2005] developed the second generation of Golden Rice (Golden Rice 2) by introgressing the biosynthetic pathway for provitamin A carotenoids (PVAC) into the Golden Rice. The beta-carotene concentration of this genetically modified organism (GMO) amounted to 1.6-35.0 microgram per gram of dry rice [Tang et al. 2009].

Using recombinant deoxyribonucleic acid (DNA) techniques, the International Rice Research Institute (IRRI) has developed a genetically modified rice event, called GR2E, which is biofortified with provitamin A [http://irri.org/]. Provitamin A Biofortified Rice Event GR2E is considered a novel food. This means the food is derived from a plant, animal or micro-organism that has been genetically modified in such a way that the plant, animal or microorganism exhibits characteristics that were not previously observed. The definition of the European Union (EU) reads as follows: novel food can be newly developed, innovative food, food produced using new technologies and production processes, as well as food which is or has been traditionally eaten outside of the EU. The novel food notion is not new. Throughout history new types of food, food ingredients or ways of producing food have found their way to Europe from every corner of the globe. Bananas, tomatoes, pasta, tropical fruit, corn, rice, a wide range of spices – they came all to Europe as novel foods.

Among the recent arrivals are chia seeds, algae-based foods, baobab fruit and physalis (Peruvian ground cherry or Cape gooseberries).

In early 2017, the Philippine Rice Research Institute together with the IRRI reached another milestone with the submission of the biosafety permit application for the direct use in food, feed, or for processing of GR2E Golden Rice. Meanwhile, in Bangladesh, the application for environmental and food safety assessment of GR2E Golden Rice was lodged with the Ministry of Agriculture on 26th November 2017 and with the Ministry of Environment and Forest on 4th December 2017, respectively. Outside of the Philippines and Bangladesh, applications for food or food and feed safety review of GR2E have been submitted to the US Food and Drug Administration (US FDA), Food Standards Australia New Zealand as well as to Health Canada. Collectively, the data presented in these application submissions have not revealed potential health or safety concerns and support the conclusion that food and/or livestock animal feed derived from provitamin A biofortified GR2E rice is as safe and nutritious as food or feed derived from conventional rice varieties. Food Standards Australia New Zealand, Health Canada and US FDA concurred with the assessment of the IRRI regarding the safety and nutrition of Golden Rice.

After more than a decade of rigorous scientific testing and extensive research trials amid violent attempts by anti-GMO groups to discredit its nutritional value and usefulness, Golden Rice is now moving closer to the marketplace. The much awaited vitamin A enriched rice variety will finally find its way onto dining tables and gradually help address the health problems associated with VAD. The first high yielding varieties containing the GR2E trait should be available to farmers at the end of this decade.

Golden orange-fleshed bananas rich in pro-vitamin A

In 2014 Jonathan O'Callaghan commented on the Queensland University of Technology project that aims to improve the vitamin A levels of bananas: ... *The world's first human trial of "super bananas" will start soon in the hope of a more nutritious source of food to Ugandans and East Africans. The bananas will be enriched in pro-vitamin A, which the human body can break down into "regular" vitamin A, to tackle the consequences of vitamin A deficiency in the regions. And, if the trial is successful, it's hoped farmers could begin growing the enhanced food by 2020...* Bananas that are enriched in pro-vitamin A are considered an extra tool in the battle against VAC, and all its multifold negative health consequences! [http://www.dailymail.co.uk/sciencetech/article-2660138/ Super-bananas-sale-2020-Fruit-laced-vitamin-A-begins-humans-trials-tackle-deficiency-Africa.html#ixzz52Hauw4v6].

Since white-fleshed Cavendish bananas that dominate the export trade are low in pro-vitamin A, it was long thought that bananas in general were poor sources of PVAC, the chemical precursors of the essential vitamin A. Fortunately, interest in vitamin A-rich bananas began in the early 2000s when highly efficient chemical analyses revealed that some orange-fleshed cultivars from the Pacific region have high PVAC levels. Highest levels were measured in a Fe'i banana from the island of Pohnpei, which belongs to Pohnpei State, one of the four states in the Federated States of Micronesia. Beta-carotene levels in the Fe'i banana are as high as ~8000 micrograms per 100 gram fresh weight [Englberger et al. 2003]. African as well as Pacific plantains and AA cultivars from Papua New Guinea also have relatively high levels, but most plantains have long intervals between cycles due to their slow sucker growth that is related to a shortage in gibberellins[21] [Swennen & Wilson 1983]. This makes them less popular for staple food production and less suitable to meet the great and urgent need for vitamin A.

Deeply concerned about the thousands of children dying worldwide from VAD, researchers from the Queensland University of Technology decided to investigate a possible way to enhance pro-vitamin A levels in bananas. Basically, they took a gene from a banana originating in Papua New Guinea, which is naturally very high in pro-vitamin A but grows in

---

21 Gibberellins (GA) are the plant hormones that promote germination, stem elongation, and leaf development; they are also instrumental in determining dormancy, sexual reproduction, and flowering. It is thought that the (albeit unconscious) selective breeding of crops strains that were deficient in GA synthesis was one of the key drivers of the "green revolution" in the 1960s [Spielmeyer et al. 2002].

small bunches, and inserted it into a Cavendish banana. The Cavendish cultivars, Williams and Dwarf Cavendish, were genetically modified in an attempt to transfer the elevated PVAC production capacity into East African highland bananas, the main staple food in Uganda. Also the Pome cultivar Lady finger was genetically modified. It was now only a matter of being able to produce and harvest PVAC-rich bananas in the field.

Paul et al. [2017] reported on the "proof-of-concept" technology required to successfully develop and grow pro-vitamin A fortified East African highland banana varieties in Uganda. It immediately became clear that the genetically modified Cavendish dessert banana, now grown in the field in Australia, produces fruits with significantly enhanced pro-vitamin A levels. This research project was supported by the Bill & Melinda Gates Foundation and by the UK Department for International Development.

We may now legitimately hope that pro-vitamin A rich bananas will soon be harvested in Africa!

Arctic apples: the jucy newcomers that have the special ability to resist browning

Last year, Amy Maxmen [2017] published the Nature News article *"Genetically modified apple reaches US stores, but will consumers bite?"*: *... the "Arctic apple" is one of the first foods to be given a trait intended to please consumers rather than farmers, and it joins a small number of genetically modified organisms to be sold as a whole product, not an ingredient. Since Okanagan Specialty Fruits in Summerland, Canada, planted its first test apples in 2003, the array of foods modified in labs has expanded to include meatless burgers, made with soya protein produced by recombinant yeast, fish fillets grown from seafood stem cells, and mushrooms whose genomes have been edited with CRISPR technology. Most of these items have not yet reached the market though...*

The slightly yellow-green flesh does not turn brown because scientists have figured out how to silence the genes that produce the browning enzyme. Growers as well as opponents of GMO have raised concerns about genetically engineered crops and the complicated technology behind it. Health Canada however has approved the sale of genetically modified apples and so has the US Department of Agriculture. And many are now keenly watching the launch of the Arctic apple for clues as to how consumers will perceive the "new" fruit.

Harvesting tasty apples is far more complicated than simply planting a seed and waiting for a tree to grow [Baker 2018]. Indeed, it is hard to predict what an apple grown from a seed will look and taste like since every seed contains a combination of genetic materials from its parents. Yet, farmers can reliably grow orchards of tasty apples by using the ancient grafting technique. After a tree that produces apples with a desirable, delicious taste has been selected, cuttings of that original tree are grafted or fused onto a rootstock. The cuttings then grow into a full-sized tree that contains exactly the same genetic material as the original one. On the other hand, new apple varieties emerge when genetic changes are allowed to occur. Traditionally, they are produced by cross-breeding existing apple varieties. This reshuffles the genetic makeup of the seeds, which are then planted to see if they grow into trees that produce valuable, new apples. Arctic apples® were created by a targeted change to the genetic material of existing varieties. The advantage is that scientists focussed on apples that were already popular with consumers, a highly efficient approach when compared to traditional and relatively random cross-breeding.

When the cells of conventional apples are damaged, which happens when they are cut, bitten into or bruised, an enzyme called polyphenol oxidase (PPO) initiates a chemical reaction that turns the flesh of the fruit brown. Due to varying levels of PPO, some apple varieties brown fast, while others have a lower degree of browning. The Arctic Apple is the world's first non-browning apple. Its flesh will retain its fresh, appealing colour even days after it has been sliced, which the producers claim will increase apple consumption and mitigate a major source of food waste. The production of PPO enzymes is blocked by simply removing their ribonucleic acid (RNA) blueprints. This was done by a tool that originates from molecular biology, called RNA interference, a natural process that recognizes and destroys specific RNA structures. By introducing RNA sequences that cause the degradation of PPO RNA, an anti-PPO gene was developed that destroys the PPO RNA before it can be used to make PPO enzymes [Baker 2018].

Arctic® Golden slices were available for the first time in 2017. A significant market presence increase is expected after the fall harvest of 2018, including the new Arctic® Granny. I can already imagine the advertising slogans: "Crisp, wholesome, great-tasting apple slices are perfect for fresh and healthy snacks. And no time wasted"!

What are genetically modified foods? And are they safe for consumption?

Genetically modified foods or GMO result from the application of recombinant DNA biotechnological procedures that allow the genetic makeup of a food product or organism to be altered in some favourable way. The recombination can be achieved by moving genes from one organism into another or by changing genes that are already present in the organism. These changes result in the expression of attributes not found in the original organisms [Schneider et al. 2017]. Examples include provitamin A enriched food crops, non-browning apples, pest-resistant as well as herbicide-tolerant crops, and many others. Genetic modifications are meant to assist food growers and manufacturers either by increasing the nutritional value of the food crops or by improving the crop yields through reduced insecticide and herbicide requirements.

GMO have their genetic material altered using one of several methods. Although traditional animal breeding and genetic modification through plant hybridization techniques are technically genetic modifications, these techniques pre-date recombinant techniques and are not considered genetic modifications. A genetically engineered organism is one that has its DNA modified, using techniques that enable the direct transfer or removal of genes in that organism. Organisms that undergo genetic engineering are often referred to as transgenic. Originally, the term "transgenic" referred to an organism that had a gene from another, different organism inserted into it. Nevertheless, especially in newspapers, magazines and on the internet, the term "transgenic" is frequently used to refer to any genetic modification, regardless of the source and recipient of genetic material.

There are three generations of genetically modified foods. First-generation crops have enhanced input traits, such as herbicide tolerance, better insect resistance, and better tolerance to environmental stress. Second-generation crops include those with added value output traits, such as nutrient enhancement. Third-generation crops include those that produce pharmaceuticals, improve the processing of bio-based fuels, or produce products beyond food and fiber [Fernandez-Cornejo et al. 2006].

The recent developments of cost-effective, high-throughput sequencing technologies have resulted in significant increases in available genomic information of fruit crop species. They have redefined the boundaries of genetic engineering and genetically modified crop plants. Since fruit and vegetable crops play a key role in the economy of both developed and developing countries, substantial efforts have been made to improve crop quality. Both conventional breeding and genetic engineering techniques were used to introduce desirable genes in fruit crops. Collective mistrust for the latter technologies, however, coupled with misleading and false information regarding nutritional efficiency and safety, have made it hard and often impossible to successfully commercialise GMO [Pussemier & Goeyens 2017].

Some twenty years ago, Hawaiian papaya farmers were in serious trouble. Ringspot virus, transmitted by insects, was destroying their crops. Farmers tried everything to eradicate the virus: selective breeding, crop rotation, quarantine. Nothing worked. One scientist however had a different idea: what if a gene, known as the coat protein, could be transferred from a harmless part of the virus to the papaya's DNA? Would the genetically modified papaya then be immune to the virus? And it was! A fierce battle broke out between GMO supporters and opponents, but in the end it was the GMO supporters who won and the papaya survived. Papayas that are resistant to ringspot virus have now been cultivated in the US for more than a decade [Kanchiswamy et al. 2015; Saletan 2015].

Groups like Independent Science News and Greenpeace argued that the approved version of Golden Rice does not have enough beta-carotene to make a nutritional difference. This has been a common criticism, even after the US FDA as well as Health Canada stated that a replacement of all rice and rice products with GR2E rice would merely result in a very small increase in beta-carotene intake. A health claim is not the same however as a nutrition statement, and the US FDA and Health Canada statements did not translate into "no nutritional value". The FDA's report stated that: *"Based on the safety and nutritional assessment IRRI has conducted, it is our understanding the IRRI concludes that human and animal food from GR2E rice is not materially different in composition, safety, or other relevant parameters from rice-derived food currently on the market except for the intended beta-carotene change in GR2E rice",* and that *"the concentration of β-carotene in GR2E rice is too low to warrant a nutrient content claim."* The US FDA, Health Canada and even Australia and New Zealand were considering overall safety and making nutritional claims for the benefit of their own, healthy populations. The VAD targeted by Golden Rice does not exist in those countries, and IRRI has no intention of introducing Golden Rice in countries that are not experiencing high levels of VAD among children and infants [Porterfield 2018].

On the whole, there seems to be more scope for marketing new genetically modified varieties, developed with novel technologies, that enhance the consumer experience (fruit crops, for example, with increased levels of antioxidants, more flavour or sweetness), in addition to other improvements such as pest and disease resistance. Moreover, when biotechnology is used to target the luxury product market, it easily gains consumer acceptance. Examples include the blue pigmented roses developed jointly in Japan and Australia, using a transgene for the expression of the blue pigment delphinidin [Katsumoto et al. 2007]. Not an unimportant chemical, since it is common knowledge that delphinidin also has strong antioxidant and anti-inflammatory properties.

The market can certainly be expected to offer a larger choice of products in the future, including genetically modified food products which in addition to environmental and societal benefits will provide novelty and enhanced quality, thereby enriching the quality of consumer experience.

Today, most transgenic fruit crop plants have been developed using *Agrobacterium*-mediated transformation. Among those that have been developed, only papaya has so far successfully been commercialised. Following the regulatory and social hurdles associated with transgenic crops, novel biotechnological tools have emerged. They allow for the insertion of specific genes that make it possible for genes to be modified or replaced at their genomic location without involving any other source of DNA [Liu et al. 2013; Araki et al. 2014]. The absence of foreign DNA and the introduction of genes derived from the same plant species should help enhance consumer acceptance of novel genetically modified plant products (food products) that were developed using those technologies [Kanchiswamy et al. 2015].

With the development and improvement of those technologies, it is now time to revisit the benefits of genetic modification and initiate the development of novel, consumer acceptable products. Recently designed tools will enable modifications or mutations of genes of interest without involving foreign DNA. As a result, plants developed using this technology could be considered as non-transgenic genetically altered plants. According to Kanchiswamy et al. [2015], this would pave the way for the development of fruit crops with superior phenotypes and allow them to be commercialised even though GM crops are currently poorly accepted, with the exception of a few products such as the super bananas that produce more vitamin A, and the non-browning apples that do not turn brown after being cut and retain their original and natural flavour and taste for long periods of time.

A list of recently engineered plants presents a number of valuable options for the future: drought tolerant corn, virus resistant plums, potatoes with fewer natural toxins, and soybeans that produce less saturated fat. A global inventory by the UN Food and Agriculture Organization discusses other projects currently in the pipeline: virus resistant beans, heat tolerant sugarcane, salt tolerant wheat, disease resistant cassava, high-iron rice, and cotton that requires less nitrogen fertilizer. The news media also provide information about ambitious scientific projects: high-calcium carrots [Park et al. 2004], antioxidant tomatoes [Verhoeyen et al. 2002], non-allergenic nuts [Robotham et al.

2009, and references herein], bacteria resistant oranges [Cardoso et al. 2010], corn and cassava loaded with extra nutrients, and a flax-like plant that produces the healthy oil formerly available only in fish [Jhala & Hall 2010].

There is a great deal genetic engineering can do for public health and the quality of our planet. We cannot afford to engage in pointless fighting over GMO, in a sterile struggle of "life and death" between an army of quacks and pseudo-environmentalists waging a war on science and a gang of corporate cowards who would rather stick to profitable weed-killing [Saletan 2015].

Honest, scientific arguments should always prevail!

Bibliography

Araki et al. [2014]. Caution required for handling genome editing technology, *Trends in Biotechnology* 32, 5, 234-237

Baker [2018]. Arctic Apples: A fresh new take on genetic engineering, *science in the news*, Harvard University, http://sitn.hms.harvard.edu/flash/2018/arctic-apples-fresh-new-take-genetic-engineering/

Cardoso et al. [2010]. Transgenic Sweet Orange (*Citrus sinensis* L. Osbeck) Expressing the *attacin* A Gene for Resistance to *Xanthomonas citri* subsp. *Citri, Plant Molecular Biology Reporter* 28, 2, 185-192

Englberger et al. [2003]. Further analyses on Micronesian banana, taro, breadfruit and other foods for provitamin A carotenoids and minerals, *Journal of Food Composition and Analysis* 16, 219-236

Fernandez-Cornejo et al. [2006]. The First Decade of Genetically Engineered Crops in the United States/EIB-11 Economic Research Service/USDA

Jhala & Hall [2010]. Flax (*Linum usitatissimum* L.): Current Uses and Future Applications, *Australian Journal of basic and Applied Sciences* 4, 9, 4304-4312

Kanchiswamy et al. [2015]. Looking forward to genetically edited fruit crops, *Trends in Biotechnology* 33, 2, 62-64

Katsumoto et al. [2007]. Engineering of the Rose Flavonoid Biosynthetic Pathway Successfully Generated Blue-Hued Flowers Accumulating Delphinidin, *Plant Cell Physiology* 48, 11, 1589-1600

Liu et al. [2013]. Advanced genetic tools for plant biotechnology, *Nature Reviews Genetics* 14, 781-793

Maxmen [2017]. Genetically modified apple reaches US stores, but will consumers bite? *Nature* 551, 149-150

Paine et al. [2005]. Improving the nutritional value of Golden Rice through increased pro-vitamin A content, *Nature Biotechnology* 23, 482-487

Park et al. [2004]. Increased calcium in carrots by expression of an *Arabidopsis* H+/Ca2+ transporter, *Molecular Breeding* 14, 3, 275-282

Paul et al. [2017]. Golden bananas in the field: elevated fruit pro-vitamin A from the expression of a single banana transgene, *Plant Biotechnology Journal* 15, 520-532

Porterfield [2018]. Anti-GMO groups draw FDA rebuke over misrepresentation of Golden Rice nutrition, *Genetic Literacy Project*, June 11

Pussemier & Goeyens [2017]. *AgricultureS & Enjeux de société*, Les presses agronomiques de Gembloux, pp. 112

Robotham et al. [2009]. Linear IgE-epitope mapping and comparative structural homology modeling of hazelnut and English walnut 11S globulins, *Molecular Immunology* 46, 2975-2984

Saletan [2015]. Unhealthy Fixation - The war against genetically modified organisms is full of fearmongering, errors, and fraud. Labeling them will not make you safer, *Slate*, July 15

Schneider et al. [2017]. Genetically Modified Food, University of Florida, IFAS Extension, http://edis.ifas.ufl.edu/

Spielmeyer et al. [2002]. Semidwarf (sd-1), "green revolution" rice, contains a defective gibberellin 20-oxidase gene, PNAS 99, 13, 9043-9048

Swennen & Wilson [1983]. La stimulation du développement du rejet baïonnette du bananier plantain (Musa sp. groupe AAB) par application de Gibberelline (A3), *Fruits* 38, 4, 261-265

Tang et al. [2009]. Golden Rice is an effective source of vitamin A, *The American Journal of Clinical Nutrition* 89, 1776-1783

Verhoeyen et al. [2002]. Increasing antioxidant levels in tomatoes through modification of the flavonoid biosynthetic pathway, *Journal of Experimental Botany* 53, 377, Fruit Development and Ripening Special Issue, 2099-2106

Witcher et al. [2001]. Corneal blindness: a global perspective, *Bulletin of the World Health Organization* 79, 214-221

Ye et al. [2000]. Engineering the Provitamin A (β-Carotene) Biosynthetic Pathway into (Carotenoid-Free) Rice Endosperm, *Science* 287, 303-305

By uncovering its genetic journey, researchers believe they can restore the flavour of the old-fashioned tomato

What is wrong with the ubiquitous and attractive supermarket tomatoes?

For many city dwellers, the delicious taste of a succulent garden tomato is little more than a distant memory. The standard grocery varieties have grown larger and blander. Indeed, the decline in flavour quality of the modern commercial tomato compared to heirloom varieties is often the cause of consumer complaints.

Internet papers, websites and the popular press often stress that the mineral nutrient compositions of vegetables, fruits and grains have considerably declined over the past 50-odd years. What should we make of these comments? Has the quality of our food deteriorated?

A frequently found quotation is: ... *A Kushi Institute analysis of nutrient data from 1975 to 1997 found that average calcium levels in 12 fresh vegetables dropped by 27%; iron levels 37%...* [Marles 2017]. These numbers appeared for the first time in an article by Jack [1998], a health writer associated with the Kushi Institute. He compared US Department of Agriculture (USDA) fresh food composition tables from 1997 with those from 1975. However, while the original source of information – the USDA food composition tables – is authoritative, a direct comparison of the values does not take into account differences in crop varieties or methods of nutrient analysis; nor does it provide information about potential causes of reported differences. The Kushi Institute report was not subjected to scientific peer review.

Yet, there can be little doubt that food composition changes have occurred. Donald Davis and his team of researchers studied USDA nutritional data from both 1950 and 1999 for 43 different vegetables and fruits. They observed significant differences but concluded that many important questions remain unanswered [Davis et al. 2004]. Are there real nutrient declines in staple food sources? Which nutrients show the greatest differences? Have declines been offset by increases in other foods or by new sources of nutrients, including fortification in some countries? A later study by Fan et al. [2008] evidenced that decreasing mineral concentrations in wheat grains are partly due to a dilution effect[22] resulting from increased yield. Moreover, changes in cultivar are key determinants of the relationship between grain yield and mineral concentrations. Yield increases in crops tend to be accompanied by an unintended and broad decline in the concentrations of minerals and some vitamins. The evidence is most compelling for cereal grains; but emerging results show that fruits and vegetables have not escaped this law of unintended consequences [Davis 2009 & 2011].

Natural tomatoes have an uneven ripening, showing darker green patches when unripe, and variable redness when ripe, traits that still show up in garden variety and heirloom breeds. However, in the late 1920s, commercial growers stumbled across a natural mutation that caused tomatoes to ripen uniformly, from an even shade of light green to an even shade of red. This mutation, known by plant biologists as "uniform ripening", has become crucial to the commercial tomato market, showing up in almost all tomatoes produced for grocery stores. The trait however reduces sugars and nutrients in the fruits. Once again, there are two sides to every coin.

To address the problem of the tasteless tomatoes that lack sweetness and flavour but look perfectly ripe, an international research team under the leadership of professor Harry Klee of the University of Florida

---

22 Yield-enhancing methods such as fertilization, irrigation, and timing tend to decrease nutrient concentrations.

performed a comprehensive study of the chemistry and genetics of tomato flavour. Tieman et al. [2017] identified the key flavour enhancing genes that have dwindled or disappeared as the tomato changed over the years.

Moreover, these scientists also believe they could return the original taste to contemporary fresh market tomatoes.

Flavour is an intricate combination of what the tongue tastes and the nose smells

The flavour of any food item can be regarded as the sum of interactions between taste and olfaction. Taste is one of the five traditional senses that belong to the gustatory system, whereas olfaction is the sense of smell[23]. For the tomato, sugars such as glucose and fructose as well as acids such as citrate and malate activate the taste receptors. On the other hand, a highly diverse set of volatile compounds including alcohols and aldehydes such as 3-methyl-1-butanol, cis-3-hexen-1-ol and hexanal activate the olfactory receptors [Tieman et al. 2012]. Organic volatiles in particular are essential for good tomato flavour.

For commercial reasons, breeders predominantly focused on yield, disease resistance, and external appearance rather than flavour quality. Also, the fruit and vegetable flavour associated volatiles are present at nano to subnano molar concentrations. They are difficult to identify and quantify and have as a result received significantly less attention. Unfortunately, over recent decades, the strong emphasis on production traits has inadvertently led to a decline in flavour quality. Several scientists have evidenced the steadily declining nutrient content in cultivated varieties [Davis 2009 & 2011, Marles 2017]. Word has spread that one would have to eat eight oranges today to derive the same amount of vitamin A as our grandparents would have ingested from

---

23 This sense enables you to perceive odours. It depends on the stimulation of sense organs in the nose by small particles carried in inhaled air. It is important not only for the detection of odours, but also for the enjoyment of food, since flavour is a blend of taste and smell. Taste registers only four qualities: salt, sour, bitter, and sweet; other qualities of flavour depend on smell [The Free Dictionnary].

one. A seriously annoying conclusion: receiving enough vitamin A, an important fat-soluble vitamin and a potent antioxidant, is absolutely essential to maintaining overall health.

Breeders have selected plants to produce huge amounts of fruit. What they want is larger fruits on the plant, but since the plant cannot cope, what happens is a substantial dilution of the flavour chemicals. Putting tastier sugar back into mainstream tomatoes is simply not feasible when you consider today's production procedures. That is because growers are not paid for flavour, they are paid per kilogram. It costs just as much to have a worker pick a small tomato as it does to pick a large one, which explains why commercially produced tomatoes are much more massive than their tiny wild ancestors.

Today, however, our first priority is no longer how well tomatoes ship and last on a shelf. The number one priority has now become to substantially increase fruit quality with minimal impact on yield.

Will scientists breed much better tomatoes by focusing on flavour genes? The answer is yes, they soon will!

Step one was to identify the chemical tomato components that most contribute to taste.

The researchers studied the alleles, i.e. the variants of a tomato gene located at a specific locus on a chromosome. Alleles induce specific traits[24]. Most genes have two alleles, a dominant and a recessive one. In a certain sense, allele differences can be likened to DNA in humans. We all have the same number of genes in our DNA, but a particular version of each gene determines the specific characteristics, i.e. how heavy we are, how tall, whether we have blue or brown eyes etc.

---

24 An allele is a variant form of a gene. Each gene resides at a specific locus (location on a chromosome) in two copies, one copy of the gene inherited from each parent. The copies, however, are not necessarily the same. When the copies of a gene differ from each other, they are known as alleles. A given gene may have multiple different alleles, though only two alleles are present at the gene's locus in any individual [Encyclopaedia Brittanica].

The aim of the study by Tieman et al. [2017] was to uncover why modern tomato varieties are deficient in those flavour chemicals, i.e. why they have lost the more desirable alleles of a number of genes. The researchers therefore had to identify the locations of the good alleles in the tomato genome. This required what is called a genome-wide assessment study.

Modern commercial tomato varieties were found to have substantially less flavour than heirloom varieties. To understand and ultimately correct this deficiency, the research team quantified flavour-associated chemicals in 398 modern, heirloom, as well as wild accessions. To include wild accessions and the closest relative of the commercial tomato provided a baseline for its chemical composition before human intervention. A subset of these accessions was evaluated in consumer panels to identify the chemicals that made the most important contributions to flavour and consumer appreciation. It was particularly obvious that modern commercial varieties contain significantly lower amounts of many of these important flavour chemicals than older varieties. The whole-genome sequencing and a genome-wide association study enabled the genetic loci to be identified that affect most of the target flavour chemicals including sugars, acids, and volatiles. Together, these results provide an understanding of the flavour deficiencies in the tomatoes we buy and the information necessary for the recovery of good flavour through molecular breeding [Tieman et al. 2017].

The scientists mapped the genes that control the synthesis of important chemicals. Once they had found them, they used genetic methodology to replace unwanted alleles in modern tomato varieties with desirable ones. So, it appears that it is possible to significantly improve our average, ordinary grocery tomatoes. If these tomatoes could be improved, it would be a big gain for consumers. Moreover, the study outlines how to do so.

Will the high-taste, high-quality, and inevitably higher-cost tomatoes sell?

Because breeding takes time, it may take three or four years before the genetic traits now being analysed are actually produced in new tomato varieties. This sounds like great news. Let us not forget, however, that a really tasty tomato is one that ripens on the vine, and that post-harvest practices such as refrigeration can irreversibly damage flavour. Moreover, super tasty tomatoes should not be transported over long distances and cannot be stored in a grocery store for many weeks without rotting.

Remember also that prime quality comes at a price.

Bibliography

Davis [2009]. Declining Fruit and Vegetable Nutrient Composition: What Is the Evidence?, *HortScience* 44, 1, 15-19

Davis [2011]. Impact of Breeding and Yield on Fruit, Vegetables, and Grain Nutrient Content, in Jenks & Bebeli (eds.) *Breeding for Fruit Quality*, John Wiley & Sons, Inc.

Davis et al. [2004]. Changes in USDA Food Composition Data for 43 Garden Crops, 1950 to 1999, *Journal of the American College of Nutrition* 23, 6, 669-682

Fan et al. [2008]. Evidence of decreasing mineral density in wheat grain over the last 160 years, *Journal of Trace Elements in Medicine and Biology* 22, 315-324

Jack [1998]. Nutrition under siege, *One Peaceful World Journal* 34, 1, 7-9

Marles [2017]. Mineral nutrient composition of vegetables, fruits and grains: The context of reports of apparent historical declines, *Journal of Food Composition and Analysis* 56, 93-103

Tieman et al. [2012]. The Chemical Interactions Underlying Tomato Flavor Preferences, *Current Biology* 22, 1035-1039

Tieman et al. [2017]. A chemical genetic roadmap to improved tomato flavor, *Science* 355, 391-394

No more worries about slaughtered animals

Imagine biting into a burger that was produced without the slaughtering

Meat grown from cultured cells is turning that vision into reality. In 2013, the world's first lab-grown burger was prepared and eaten at a news conference in London. Scientists at Maastricht University in the Netherlands, led by Professor Marc Post, took cells from a cow and turned them into strips of muscle that they combined to make a patty. Since then, several start-ups have been developing lab-grown beef, pork, poultry and seafood. This new field of application attracts millions in funding: Memphis Meats [http://www.memphismeats.com/], for instance, took in 17 million dollars in 2017 from sources that include Bill Gates and the agricultural company Cargill.

Also, consumers have expressed a growing uneasiness over some of the consequences of meat production. Reports on Bovine Spongiform Encephalopathy or Mad Cow Disease outbreaks [Ruth et al. 2005], *Escherichia coli, Salmonella* and other microorganism contaminations that often required hospitalizations [Omer et al. 2018], Horsegate [Brooks et al. 2017], and in particular reports on the contribution of livestock production to global warming [Koneswaran & Nierenberg 2008] have added to the increasing consumer concern regarding meat production and processing. Moreover, if widely adopted, lab-grown meat, also called cultured meat, cell-based meat, *in vitro* meat or clean meat, could eliminate much of the harsh and unethical treatment of animals that are raised for food. Upton Sinclair (1878-1968) should never be forgotten. He had already exposed the appalling working conditions and cruelty inflicted upon animals in the meat-packing industry in *The Jungle*, his sensational novel published in 1906. Several years later, the publication of *Animal Liberation: A Personal View*, the most widely-read work by the Australian moral philosopher Peter Singer [1975], had confronted millions of readers with the shocking abuse of animals and inspired a worldwide movement to improve human attitudes to animals and eliminate the cruelty we subject them to. I cannot imagine that some people are still claiming that the animals commonly used in factory farming are not sentient creatures with their own consciousness, emotions, and ability to feel pain.

Just imagine you could grow enough meat in a laboratory to satisfy at least some of the world's appetite for meat, while at the same time solving most of the issues of animal welfare and environmental quality degradation. What earthly reason would there be for not doing it? Let's not fire up the grill quite yet, however. Between what we have now and a lab-grown chicken in every pot, there is still a long way to go.

Even Winston Churchill thought in vitro meat was a good idea

He once said *We shall escape the absurdity of growing a whole chicken in order to eat the breast or wing by growing these parts separately under a suitable medium* [Churchill 1932]. Winston Churchill (1874-1965): an inspired and erudite man! He was among the first to recognize and promote the advantages of lab-grown meat. The production of cultured meat can provide the benefit of improved food security[25] and of reduced real and/or perceived health problems (e.g. less harmful saturated fat levels, reduced food borne illnesses, etc.). Many publications also refer to the growing human population and inherently increasing demand for meat, while citing lab-grown meat as a solution to the global food crisis. It is hard to come up with arguments against these benefits, which are

---

25 Food security is defined by the United Nations' Committee on World Food Security as the condition in which all people, at all times, have physical, social and economic access to sufficient safe and nutritious food that meets their dietary needs and food preferences for an active and healthy life.

future-oriented and could reasonably affect every segment of the world population. Lab-grown meat is very often suggested as a solution for feeding the growing global population [Edelman et al. 2005; Goodwin & Shoulders 2013].

Another obvious benefit is the reduced environmental impact, e.g. reduced greenhouse gas (GHG) emissions, significantly better water footprints, etc. Lab-grown meat could considerably reduce the elevated environmental costs of meat production [Pussemier & Goeyens 2017], since resources would be needed only to generate and sustain cultured cells, not entire organisms from birth. Tuomisto & Teixeiro de Mattos [2011] found that the lab-grown meat production process would consume 35 to 60 % less energy, ~98 % less land, and produce 80 to 95 % less GHG than conventional animal husbandry.

Additionally, concerns regarding animal welfare may be significantly less pronounced with a meat alternative such as cultured meat. Hopefully, at some stage, there will be a change of attitude and the elimination of the misery suffered by billions of animals. No more castration without anaesthetics; no more chopped chicken beaks; and no more insalubrious, overcrowded sheds for pigs and chickens. No more unhealthy fish hatcheries. Don Staniford, who runs the Global Alliance Against Industrial Aquaculture, called fish farms "toxic toilets". He warned that diseases were rife, waste was out of control and that the use of chemicals was growing fast [The Global Alliance Against Industrial Aquaculture 2017, http://www.gaaia.org/]. Concentrated fish mean concentrated waste and the emergence of antibiotic resistant bacteria. Today countless fish live in very limited amounts of space. They are are fed on oil and smaller fish, ground-up feathers, genetically modified yeast, soybeans and chicken fat. They are "protected" by an excess supply of chemicals to combat parasites, e.g. sea lice that can attach themselves to the fish and eat its blood and skin [Urbina et al. 2019]. As you may imagine, these conditions affect both the quality of the fish as well as the health of the oceans.

10 cells could grow into 50000 metric tons of meat in just 2 months

The meat is made by first taking a muscle sample from a pig, cow, chicken, fish or other animal. Technicians collect stem cells[26] from the tissue, multiply them dramatically and allow them to differentiate into primitive fibres that then bulk up to form muscle tissue. It couldn't be simpler. Or so it would appear ...

In 2002, Morris Benjaminson, now a professor emeritus at Touru University California, received a small grant from NASA to explore the possibility of lab-grown meat, with the idea that future astronauts might use the technology to enjoy steak nights in space [Bartholet 2015]. In a rather grisly experiment, Benjaminson and his colleagues excised chunks of goldfish muscle from live fish and dunked them in vats of foetal bovine serum, a nutrient-rich cocktail brewed from the blood of unborn calves. After about a week, the severed fish chunks had grown in size by 14 % and resembled small filets [Benjaminson et al. 2002]. An associate of Benjaminson briefly marinated the explants in olive oil, chopped garlic, lemon and pepper, covered them in bread crumbs and deep-fried them. A panel of female colleagues gave it a visual and sniff test: it looked and smelled pretty much the same as any fish you could buy at the supermarket. NASA, however, that was apparently convinced there were easier ways to provide astronauts with protein on long deep-space voyages, decided to stop funding the research.

In the Netherlands, three universities joined their efforts, with each studying a different aspect of *in vitro* meat production. Scientists at the University of Amsterdam focused on producing efficient growth media; a group at Utrecht worked on isolating stem cells, making them proliferate and coaxing them into muscle cells; and their colleagues at Eindhoven University of Technology attempted to "train" the muscle cells to grow

---

26　A stem cell is a cell defined by its ability to self-renew or differentiate into another cell type in the body; in addition, in many tissues they serve as a sort of internal repair system, dividing essentially without limit to replenish other cells as long as the person or animal is still alive [National Institutes of Health, https://stemcells.nih.gov/info/basics/1.htm].

larger [Bartholet 2015]. The scientists were able to grow small, thin strips of muscle tissue – something that looks like bits of scallop and has the chewy texture of squid – but several obstacles stood in the way of commercial scale production. In 2011, Professor Marc Post pursued the project by launching the ambitious attempt to culture enough beef to make a hamburger.

Tissue engineering turned out to be more difficult than had originally been thought

Producing 50000 metric tons of meat in just 2 months is possible, but it is difficult and expensive. In an animal, single myotubes[27] will align and form myofibrils[28], muscle fibres, fibre bundles, and finally muscle. However, re-creating this process in a test tube is not that simple.

Meat growth occurs in three main phases: proliferation, fusion, and polishing. First, laboratory technicians would isolate embryonic or adult stem cells from a farm animal. Then they would grow those cells in bioreactors, using specialized media containing morphogens[29] that will allow for self-renewal of the cells. The stem cells would divide and re-divide for months on end. Once enough cells have been produced, they are transferred to a separate apparatus in a new medium that will promote the production of myocytes as well as their fusion into myotubes, i.e. the experts would "instruct" the cells to differentiate into muscle (rather than, say, bone or brain cells). This fusion process may be aided by nano-patterned plastics or other scaffolding materials, substrates, or biomaterials, which will promote myotube maturation and provide tensile points of attachment. Once mature myotubes have been

---

27 A developmental stage of a muscle fibre composed of a syncytium formed by fusion of myoblasts; a syncytium is a multinucleate mass of cytoplasm resulting from the fusion of cells [Merriam-Webster].

28 The longitudinal parallel contractile elements of a muscle cell [Merriam-Webster]

29 Morphogens are signaling molecules that emanate from a restricted region of a tissue and spread away from their source to form a concentration gradient; as the fate of each cell in the field depends on the concentration of the morphogen signal, the gradient prefigures the pattern of development [Tabata & Takei 2004].

produced, they can be harvested and polished into the final product, meaning the muscle cells need to be bulked up in a fashion similar to the way in which animals build their strength by physical exercise. This entire process could indeed take place within a month or two with the final product consisting of up to dozens of billions of cells starting from a few thousand. In theory, one single cell line would be sufficient to literally feed the world. Moreover, proponents of lab-grown meat look forward to the day when governments will levy special environmental taxes on meat produced from livestock and when consumers will be able to opt for *in vitro* meat that is labelled "cruelty-free". Hence, it seems quite logical that we will not only rely on old fashioned farm animal husbandry in the future.

Today, tissue engineers still face multiple problems [Bartholet 2015]. When stem cell lines proliferate for long periods, many of the cells "decide" to differentiate on their own, and many do not turn into muscle, which drastically reduces the yield. The procedure was also not acceptable to vegetarians, because the nutrient baths were derived from foetal calf or horse serum taken from slaughtered animals. But scientists have since developed recipes for chemical media that include no animal products. They have also been able to genetically engineer plant cells to produce animal proteins that could be used to grow the meat. Nowadays, both these types of media still remain prohibitively expensive, however.

The Utrecht University researchers tried to extract and develop embryonic stem cell lines from pigs. They were expected to duplicate every day for very long periods, meaning that a small number of cells could grow into a staggering amount of potential meat in just a few months. Culturing embryonic stem cells would be ideal for this purpose, since they have an (almost) infinite self-renewal capacity, according to the report by the Dutch team [Haagsman et al. 2009]. And embryonic stem cell lines had been developed from mice, rats, rhesus monkeys and humans. But, embryonic cells from farm animals have a tendency to differentiate quickly – and of their own accord – into specialized cells. The Utrecht team's porcine cells often veered toward a neural lineage [Bartholet 2015]. Brains, rather than bacon!

The research team of Maastricht University [Boonen & Post 2008] chose to work with adult stem cells, called muscle satellite cells[30], which exist within skeletal muscle and are largely pre-programmed to replace muscle fibres when they are injured or die off. Satellite cells do not proliferate as readily as embryonic cells do, but they produce muscle more reliably.

The cost of all this still constitutes a real obstacle to its application. The culture used to grow stem cells of every kind is very expensive. An algae-based medium may eventually work best because algae can produce the proteins and amino acids necessary to sustain cell life. But this is seen as far too expensive – at least for now. Post optimistically estimated that large-scale production of in vitro meat could lower the price. Moreover, once researchers are able to produce a big supply of muscle cells, they will need to keep them alive and bulk them up. It is possible now to assemble cells into a thin strip of tissue, but when the layer grows to more than a few cell layers thick, parts of it start to die off. The cells require a constant flow of fresh nutrients to stay alive. In the body, these nutrients are delivered by the bloodstream, which also removes waste. Post is now trying to develop a three-dimensional system that delivers the nutrients.

He achieved some success with a different approach, providing sticking points (made of Velcro) to which the developing tubules of muscle can attach. When anchored on either end, the fibres develop tension on their own and expand in size. But at this stage, he says, the objective is not to generate Schwarzenegger muscle cells.

Moreover, Post has described another, more complex method that might work even better. The body naturally stimulates muscle growth with micro-pulses of acetylcholine and other chemicals — which are inexpensive to supply. To generate very short pulses of chemicals is a technological hurdle rather than a scientific one.

---

30 Satellite cells are considered to be adult skeletal muscle stem cells.

How will the consumers react?

Makers of lab-grown meat claim their products will taste exactly like the real thing, because they *are* the real thing. Some meat industry groups oppose the use of the word "meat", even if everybody is well aware that both in vitro meat and meat from slaughtered animals are muscle cells. This leaves consumers free to make their own decision based on factors other than taste; and lab-grown meat definitely has advantages.

Some advantages are obvious, e.g. the animal welfare issue. Take the animals out of the equation and the welfare problems diasppear. No more slaughterhouses[31]; no more cageing, crating, and crowding of animals; no more cases of outright abuse; and a much easier and more efficient approach than official controls to guarantee animal welfare.

Then there is the issue of foodborne illnesses. Since the meat is grown in a closed vessel in a sterile environment – as opposed to, say, a cowshed, stable or a huge windowless shed for thousands of chickens – the expectation is that there would be much less opportunity for pathogens to sneak in. That is also highly relevant for antibiotics. In standard cell cultures, a near-sterile environment is obtained through the use of culturing cells and tissues in plastic dishes, which keep bacteria or spores in the air from getting in. Replacing the medium for the cells is achieved in a biosafety cabinet which controls the environment through air regulation and filtration. Through standard cell culture practices, the possibility of outside contamination is largely eliminated. And although drugs/chemicals can theoretically be used in the lab-grown process, a sterile environment means they would not be required and so the issue of antibiotic-resistant bacteria disappears.

Finally, there is the environmental impact. Maintaining animal populations takes a massive toll on the environment, arable land, and water availability [Pussemier & Goeyens 2017]. Taking the animals out of the industry drastically reduces land and water use and will certainly

---

31 The Federation of Veterinarians of Europe believes a Regulation must ensure that stress during the slaughter process should be kept to a minimum and where possible distress and pain should be eliminated.

help reduce GHG emissions. Animal agriculture is responsible for significant GHG productions, mostly from enteric methane burped up by ruminants like cows and goats. No cows, no methane, and no more need to destroy tropical forests to make way for new ranches or new maize fields. But the concept of farming animals for food will likely always exist and markets for "high quality" meat seem likely to remain for the foreseeable future. What *in vitro* meat essentially provides is an opportunity to eliminate the need for animals altogether, and so there is always the possibility that technological maturity will some day eliminate the need for traditional animal farming.

But what about the ick factor? Some see social acceptance as the biggest obstacle of all. Scientists seem to think producing in vitro meat on a commercial scale it is a great idea. Non-scientists however may not agree. Lab-grown meat sounds scary, even if it is basically the same as the meat we are used to. Lab-grown meat is no more than muscle cells. It is simply produced differently. People often associate cultured meat with two other issues: genetically modified foods – which in Europe are often seen as a dangerous corporate scheme to dominate or control the food supply – and negative perceptions of the meat industry in general, with its factory farms, diseases (e.g. mad cow disease, bird flu, African porcine fever, etc.) and mistreatment of animals, and fraudulent practices (e.g. the horsegate scandal, the Belgian dioxin crisis, the recent fipronil egg contamination, etc.).

Once people come to realize that cultured meat is not genetically modified and can provide a clean, animal-friendly alternative to factory farmed meat, the reticent and very negative reactions tend to diasppear.

Bibliography

Bartholet [2015]. Inside the meat lab, *Scientific American 304, 6, 64-69.*
Benjaminson et al. [2002]. In vitro edible muscle protein production system (MPPS): Stage 1, fish, *Acta astronautica* 51, 12, 879-889
Boonen & Post [2008]. The Muscle Stem Cell Niche: Regulation of Satellite Cells During Regeneration, *Tissue Engineering Part B* 14, 4, 419-431

Brooks et al. [2017]. Four years post-horsegate: an update of measures and actions put in place following the horsemeat incident of 2013, *npj Science of Food* 1, 5, pp. 7

Churchill [1932]. *Thoughts and Adventures*, Thornton Butterworth Limited, London, pp. 328

Edelman et al. [2005]. In vitro cultured meat production, *Tissue Engineering* 11, 5/6, 659-662

Goodwin & Shoulders [2013]. The future of meat: A qualitative analysis of cultured meat media coverage, *Meat Science* 95, 445-450

Haagsman et al. [2009]. *Production of animal proteins by cell systems*, University Utrecht, Faculty of Veterinary Medecine, pp. 58

Koneswaran & Nierenberg [2008]. Global Farm Animal Production and Global Warming: Impacting and Mitigating Climate Change, *Environmental Health Perspectives* 116, 578-582

Omer et al. [2018]. A Systematic Review of Bacterial Foodborne Outbreaks Related to Red Meat and Meat Products, *Foodborne pathogens and disease*, in press

Pussemier & Goeyens [2017]. *AgricultureS & Enjeux de société*, Presses Universitaires de Liège - Agronomie, Gembloux, pp. 112

Ruth et al. [2005]. Framing of Mad Cow Media Coverage, *Journal of Applied Communications* 89, 4, pp. 18

Sinclair [2015]. *The Jungle (first edition 1906)*, Signet Classics, Penguin Group, New York, pp. 400

Singer [2009]. *Animal Liberation (first edition 1975)*, HarperCollins Publishers, New York, pp. 311

Tabata & Takei [2004]. Morphogens, their identification and regulation, *Development* 131, 703-712

The Global Alliance Against Industrial Aquaculture [2017]. *Toxic Toilets – Salmon Farms Pollute Scotland's Lochs*, http://donstaniford.typepad.com/files/pr-toxic-toilets-26-feb-2017.pdf

Tuomisto & Teixeiro de Mattos [2011]. Environmental Impacts of Cultured Meat Production, Environmental Science and Technology 45, 14 6117-6123

Urbina et al. [2019]. Effects of pharmaceuticals used to treat salmon lice on non-target species: Evidence from a systematic review, *Science of The Total Environment* 649, 1124-1136

Providing food security while remaining within the safe operating space of planetary boundaries

The chilling Intergovernmental Panel on Climate Change report

It has become clear now that greenhouse gas (GHG) emissions[32] generated by human activities are the main cause of global warming. There can no longer be any doubt about it. Global warming has occurred at a rate of 0.17° Celcius (C) per decade since 1950. So, at the current rate, the world is liable to face a rise in average temperature of 1.5° C between 2030 and 2052. In 2017-2018, there has already been a 1° C rise since pre-industrial times. The report recently issued by the Intergovernmental Panel on Climate Change (IPCC) raises the question whether the objective of the Paris Agreement, i.e. to strengthen the response to the threat of climate change by keeping the global temperature rise this century well below 2° C above pre-industrial levels and to pursue efforts to limit the temperature increase even further to 1.5° C, can be achieved [IPCC 2018].

The objective of the Paris Agreement was no unanimously given a warm welcome. The European employers' lobby wanted to "minimize"

---

32 Greenhouse gases refer to carbon dioxide, nitrous oxide, methane, ozone and chlorofluorocarbons occurring naturally and resulting from human activities, and contributing to the greenhouse effect or global warming [https://stats.oecd.org/glossary/detail.asp?ID=1152].

climate efforts. A leaked internal memo unveiled by EURACTIV offers a rare glimpse into the communication strategy of Europe's main business lobby group. The memo recommends opposing a new increase in the climate ambition of the European Union (EU) by resorting to the usual arguments that Europe cannot take action on its own and should seek a level playing field with global competitors before making any moves in isolation. The worrying BusinessEurope memo has 4 recommendations for advocacy and communication stategy. Their members are asked to adhere to the prescribed approach: ... *They should be rather positive as long as it remains as a political statement with no implications on the range of 2030 EU legislation, and oppose the new increase of ambition* (Mr Miguel Arias Cañete, the EU climate action commissioner, suggested updating the EU's greenhouse gas reduction target for 2030) ... *They should also challenge the process, such as the need for more transparency on the calculations, and "minimise" the issue arguing that the formation of a "de facto" extra ambition is not what matters most* ... [the BusinessEurope's discussion note for the energy and climate WG meeting on 19/09/2018, as available on EURACTIV, https://www.euractiv.com]. Who then will be brave enough to be seen as a trendsetter and take the lead in the struggle for ambitious climate targets? The European lobby group BusinessEurope has chosen to turn a deaf ear to climate concerns. In fact, the group is prepared to undermine climate targets. This is certainly a very unwise attitude, now that it has been demonstrated that the world is closer than previously thought to exceeding the budget for the long-term target of the Paris Climate Agreement [Gasser et al. 2018].

The environmental issues are not low-profile and neither are the inherent public health threats. You might think that policymakers would be aware of the problems and deliver robust decisions. However, we continue to receive disappointing news. On October 8, 2018 the executive director of the International Energy Agency, Dr. Fatih Birol, told The Guardian: ... *When I look at the first nine months of data, I expect in 2018 carbon emissions will increase once again...* A most alarming message for our climate goals.

The beverage industry does not want to pay for the plastic waste clean-up: another unwise decision! Researchers at the Environment

Agency Austria and the Medical University of Vienna have found evidence that microplastics – the ubiquitous, and extremely small pieces of plastic beads, fibres, or fragments – accumulate in human faeces. About 18 billion pounds of plastic flow into the world's oceans each year. After sea animals consume some of this plastic, humans are likely to ingest it through tuna, shrimp, lobster, and many other gourmet foods from the ocean. In addition, humans are likely to consume more plastic in their daily meals from food processing and packaging systems. The occurrence of microplastics in our daily food was to be expected [Catarino et al. 2018]. Now, research data evidence the presence of plastics in the human gut. This then is yet another frightening piece of news coming just a few months after the World Health Organization (WHO) announced it planned to investigate the potential effects of plastic on human health. This up-to-the-minute information will be presented at a United European Gastroenterology conference in Vienna and afterwards published in a peer reviewed journal.

Agriculture (for food as well as feed production) will also have to make an effort. Luckily, many excellent collaborative efforts have already arrived at fruition [Pussemier & Goeyens 2017]. Not all is rosy, however. The investigation unit of Greenpeace France has revealed that a Monsanto lobby has allegedly created groups of "fake farmers" to vote for glyphosate. The purpose of these alleged fake groups is to make out that farmers considered the chemical glyphosate to be safe. The source of the story was published in the French weekly magazine L'Obs on October 17, 2018. Does the multinational have something to hide? Is it prepared to lie to consumers? To misrepresent and conceal relevant information? It is clear that in a society where everyone considers resorting to such extremities, the notion of promise would lose its meaning. In addition, if everyone lies, it is the very possibility of any reliable exchange of information that is destroyed – which is why lying is immoral.

How do we provide enough food to 9 billion people and more?

The fundamental question that the agricultural industry seeks to answer is how do we provide quality food to all people at a decent price and without negatively impacting the environment.

The world population – there are now ~7 billion people on Earth – is projected to reach ~9 billion or more by 2050 [Gerland et al. 2014]. So, the challenge really is daunting. We shall have to produce approximately twice as much food as we do now knowing full well that all readily arable land has run out. And if we cannot rely on more fields, we shall have to enhance the productivity of those we have now. That is much more easily said than done. All the simple things – finding new land, clearing it, growing more crops, and breeding more animals – were done over the last 100 years. Today we have to think a lot harder about how to maximise productivity. And at the same time we should be careful not to damage our environment. The ICPP message is clear on this point. Agriculture as well as agricultural science and research have to account for food production issues, but at the same time for environmental issues and social issues related to food (and feed) production.

Tomorrow's agriculture will be ecological and multiple, or it will cease to be [Pussemier & Goeyens 2017]. Modern-day agriculture already occupies a very large part of the planet Earth and even of the World's Oceans if fisheries and aquaculture are taken into consideration. Cultivating more land and breeding more fish and crustaceans has become a huge, worldwide problem. We cannot endlessly continue to deplete our resources, to produce GHG and lose biodiversity. Agricultural activities are already responsible for 13.5 % of the global GHG emission through the generation of methane (from livestock and soil), nitrous oxide (because of nitrogen fertilization and manure management) and carbon dioxide (through energy consumption). The intensive industrial agriculture is fueling climate change and even causing it to accelerate. Cultivation of new land is done at the expense of virgin regions, which were and remain vital carbon sinks. Industrial farming and the enormous use of mineral nitrogen fertilizer are responsible for dramatic GHG emissions. The combination of deforestation with intensive agriculture and livestock farming has serious consequences in terms of global warming (monstrous wildfires, record high temperatures, heatwaves and unprecedented flooding across the globe have become facts of life). This is not rocket science! The Earth is overheating and we are going to have more extreme high temperatures as well as longer periods of extreme heat. That is what we are witnessing already!

Obviously, tomorrow's agriculture will have to be sustainable. Sustainability, in my opinion, means that we must have the highest level of respect for the laws of ecology. Ecological balances are crucial for sustainable agriculture. Tomorrow's agriculture should rely on multiple aspects. Several approaches will coexist and even complement each other. The facts clearly illustrate that different types of agriculture must be allowed to develop. The smallholders in the third world differ significantly from the great landowners in the western world. The eating habits vary from one continent to another and even within individual regions. Furthermore, consumer needs are guided by various motivations. Some families predominantly focus on purchasing sufficient food with the available financial resources, while some will privilege the nutritional quality or organoleptic properties of the food, and others will be most sensitive to the ethical aspects or to the impact of food production on the harmonious development of the local community.

An ecological agriculture can assume various forms [Pussemier & Goeyens 2017]. Organic agriculture, permaculture, biodynamics, urban or peri-urban agriculture, diversified ecological agriculture, intensive ecological agriculture – all have common and overlapping properties. They focus on biodiversity, not least through crop selection. Their circular economy approach prevails, especially with respect to nitrogen fertilization. Good management of nitrogen and energy plays a central role in the efforts required for a drastic reduction in GHG emissions. If we are to overcome the challenges ahead, we will have to combine all efforts. All stakeholders, including citizens as well as consumers, will have to pursue the same objective(s). These priorities are well known: (1) improve the biodiversity within the ecosystems; (2) favour all sources of fertilization and reduce mineral fertilization; (3) innovate through genetics and develop new cultivars more likely to resist the various forms of stress.

Criss-crossing the Belgian countryside, you will observe striking changes in the farmers' interest for culture systems which favour good soil health and respect for the environment. In addition to traditional field crops such as wheat, beetroot, and potato, many crops that were neglected during the last decades of the 20th century are now reappearing. Gardeners who practice organic farming have introduced numerous crops from warmer climate, such as artichokes, tomatoes, peppers and a multitude of cucurbits. Many efforts have also been made to revive many kinds of conventional crops such as beans, peas, carrots, and onions. And among the non-food crops, there are cultivations of flax, rapeseed and even miscanthus, which has been trialed as a biofuel in Europe since the early 1980s. Moreover, hemp, chia and quinoa have followers in France and why shouldn't they be grown in neighbouring countries.

Industrial livestock farming is still very common. However, Belgian livestock breeding has some striking examples of more extensive breeding systems and less common cattle breeds than the Belgian blue white or the Holstein are now found. Moreover, ecological livestock feeding does not lag behind. Many farmers have grassland and meadows to graze their herds. They also produce their own forage maize and hay. The alfalfa and faba bean fields they need for winter fodder have brought a touch of colour to the landscape and often alternate with special strips for the benefit of wildlife. There is no denying that ecological farming is well underway in our countries. The diversity of living organisms makes our countryside more attractive. Many farmers care passionately about their crops and livestock and at the same time about the environment and animal welfare.

And the changes are not only seen in the fields …

Vertical farming: eco-friend or foe?

We realize only too well that traditional agriculture is highly resource-intensive. It requires a great deal of land, water and energy to produce food crops. This is something we must change. Without enhanced, environment-friendly agricultural productivity the world population is heading for a food crisis. The world has witnessed changes in agricultural practices before in response to growing population and changing society. During the Green Revolution of the 1960s, new technologies resulted in marked increases in production. But today, agricultural production has plateaued and sometimes even declined. Current agricultural practices face decreasing land and water availability in many parts of the world. We must come up with innovations that enable us to produce more food (about twice as much food) with less reliance on resources.

In vertical farms?

A vertical farm at its most basic is a crop production building [Cuello 2018]. Shelves are stacked, one on top of the other, full of fast growing crops. A true vertical farm is completely enclosed, like a warehouse, and can be operated year-round. In Japan, where vertical farming has been pioneered, the name plant factory is typically used [Ono & Watanabe 2006].

Vertical farms are independent of geography, climate or season. Inside, every ingredient is carefully managed and controlled in contrast to the relative unpredictability of traditional agriculture, which is highly dependent on the weather. In vertical farms, productivity is optimized or maximized, and it is consistent. Everything the plants need to thrive – basically crops require light, water, clean air and especially carbon dioxide, nutrients, etc. – are supplied in optimal concentrations, resulting in a high level of sustainability. Instead of soil, crops are grown hydroponically[33] in nutrient-rich water. Sunlight is replaced by efficient fluorescent lamp or light-emitting diode (LED) lighting. The temperature and relative humidity are controlled, and in many cases the carbon dioxide content of the air is enriched to promote photosynthesis. And it is all done with the help of artificial intelligence (AI)[34].

---

33 Hydroponics is a method of growing plants in a water based, nutrient-rich solution; it does not use soil, instead the root system is supported using an inert medium such as rockwool, for example.

34 AI works by combining large amounts of data with fast, iterative processing and intelligent algorithms, allowing the software to learn automatically from patterns or features in the data.

The commercial development of vertical farms began in the 1980s in Japan. With the technology improvements achieved over the years, more particularly the LED revolution, the production capacity of vertical farms has steadily risen. The concept of modern skyscraper vertical farms [Despommier 2010] was introduced by Dickson Despommier, now an emeritus Professor of microbiology and public health at Columbia University. Owing to the subsequent association of the vertical farm concept, fairly or unfairly, with grand architectural designs of awe-inspiring and often futuristic looking edifices, the prospects for vertical farms in recent years were significantly diminished as a result of their projected high costs. So, to devise a new strategy for designing and developing vertical farms that can achieve economic feasibility, it was crucial to decouple the concept of vertical farms from the conventional buildings with which vertical farms have become inadvertently intertwined.

The Vertical Greenbox Solution (VGS) was introduced as a new strategy for designing vertical farms to achieve economic feasibility [Cuello, 2014]. The VGS pertains to vertical farms constructed without using standard or conventional buildings. It prescribes the following three critical architectural features [https://abe.arizona.edu/content/vertical-green-box].

- First, it should be minimally structured, meaning that it should be characterized by reduced load-bearing requirement, reduced materials, limited total weight, and few plumbing and electrical services.
- Secondly, it should be modular with uniformity of growing space, consistency of operational procedures, and interchangeability of units. Wall types, e.g., could conceivably vary from solid and non-transparent to transparent plastic material. The size range for a module could range from that of a used shipping container to that of a sizable warehouse.
- And finally, it should be prefabricated. Any VGS should allow for off-site construction and assembly of modules at significantly lower costs of both construction and labour. It should be possible

96

to vertically stack the individual, modular boxes or to arrange them in geometric configurations to optimise the crop growing operations.

Vertical farming, together with several other forms of urban farming such as community gardens on vacant lots, rooftop gardens or greenhouses, also helps building social capital in cities and communities in which they are located [Cuello 2016]. Obviously, a series of high-profile food contamination cases that have scandalised the consumers in recent years, fuel the demand not only for fresh produce, but also for scalable crop production systems that are demonstrably safe. Hence, the emergence of vertical farms and other forms of urban agriculture around big cities has attracted many consumers because they can observe how the crops are cultivated in fully or semi-controlled environments. The consumers perceive this to be not only efficient, productive and promoting premium crop quality, but also safe. Moreover, vertical farms help collapse the distance fresh crops travel from the farm to the dinner table. They also foster community cohesion, building and strengthening by encouraging community participation and involvement in their production operations. Social farming applied to vertical farming constitutes one notable example [FAO 2014]. The specific type of vertical farm employed in a community could also spur and enable members of the community to cooperate as well as to participate in vertical farming as a business enterprise. For instance, the modular VGS type is certainly more affordable to community associations or cooperatives than conventional greenhouse buildings which are (too) costly to build. A conceivable scenario is for a city to build the modular units of vertical farms and then lease or rent the modular units to various community groups, including neighbourhood associations, student groups and even schools [Cuello 2018].

"Bigger is better" has outperformed

To date, farmers have adopted more and better technologies and more sophisticated tools in their pursuit of greater yields (larger fields and heavier machines). The belief that "bigger is better" came to dominate farming, rendering small-scale operations impractical. Today, this accepted pillar of agricultural wisdom is seriously challenged. The economies of scale and the bulkiness of farm machinery has meant that huge fields of one single crop[35] is the most efficient way to farm; and the bigger the machines, the more efficient the process. This concept has had its day. For example, some of the heavier harvesters weigh ~60 tonnes; they leave a trail of soil compaction in their wake that can last for years. Today, however, when the human component is removed, size becomes irrelevant. Robotics and autonomous systems (RAS) can take over part of the farmer's job and of course, they do not crush the soil [King 2017]. In fact, farmers have already started using them. The opportunities for RAS in the field include: the development of field robots that can assist workers by carrying payloads and conduct agricultural operations such as crop and animal sensing, weeding and drilling, integration of autonomous systems technologies into existing farm operational equipment such as tractors, robotic systems to harvest crops and conduct complex precision work. Moreover, the use of soft robotics to drive productivity beyond the farm gate into the factory and retail environment has come into being. And finally, RAS can reduce the reliance on human labour and skills, e.g. in farming management, planning and decision making [UK-RAS 2018].

The 21st century robotics and sensing technologies have the potential to solve problems that are as old as farming itself. It is now believed that relying on a robotic agricultural system can make crop production significantly more efficient and especially more sustainable [Bac et al. 2014; Berckmans 2014; Pussemier & Goeyens 2017; Fernández-Quintanilla et al. 2018; Roldán et al. 2018]. In greenhouses intended for fruit and vegetable production, engineers are exploring automation as

---

35 In contrast with polyculture, monoculture is the practice of producing or growing one single crop, plant, or livestock species, variety, or breed in a field or farming system at a time. There are many downsides to this form of plant growing: reusing the exact same soil instead of rotating three or four different crops following a pre-determined cycle can lead to plant pathogens and diseases that adapt to the soil and attack the crops so that the quantity produced eventually decreases.

a way to reduce costs and boost quality. Devices to monitor vegetable growth as well as robotic pickers are currently tested. Moreover, in the arable sector several efforts are underway to improve monitoring and maintenance of soil quality and to eliminate pests and diseases without resorting to abundant and indiscriminate use of agrichemicals. For livestock farmers, on the other hand, sensing technologies are being developed to manage the health and welfare of their animals. Smart collars – a bit like the very fashionable devices designed to track human health and fitness – have been used to monitor the herds for the last 8 to 10 years.

King [2017] distinguishes between two highly important fields of application: the elimination of enemies and the soil saviours. The Food and Agriculture Organization (FAO) of the United Nations estimates that 20 to 40 % of global crop yields are lost to pests and diseases, despite the application of some three million and more tonnes of pesticide [Zhang 2018]. It goes without saying that the chemical industry will never kill this golden goose. Others will have to take the necessary initiatives. Intelligent devices, such as robots and drones, could however help farmers to slash the use of chemicals by spotting crop enemies as they appear and spray chemicals or apply any other pest removal exclusively on the vulnerable spot. Imagine drones, equipped with Red-Green-Blue or multispectral cameras, taking off every morning before the farmer gets out of his bed, and identifying where in the field there is a pest or for that matter any other problem. Companies also supply drones and software that use near-infrared images to map unhealthy vegetation patches in large fields. Modern technology, that can target essential pesticides and/or fertilizers and autonomously eliminate pests will reduce collateral damage to wildlife, lower resistance to agrichemicals and cut costs. Rather than spraying a whole field, pesticides could precisely be applied to the right spot with adequate consideration of action and required concentrations. The potential reductions in pesticide use are impressive. Several studies [Pérez-Ruiz et al. 2015; Malneršič et al. 2016] highlight that targeted spraying consumes considerably less of the herbicide volume necessary for conventional, "voracious" blanket spraying.

On the other hand, robotics and autonomous machines considerably help protect the soil quality. The most important resource for arable farmers is the soil they cultivate. But large harvesters damage and compact soils, and overuse of chemical ingredients such as nitrogen fertilizer and pesticides are harmful to both environmental quality and the biodiversity. Data from drones are now used for smarter application of nitrogen fertilizer. The ratio of red to near-infrared bands on a multispectral image can be used to estimate the chlorophyll concentrations and so, map the biomass. This determines where interventions such as fertilization are required after damage caused by weather or pests for example. Moreover, car-sized robots can measure plenty of other soil quality indicators using various sensors and modules, including a moisture sensor and a penetrometer[36]. Soil mapping also paves the way for the sowing of different crop varieties in one field to better match the shifting soil properties such as water availability and infiltration. Growing multiple crops together could then lead to smarter and reduced use of agrichemicals.

In fact, Mother Nature hates monocultures. Our currently predominant food production and farming systems continue to create dry, dead ends. All too often we still have to do with agricultural practices characterised by industrial-sized cultivation of a single plant or monoculture, genetically engineered crops (monocultures) and repeated, lavishly toxic pesticide infusions in combination with the application of synthetic fertilisers.

All of these characteristics directly or indirectly harm people and the farming ecosystems they depend on. There are tools to improve the situation, however, and we know what they are. Why not then grasp the opportunities that emerge?

---

36 Device used to assess soil compaction.

Over the last 30 years, the consumption of meat, milk and eggs has more than tripled

Population growth, urbanization, income gains and globalization continue to fuel the livestock revolution[37], offering business opportunities for many livestock producers. According to the latest FAO projections, under a business-as-usual scenario, meat demand in low- and middle-income countries (LMICs) will increase by a further 80 % by 2030 and by over 200 % by 2050 [FAO 2018]. Livestock agrifood systems are cranking up production to meet this demand and adapting to satisfy the changing food preferences. However, such a rapid growth in production and trade does not only offer opportunities. It also entails worrying threats for mankind. The global picture now dominates the policy debate, but policymakers and development practitioners should be careful not to generalize global data and developing policies and strategies without first carrying out detailed land surveys and analyses [Pico-Ciamarra & Otte 2009]. Growth is not an even process. Most of the growth can still be seen to occur in intensive cattle farming systems with relatively little contribution from smallholder producers. The risks include concerns over food and nutrition security and safety, livelihoods and equity, health and animal welfare, as well as environmental quality [FAO 2018].

It is hard to believe that the FAO still had to reiterate that animal welfare deserves more attention. Upton Sinclair's vivid depiction of the horrors of Chicago's stockyards and slaughterhouses was already a plea for public attention in 1906 [Sinclair 2015]: ... *And yet somehow the most matter-of-fact person could not help thinking about the hogs; they were so innocent; they came so very trustingly; and they were so very human in their protests – and so perfectly within their rights! They had done nothing to deserve it, and it was adding insult to injury, as the thing was done here, swinging them up in this cold-blooded, impersonal way, without a*

---

37 The basic tenet of the Livestock Revolution paradigm is that the combination of population growth, rising per capita incomes, and progressive urbanization are creating an unprecedented growth in demand for food of animal origin in developing countries, giving rise to major opportunities and threats for mankind [Pico-Ciamarra & Otte 2009].

pretence at apology, without the homage of a tear... If slaughterhouses had glass walls, there would be no need to advocate for animal welfare-friendly practices!

Depending on the context, livestock can serve a variety of functions. So, adding their contribution to the 2030 Agenda for Sustainable Development will require interventions that are tailored to the specific needs of diverse livestock agri-food systems. Livestock are broadly divided into ruminants, which through enteric fermentation[38] have the capacity to digest rough plant material, and monogastric species whose dietary needs are more similar to our own. The main ruminant species are cattle and buffaloes, which may be multi-purpose or specialized for beef, dairy or draft power. Camelids have been domesticated by humans for ~5000 years. Llamas, alpacas, vicuñas, and guanacos have been important for communities in South America since the first humans arrived on the continent. Both their milk and meat are rich in protein and their fur is used to weave very fine woollen garments. Globally, camelids can be found in ~90 countries in South America, Africa and Asia. There is also a small community in Australia, where camels were once introduced and used for transportation and to access very remote areas. Finally, the smaller ruminants such as sheep and goats are important sources of meat, milk, wool and hides. Monogastric species[39], on the other hand, include pigs which are predominantly raised for meat and a range of poultry species such as chickens, ducks and turkeys, which are raised for meat, eggs and feathers.

Think of a farm and what comes to mind? Lambs leaping through a field, pigs rolling around in the mud and cows chomping on lush grass.

---

38 Enteric fermentation takes place in the digestive systems of ruminant animals that have a large "fore-stomach" or rumen, within which microbial fermentation breaks down food into soluble products that can be utilized by the animal; the microbial fermentation that occurs in the rumen enables ruminant animals to digest coarse plant material that monogastric animals cannot digest. Moreover, methane is produced in the rumen by bacteria as a by-product of the fermentation process; it is exhaled or belched by the animal and accounts for the majority of GHG emissions from ruminants.

39 Monogastric organisms have a simple single-chambered stomach, their ability to extract energy from cellulose digestion is less efficient than in ruminants.

Sadly, that vision no longer corresponds to the real world situations. Farm animals disappeared from our fields as the production of food became a global industry. We may have some idea of the extent to which things have changed, but we probably still prefer to believe that chickens scratch around in the farmyard, that pigs snooze and snort in muddy pens, that happy cows chew their cud, etc. Almost without our noticing, animals disappeared from fields and meadows and were moved into cramped hangars and barns. Why does big mean bad? Why have mixed farms all too often been replaced by farms that specialize in only one thing, whether the production of milk, eggs, chicken, turkey, pork or beef? Animals that are raised for meat are fattened up for slaughter as fast as possible and by all possible means. Admittedly, issues relating to the welfare of farm animals have today become increasingly important within the EU. Deep consumer concerns are expressed and are taken into account by an increasing amount of EU Legislation designed to improve the welfare of farm animals. The Commission has adopted the EU animal welfare strategy with the aim of ensuring that existing animal welfare standards are consistently applied and enforced across the EU and that the animal welfare policy is well coordinated with the Common Agricultural Policy (CAP). Responsibility for enforcing animal welfare legislation and managing the CAP is shared between the European Commission and the Member States [European Court of Auditors 2018].

Methane from cows, rubbish tips and rice fields is warming the Earth. Car exhausts may help the process. But methane from the Arctic tundra could be most damaging of all. This outcry by Fred Pearce [1989] did not attract a great deal of support. Some 30 years ago, public concern about the greenhouse effect and its potential to warm the Earth's atmosphere focused on carbon dioxide. However, bacteria that break down cellulose[40] in the guts of cattle convert approximately 3 to 10 % of the food that cattle eat into methane. Nobel Prize-winning atmospheric chemist,

---

40 Wherever bacteria break down organic matter in the absence of oxygen, they produce methane; when the same process occurs in the presence of oxygen, carbon dioxide is produced.

Paul Crutzen[41], warned about the consequences of livestock expansion – especially, the intensive breeding of ruminants – to meet the world's evergrowing demand for meat [Crutzen et al. 1986].

The FAO report extends the argument of Frances Moore Lappé's well known bestseller *Diet for a Small Planet* [Lappé 1971] that feeding a population on a diet of animal protein more farmland than does a diet of plant protein. The FAO [2006] report focuses specifically on the current and future effects of livestock production on the world's environment and climate. It emphasizes that the world's livestock sector, which provides the livelihoods of ~1.3 billion people, is growing faster than other agricultural subsectors. The increase is projected to occur mainly in LMIC. Livestock currently use almost a third of the world's entire land surface, mostly permanent pasture, but also including the third of the world's arable land that provides livestock feed [McMichael et al. 2007]. Given the projected global livestock production increases and inherent GHG emissions, urgent attention needs to be paid to finding ways of reducing the demand for animal products as well as the energy intensity of their production. Since rapid reductions in GHG emissions per unit of livestock production seem to be technically and culturally difficult in the short term. The prime objective must be to reduce (sometimes excessive) consumption of animal products in high-income countries and thus lower the ceiling consumption level to which LMIC would then converge. The main options for reducing GHG emissions per unit of animal production include: (1) sequestering carbon and mitigating carbon dioxide emissions by reducing and reversing deforestation arising from agricultural intensification and by restoring organic carbon to cultivated soils and degraded pastures; (2) reducing methane emissions from enteric fermentation in ruminants through improved efficiency and diets; (3) increasing the proportion of chickens, monogastric mammals and vegetarian fish grown for human consumption; (4) mitigating emissions of methane through improved management of manure and biogas; and (5) mitigating emissions of nitrous oxide via more efficient

---

41   Paul Crutzen was awarded the Nobel prize in Chemistry in 1995 for his work on the hole in the ozone layer.

use of nitrogenous fertilisers [McMichaels et al. 2007; Pussemier & Goeyens 2017]. This comes at a price, however. Recent reviews suggest that available moderation technologies could reduce emissions per unit of animal product by ~20 % at fairly low cost. But, reductions beyond that level are not currently available at realistic prices [McMichaels et al. 2007].

FAO [2018] defines three broad livestock systems. Extensive systems are characterized by low labour and capital inputs. Labour-intensive systems are typically smallholder farms with low returns and a surplus of labour and often constrained by land as well as capital scarcity. Capital-intensive systems are usually associated with highly modified environments, where arable land and labour inputs require substantial capital investments.

On a global level, extensive livestock systems are typically pastoralist [Clutton-Brock 2015]: ~180 million pastoralists benefit directly from these systems characterized by livestock grazing large expanses of marginal rangelands. With few inputs beyond basic animal health care, these systems are efficient but of low productivity. They tend to occur in areas that are unsuitable for crop growth and therefore do not compete with direct food production; they make use of environments that would otherwise not contribute to feeding the world's population. While generally inefficient in terms of GHG emissions, they account for only a small proportion of global agricultural emissions. Conversely, if degraded rangelands are restored to health, they hold great potential to sequester soil organic carbon.

Labour-intensive systems are typically smallholder-based and mostly occur as part of mixed crop-livestock farms. They include arable crops, aquaculture, and also tree crops, and are typified by the smallholder systems of Central America, Africa and Asia. The majority of labour-intensive systems are family farms with a focus on producing staple foods for subsistence. Surpluses may be sold or exchanged locally. Sometimes these systems are well organized and linked to national and international markets, e.g. the smallholder dairy production in East Africa and South Asia. For the poor, farming families, livestock are an important source of nutritious food. They also provide an important source of food for people outside farming households: smallholders produce by far the largest share of milk in developing countries. The production of livestock in these systems is generally inefficient compared to both the extensive and capital-intensive systems. However, there are other efficiencies that must be accounted for, particularly in relation to nutrient cycling, giving value to crop residues and providing draft power. Today, organic agriculture[42] is making an important contribution to the agro-ecological transition process underway in Africa. Organic systems are labour-intensive, and as such can be a source of employment for young people in rural areas. However, to ensure the fledgling initiatives develop, research should contribute to appropriate public policy making at different levels [De Bon et al. 2017].

Capital-intensive systems mainly produce beef, dairy, pork and poultry. Highly mechanized and extremely productive mega-dairy farms, e.g., are becoming more and more prevalent. Half of America's milk now comes from farms with more than 1000 cows and this number is increasing every year [Weber 2018]. Pigs and chickens in particular lend themselves to industrial production. These are the mainstay in high income countries, but are becoming more prevalent in LMIC as well. Capital-intensive livestock systems are highly efficient despite relying on large amounts of inputs, particularly in terms of grown feed, which often has negative effects in remote locations. Such effects include deforestation, disruption of nutrient cycles, and environmental pollution with pesticides and chemical fertilizers. With so many animals in such high densities, dealing with manure is a challenge for these systems and a major source of soil and water pollution. Capital-intensive systems also use large amounts of antimicrobials and foster ideal conditions for the emergence of resistant microbes that are hard to treat.

---

42 Organic agriculture reduces the adverse environmental and health impacts of agriculture, particularly because it uses no synthetic chemical inputs; moreover, it improves the resilience of agricultural systems [De Bon et al. 2017; Pussemier & Goeyens 2017].

Each has its own advantages and disadvantages

Who says agriculture and nature are incompatible? Who says they are for ever and ever in competition? Before the adoption of widespread mechanization in farming and biotechnical advances in breeding animals, most farming practices were designed to maintain biological diversity and enhance agricultural sustainability [Robinson 2018]. Crop rotations were integral to the diversity within farming systems. They enabled soils to remain healthy without the need for synthetic fertilizers. Without a massive input of chemicals, gigantic single-crop productions – endless monocultures of corn, for example – could be more vulnerable to attack by insects, disease micro-organisms, nematodes, and weeds. This is one of several arguments for the maintenance of diverse cropping systems and the wider claim that agricultural diversity generates a range of benefits. There are several arguments for maintaining agricultural diversity [Robinson 2018 and references herein].

- Preserving genetic diversity for current and future use.
- Maintaining diversity in the field at all levels. This includes the heterogeneity of the crop variety or animal breed; mixtures of varieties and species within and between crops; differences between crops on a farm and across agro-ecological niches; and diversity of crops and farming practices across a region/country, leading to functional heterogeneity.
- Different crops and animals can thrive under variable pest, environmental or input conditions, including the production of crops that are less dependent on external inputs.
- Different crops or animals will receive different market prices or more effectively secure subsistence production.
- Agro-biodiversity provides opportunities for humanity to exploit genetic material, varieties, and species for future use.
- Diversity of ownership and marketing of seeds and food rather than exclusive contracts going to the chemical industry.
- Marketing of unique products for niche markets.

- Targeted state, community, or private support for agro-biodiversity conservation as an alternative income stream, particularly in the margins.

Organic farming is generally regarded as synonymous with sustainable agriculture though it can assume various forms. It is an approach that emphasises environmental protection, animal welfare, food quality and health, sustainable resource use and social justice objectives, and which utilises the market to help support these objectives and compensate for the internalisation of externalities [Lampkin 2003; Stolze & Lampkin 2009]. There is however no single combination of practices that works across all climatic and terrestrial conditions. So there is a strong need for region-specific and even field-specific strategies in tillage and cropping management based on the specific requirements and characteristics of the target field [Rigby & Cáceres 2001; Ceylan 2018].

The growth in retail sales of organic foods has slowed down in recent years, reflecting deterrents to purchasing organic foods, such as high prices, poor product distribution, little obvious difference in quality, insufficient information about organic products, and doubts about the integrity of products [Reganold & Wachter 2016; Robinson 2018]. Conversion from conventional to organic farming has also proved problematic. Issues include insufficient premium prices for organic produce, higher costs as well as more labour input and the need to engage with certification bodies who enforce key standards to be reached. Yet, it is certainly the case that there are environmental gains to be achieved through organic farming, e.g. the generation of increased and diversified populations of insects, wild flowers, mammals and birds, as well as the enhanced soil structure and reduced soil erosion. These benefits however have sometimes been overstated [Hole et al. 2005].

One argument commonly deployed against organic farming is that it produces lower yields than conventional agriculture. This may be true, but it depends greatly on the local context, farming system, and site characteristics. With good management practices, suitable crop types and growing conditions, organic systems nearly match conventional yields [Seufert et al. 2012]. Higher prices for organic produce may compensate for lower outputs per hectare, and its labour intensity may support more farm workers, which can add to sustainability.

Organic farming is often not a radical alternative to globalized large-scale commercial enterprises selling to the mass consumption market. But there is an increased tendency for organics to be subsumed within the conventional agrifood system. And even if certification is not always the first priority of the farmers, it is obvious that ecological farming is doing well in our countries. The diversity of living organisms contributes towards making our fields colourful, and the care with which our farmers tend to their crops and livestock today more than ever before reflect respect for both the environment and animal welfare.

Bibliography

Bac et al. [2014]. Harvesting robots for high-value crops: state-of-the-art review and challenges ahead, *Journal of Field Robotics* 31, 6, 888-911

Berckmans [2014]. Precision livestock farming technologies for welfare management in intensive livestock systems, *Revue scientifique et technique (International Office of Epizootics)* 33, 1, 189-196

Catarino et al. [2018], Low levels of microplastics (MP) in wild mussels indicate that MP ingestion by humans is minimal compared to exposure via household fibres fallout during a meal, *Environmental Pollution* 237, 675-684

Ceylan [2018]. *Field-specific Strategies in Tillage and Cropping Management for Conserving Soil and Water Recourses and Improving Soil Quality*, pp. 4

Clutton-Brock [2015]. *The walking larder: patterns of domestication, pastoralism, and predation* (first edition in 1989), Routledge, London and New York, pp. 367

Crutzen et al. [1986]. Methane production by domestic animals, wild ruminants, other herbivorous fauna, and humans, *Tellus B: Chemical and Physical Meteorology* 38, 3-4, 271-284

Cuello [2016]. Twin Strategies to Achieve Sector Sustainability for the Vertical Farming Industry in the Next Five to Ten Years, *Agritecture*, https://www.agritecture.com/

Cuello [2018]. Mediterranean cities and vertical farming: fostering sustainable local food production and building neighbourhood esprit de corps, in

Woertz (ed.) *"Wise Cities" in the Mediterranean? Challenges of Urban Sustainability*, CIDOB edicions, Barcelona, 123-133

Cuello & Liu [2014]. Re-Imagineering the Vertical Farm: A Novel Strategy in the Design and Development of Vertical Farms, *Urban Agriculture Magazine* 28, 61

DeAngelo et al. [2006]. Methane and nitrous oxide mitigation in agriculture, *The Energy Journal*, 89-108

De Bon et al. [2017]. Organic agriculture in Africa: A source of innovation for agricultural development, *Perspective (Édition française)* 48, 1-4

Despommier [2010]. *The Vertical Farm: Feeding the World in the 21st Century*, St. Martin's Press, New York City, pp. 304

European Court of Auditors [2018]. *Background paper – Animal welfare in the EU*, pp. 13

FAO [2014]. Social farming (also called care farming): an innovative approach for promoting women's economic empowerment, decent rural employment and social inclusion. What works in developing countries?, *Global Forum on Food Security and Nutrition*, http://www.fao.org/fsnforum/activities/discussions/care-farming

FAO [2006]. *Livestock's long shadow. Environmental issues and options*, Rome, pp. 416

FAO [2018]. *Shaping the future of livestock*, The 10th Global Forum for Food and Agriculture (GFFA), Berlin, 18-20 January, pp. 20

Fernández-Quintanilla et al. [2018]. Is the current state of the art of weed monitoring suitable for site-specific weed management in arable crops?, *Weed Research* pp. 14

Gasser et al. [2018]. Path-dependent reductions in CO_2 emission budgets caused by permafrost carbon release, *Nature Geoscience* 1

Gerland et al. [2014]. World population stabilization unlikely this century, *Science* 346, 6206, 234-237

Hole et al. [2005]. Does organic farming benefit biodiversity?, *Biological Conservation* 122, 113-130

IPCC [2018]. *GLOBAL WARMING OF 1.5 °C - an IPCC special report on the impacts of global warming of 1.5 °C above pre-industrial levels and related global greenhouse gas emission pathways, in the context of strengthening the global response to the threat of climate change, sustainable development, and efforts to eradicate poverty*, pp. 34

King [2017]. The future of agriculture, *Nature* 544, S21-S23

Lampkin [2003]. From conversion payments to integrated action plans in the European Union, in OECD (ed.) *Organic Agriculture: Sustainability, Markets and Policies* CABI Publishing, Wallingford, 313-328

Lappé [1971]. *Diet for a small planet*, Ballantine Books, New York, pp. 301

Malneršič et al. [2016]. Close-range air-assisted precision spot-spraying for robotic applications: Aerodynamics and spray coverage analysis, *Biosystems Engineering* 146, 216-226

McMichael et al. [2007]. Food, livestock production, energy, climate change, and health, *The lancet* 370, 9594, 1253-1263

Ono & Watanabe [2006]. Plant factories blossom: production in Japan steadily flowers, *Resource: Engineering and Technology for a Sustainable World*, American Society of Agricultural and Biological Engineers

Pearce [1989]. Methane: the hidden greenhouse gas, *New Scientist* 122, 1663, 37-41

Pérez-Ruiz et al. [2015]. Highlights and preliminary results for autonomous crop protection, *Computers and Electronics in Agriculture* 110, 150-161

Pico-Ciamarra & Otte [2009]. The 'Livestock Revolution': Rhetoric and Reality, *Outlook on agriculture* 40, 1, 7-19

Pussemier & Goeyens [2017]. *AgricultureS & Enjeux de société*, Presses Universitaires de Liège - Agronomie, Gembloux, pp. 112

Reganold & Wachter [2016]. Organic agriculture in the twenty-first century, *Nature plants* 2, 2, 15221

Rigby & Cáceres [2001]. Organic farming and sustainibility of agriculura systems, *Agricultural Systems* 68, 21-40

Robinson [2018]. Globalization of Agriculture, *Annual Review of Resource Economics* 10, 133-160

Roldán et al. [2018]. Robots in Agriculture: State of Art and Practical Experiences, in *Service Robots*, INTECH open science | open minds, pp. 24

Seufert et al. [2012. Comparing the yields of organic and conventional agriculture, *Nature* 485, 7397, 229-232

Sinclair [2015]. *The Jungle* (first edition in 1906), Penguin Group, New York, pp. 400

Stolze & Lampkin [2009]. Policy for organic farming: Rationale and concepts, *Food Policy* 34, 237-244

UK-RAS [2018]. *Agricultural Robotics: The Future of Robotic Agriculture*, pp.36

Weber [2018]. *Manufacturing the American way of farming: Agriculture, agribusiness, and marketing in the postwar period*, PhD thesis Iowa State University, Graduate Theses and Dissertations. 16485, pp. 319

Zhang [2018]. Global pesticide use: Profile, trend, cost / benefit and more, *Proceedings of the International Academy of Ecology and Environmental Sciences* 8, 1 1-27

FOOD PROCESSING
AND PACKAGING

Cinnamon, one of the most delicious and healthiest spices on the planet

Cinnamon has been known since ancient times

It received much attention in China as is witnessed by its entry in the ancient books on Chinese botanical medicine (dated ~2700 AD), attributed to the mythical Chinese sovereign Shennong. In Ayurveda, the Hindu health doctrine from India, cinnamon is recommended for the treatment of diabetes and indisposition. Ancient Egyptians used it for beverage flavouring and in medicines, but also as an ingredient for the preparation of embalming agents. It was treasured and considered even more precious than gold.

As described in the Old Testament, cinnamon was also an essential ingredient of a holy anointing oil for the tabernacle: ... *The Lord said to Moses "Take the finest spices: of liquid myrrh 500 shekels, and of sweet-smelling cinnamon half as much, that is, 250, and 250 of aromatic cane, and 500 of cassia, according to the shekel of the sanctuary, and a hint of olive oil. And you shall make of these a sacred anointing oil blended as by the perfumer; it shall be a holy anointing oil...* [Exodus 30, 22-29].

Cinnamon was so highly prized among ancient cultures that it was regarded as a gift fit for monarchs and even for a god. The Roman Emperor, Nero, ordered an entire year's supply of cinnamon to be burnt as a sign of remorse after he had murdered his wife. And during the first century AD, the Roman author Pliny the Elder wrote of 350 grams of cinnamon as being equal in value to over five kilograms of silver.

Years ago, I came across an article on the preservation of peaches with cinnamon

Montero-Prado et al. [2011] demonstrate how the processing of cinnamon essential oil (EO) into plastic packaging and labelling materials extends the shelf life of the succulent, yellow Calanda peach. Peaches with Calanda Peach Certificate of Origin owe their market fame to their exceptional flavour and sweetness. Every single peach is bagged on the tree for the last 2 months of growth to allow the fruit to ripen inside a protective "pouch". This guarantees its purity since the bag virtually prevents any contact between the fruit and phytosanitary or other chemical agents. Moreover, "cinnamon-rich" packaging can achieve a significantly longer shelf life. For my tutorials I have used this application to illustrate the active packaging concept.

The protective role of a simple packaging is predominantly passive: packaging is a physical barrier between the food and its surrounding atmosphere, and the external environment. There are some exceptions, such as fresh produce, for which highly gas permeable or perforated packaging is used to allow for gas exchange through the packaging material [Hussein et al. 2015]. Those packaging systems are limited in their ability to further extend the shelf life of the packaged food, however.

Over recent decades, consumer concern about food safety and quality has received much attention. There is an increasing trend to natural, high quality foods, which are non-processed or minimally processed, do not contain synthetic preservatives, and have acceptable shelf lives. The protective function of packaging has been refined and improved leading to the development of new, advanced packaging technologies, such as modified atmosphere packaging, active packaging, and intelligent packaging [Janjarasskul & Suppakul 2018; Yldirim et al. 2018]. Additionally, there is a great deal of interest in applications of nanomaterials [Bumbudsanpharoke et al. 2015].

Active packaging is an innovative approach to maintain and/or increase the shelf life of food products while ensuring their quality, safety, and integrity. As defined in the European regulation (EC) No 450/2009 on active and intelligent materials and articles liable to come into contact with food, *active materials and articles means materials and articles that are intended to extend the shelf life or to maintain or improve the condition of packaged food; they are designed to deliberately incorporate components that would release or absorb substances into or from the packaged food or the environment surrounding the food.* So, active packaging systems can be divided into active scavenging systems or absorbers and active releasing systems or emitters. Whereas the scavengers remove undesired compounds from the food and its environment, the emitters add (chemical) compounds to the packaged food or into the headspace. Examples are the removal of moisture, carbon dioxide, oxygen, ethylene, etc... or the addition of antimicrobial compounds, antioxidants, flavours, ethanol, and many more.

The addition of active substances such as antimicrobials and antioxidants through the use of active packaging may decrease the amount otherwise required for direct addition into the food. Traditionally, active substances are added to the bulk of the food, whereas for most fresh and processed food, food degradation or microbial growth occurs at its surface. Furthermore, the activity of the active substances directly added to the food may be reduced or inhibited as a result of the chemical interactions between the active substances and the food components. Hence, additions of active substances via active packaging are more effective than additions into the bulk of the food.

Our recent interest in environmentally friendly additives for food preservation has led to the application of natural additives. EO are secondary metabolites and play an important role in plant defence. Hence, many of them possess strong antimicrobial and antioxidant properties [Ribeiro-Santos et al. 2017a] and, as a result, EO have been extensively studied as additives in bio-based emulsified films and coatings. Some studies have demonstrated the effectiveness of EO enriched packages containing food. Cinnamon EO is among the most studied in active materials [Manso et al. 2013; Ribeiro-Santos et al. 2017b].

Since first reading about cinnamon and the Calanda peaches, I have been fascinated by the exceptional properties of the spice and its many beneficial applications.

Cinnamon flavoured food, a spicy way to strengthen our body

The unique healing abilities of cinnamon EO come from three major chemical components, i.e. cinnamaldehyde, cinnamyl acetate and cinnamyl alcohol. However, since EO are highly complex, multi-component mixtures, it is quite possible that a wide range of other volatile substances adds to the favourable health effects [Bakkali et al. 2008].

The health benefits of cinnamaldehyde for blood thinning have well been studied. Blood platelets are constituents of blood that clump together under physical injury circumstances to stop the bleeding. When clumping becomes excessive the platelets can turn the blood flow inadequate, however. Cinnamon EO, and more particularly the major component cinnamaldehyde, helps to prevent the unwanted clotting of blood platelets, and this puts cinnamon into the category of "anti-inflammatory" food products or food additives for both humans and animals [Tung et al. 2010; Alamgir 2018; Saeed et al. 2018]. This anti-inflammatory characteristic can help relieve arthritis as well as pain and stiffness in muscles and joints.

Cinnamaldehyde has powerful anti-neuro-inflammatory capacity. However, synergistic or additive effects can possibly exist among different constituents such as 2-methoxy-cinnamaldehyde in combination with cinnamaldehyde [Ho et al. 2013]. Moreover, the positive health effects associated with the consumption of cinnamon are partly attributed to its phenolic composition [Lv et al. 2012; Gunawardena et al. 2014]. These natural compounds express anti-inflammatory activity by modulation of pro-inflammatory gene expression such as cyclooxygenase, lipoxygenase, nitric oxide synthases and several pivotal cytokines. The potential molecular mechanisms of their anti-inflammatory activities have also been suggested to include the inhibition of the enzymes related to inflammation [Chao et al. 2008]. Proanthocyanidins are the major polyphenolic component in commercial cinnamon. They are mixtures of oligomers and (small) polymers composed of flavan-3-ol[43] units; cinnamon bark contains dimeric, trimeric, and oligomeric proanthocyandins with doubly linked bis-flavan-3-ol units [Gunawardena et al. 2014].

Furthermore, given the growing awareness of the harmful effects of food poisoning, there is considerable interest in ways of reducing their incidence or — better even — of preventing them altogether. One area of research is the development of new and improved methods of food preservation. Because of negative consumer perceptions of synthetic preservatives, attention is shifting towards alternatives which the consumers consider as natural, and in particular towards plant extracts including plant EO and essences. The use of EO as antimicrobial agents was first described over 100 years ago with the phenol coefficient method, originally proposed by Samuel Rideal (1863-1929) and J. T. Ainslie Walker (1868-1930) as a means of standardizing disinfectants [Rideal & Walker 1903]. The phenol coefficient of a given chemical compound is a measure of its disinfectant activity (bactericidal activity) in relation to phenol. It indicates how many times weaker or stronger a bactericide effect is when compared with phenol; equal bactericidal activity results in a phenol coefficient of 1.

Cinnamon has been found to be an efficient means of dealing with *Candida albicans*, a fungus responsible for yeast infections. Its antifungal activity was known as early as 1974 [Bullerman 1997]. In an experiment carried out at the Department of Food Science and Technology at the University of Nebraska, slices of white, raisin, rye and whole wheat breads, all baked without the usual mould inhibitors, were subjected to various aflatoxin[44] producing moulds. The latter grew vigorously on all types of breads except raisin bread where growth was described as being *scant or not visible at all*. In trying to identify whether the raisins or the cinnamon was responsible, food scientists discovered that as little

---

43 Flavanols are a class of flavonoids containing a ketone group; they are not to be confused with flavonols that have the 3-hydroxyflavone backbone [Wikipedia].

44 Aflatoxins are toxic metabolites produced by the fungi. The main fungi that produce aflatoxins are *Aspergillus flavus* and *Aspergillus parasiticus*, which are abundant in warm and humid regions of the world. Aflatoxins are carcinogenic to humans (Group 1).

as 2 % or 20 mg of cinnamon per ml of a yeast extract and sucrose broth inhibited 97-99 % of the moulds.

And there is also exciting news for Wrigley's Popular Chewing Gum and Confections! Remember the commercial slogan *Big Red, an American classic from Wrigleys ... Cinnamon flavoured gum which, whilst refreshing like a regular gum, delivers a warm wintery heat*? Well, a research team at the University of Illinois at Chicago has discovered that the commercially available sugar-sweetened cinnamon chewing gum may actually help remedy halitosis or chronic bad breath by reducing volatile sulphur compounds producing anaerobes in the oral cavity [Zhu et al. 2011].

Cinnamon may reduce blood sugar by lowering insulin resistance

Using cinnamon to season foods which are high in carbohydrates (and also high on the glycemic index and therefore harder for the body to burn off) can help lessen their impact on blood sugar levels. Cinnamon slows down the gastric emptying rate[45] and thus reduces the rise in blood sugar after eating. Cinnamon supplementation is considered an additional dietary supplement option to regulate blood glucose and blood pressure levels along with the conventional medication used to treat type 2 diabetes melitus. Several studies [Akilen et al. 2010; Van Hul et al. 2017; Shikha & Alka 2018] support the hypothesis that the inclusion of water soluble cinnamon compounds in the diet can reduce risk factors associated with diabetes and cardiovascular diseases.

The incidence of diabetes worldwide is rapidly increasing as people adopt more sedentary lifestyles. People in developing countries are also consuming more high-calorie sweeteners, vegetable oils and foods of animal origin (such as meat, poultry, fish, eggs and dairy products). The combination of changes in lifestyle and diet has paved the way for a public health disaster, with obesity leading to an explosive upsurge in diabetes, heart disease and other illnesses. It is frightening to note that

---

45 Gastric emptying rate is the rate at which the stomach empties after the meals.

the earth's ~1.6 billion overweight people significantly outnumber the ~800 million who are undernourished [Popkin 2009].

Cinnamon may significantly help people with type 2 diabetes improve their ability to respond to insulin, thereby normalizing their blood sugar levels. Both test tube and animal studies have shown that compounds in cinnamon EO not only stimulate insulin receptors, but also inhibit the enzyme that renders them inactive. In other words, the EO markedly improved the ability of the cells to use glucose.

Convincing data from Asia

Economic, dietary and other lifestyle changes have been occurring rapidly in most South Asian countries, making their populations more vulnerable to type 2 diabetes and cardiovascular diseases. Recent data show a significant increase in the number of people affected by these diseases in urban as well as in semi-urban and rural areas. Prime determinants for type 2 diabetes in South Asian populations include physical inactivity due to urbanisation and mechanisation, imbalanced diets, abdominal obesity, excess hepatic fat and inadequate perinatal and early life nutrition [Misra et al. 2014].

Metabolic syndrome is a cluster of conditions – including increased blood pressure, high blood sugar, excess body fat around the waist, and abnormal cholesterol or triglyceride levels – that seriously increases the risk of heart disease, stroke and diabetes. Individuals with metabolic syndrome are 5 times more at risk of developing type 2 diabetes and 3 times more likely to suffer a heart attack or stroke compared to people without the syndrome [Paoletti et al. 2006]. These individuals are also twice as likely to die from type 2 diabetes and a heart attack or stroke. Metabolic syndrome affects 20 to 30 % of urban city dwellers in India.

The question, then, is: could there be a simple affordable solution? The recent publication by Jain et al. [2017] includes a strong, positive message: *cinnamon supplements alleviate metabolic syndrome.*

According to a trial led by the University of Delhi, regular cinnamon supplementation counters all aspects of metabolic syndrome in Indian adults. Previous investigations suggested the potential role of cinnamon and its components in improving insulin sensitivity. For example, it has already been reported that cinnamate, a phenolic compound found in the inner bark of cinnamon trees, provides protection against lipemic-oxidative disorder. Moreover, it acts as a hypocholesterolemic (cinnamon lowers the cholesterol levels), and hepatoprotective (cinnamon suppresses lipid peroxidation by enhancing antioxidant enzyme activity in the liver) agent in laboratory rats on a high-fat diet [Amin et al. 2009].

A 16-week randomised controlled trial was conducted with 116 Asian Indian subjects (64 men and 52 women), who had metabolic syndrome. They were divided into two groups. Participants in the first group were given 2.5 g of a wheat flour each day as a placebo, and in the second group, each participant received 3 g of powdered cinnamon daily. Both the wheat flour and the cinnamon were administered in capsule form. Compared to the placebo group, the subjects of the cinnamon intervention group experienced greater weight loss and greater high-density lipoprotein (HDL or good) cholesterol increase as well as a pronounced decrease in waist circumference, low-density lipoprotein (LDL or bad) and total cholesterol, systolic and diastolic blood pressure, and body fat percentage. Additionally, the aqueous extract of cinnamon stem bark has been shown to reduce sucrose-induced elevation in systolic blood pressure of spontaneously hypertensive rats and to lower diastolic and systolic blood pressure in pre-diabetic and diabetic humans.

The results of the latter study are very promising. Jain et al. [2017] evidenced obvious decreases in measures of glycemia, adiposity including abdominal obesity, lipids, and blood pressure. The percentage of individuals with metabolic syndrome was significantly decreased with a single cinnamon nutrient intervention.

Cinnamon adds depth and warmth to sweet and savory dishes

Cinnamon quills or sticks are prominently present in cookbooks and kitchen bibles. Everyone is familiar with the essential ingredient of cinnamon rolls, apple stuffed chicken breast, cinnamon pork loin, nectarine chutney, acorn squash stuffed with apples, banana cake with cinnamon glaze and hundreds of other recipes.

Without cinnamon sticks, no delicious creamy rice pudding in Belgium!

Cinnamon is a prime ingredient in sweets and baked dishes. It is also an unobtrusive, but much appreciated addition to marinades, beverages, dressings, meat and fish. Guyana's national pepper pot is a stewed beef dish, strongly flavoured with cinnamon, hot peppers and cassareep, a special sauce made from the Cassava root. Egyptian Luqmat al-Qadi are small, round and crunchy donuts served with dusted cinnamon and powdered sugar. In Mexico, cinnamon is added as a flavouring agent to chocolate.

Many exclusive liqueurs and bitters also contain cinnamon. It is said that the monks of the Benedictine Abbey of Fécamp in French Normandy have developed a medicinal aromatic herbal beverage. In fact, it was Alexander the Great who invented the recipe himself, with the help of a local chemist [Wikipedia]. The exact list of herbs and their proper proportions are closely guarded trade secrets, but cinnamon is obviously one of the ingredients of the herbal drink Bénédictine.

Cinnamon's popularity has continued throughout history; it became a commonly used spice in Medieval Europe. Cinnamon has a very pleasant flavour and a warm smell, which has made it very popular in cooking, baking, curries and all kinds of drinks. Because of high demand for the spice, cinnamon was one of the first commodities to be traded regularly between the Near East and Europe. Ceylon cinnamon is produced in Sri Lanka, India, Madagascar, Brazil and the Caribbean, while *Cassia* is mainly produced in China, Vietnam and Indonesia. It is obtained from the inner bark of several trees of the genus *Cinnamomum*. More than one single species is sold as cinnamon: *Cinnamomum verum* or "True cinnamon", Sri Lanka cinnamon or Ceylon cinnamon; *Cinnamomum burmannii* or Indonesian cinnamon; *Cinnamomum loureiroi* or Vietnamese cinnamon and, finally, *Cinnamomum aromaticum* or *Cassia* [Wikipedia].

Should preference be given to cinnamon-rich dishes?

While the results of the study by Jain et al. [2017] are very promising, they should be tested in a larger sample over a longer period of time. Clearly, the end of the chosen path is not yet in sight. It would be a serious mistake, however, to disregard such an interesting and promising development.

This being said, I would certainly not recommend consuming large quantities of cinnamon. Cinnamon can have several dangerous medical side effects, because of the coumarin it contains, which when ingested in excessive amounts could cause serious health problems [Iwata et al. 2016]. Coumarin is a naturally occurring flavouring substance in cinnamon and many other plants. It is known that coumarin can cause liver toxicity in several species and it is considered a non-genotoxic carcinogen in rodents. Fotland et al. [2011] established a new Tolerable Daily Intake (TDI) for coumarin of 0.07 mg per kg of body weight. By using cinnamon on oatmeal or other cereals just a few times a week, it was estimated that the TDI in children and adults can be greatly exceeded. Moreover, these scientists claim that even a few weeks of ingesting high amounts of coumarin can have serious adverse effects.

Other undesirable substances in cinnamon are safrole and styrene. Normally, only traces of safrole are found in cinnamon. Higher concentrations are however common in oils from cinnamon leaves, which may be used for blending purposes with other cinnamon oils. Styrene is formed in cinnamon under unfavourable transport and storage conditions.

All the same, there is reason enough to pursue the research

Research is four different things: brains with which to think, eyes with which to see, machines with which to measure and fourth, money [Albert Szent-Gyorgyi, Nobel prize in Physiology or Medicine in 1937]. This can only come about through efficient co-operation between all actors: scientists, decision makers, industrialists and consumers.

So, let us hope that all the thinking, seeing, measuring and financing will confirm the beneficial effects of cinnamon on human health!

Bibliography

Akilen et al. [2010]. Glycated haemoglobin and blood pressure-lowering effect of cinnamon in multi-ethnic Type 2 diabetic patients in the UK: a randomized, placebo-controlled, double-blind clinical trial, *Diabetic Medecine* 27, 1159-1168

Alamgir [2018]. Secondary Metabolites: Secondary Metabolic Products Consisting of C and H; C, H, and O; N, S, and P Elements; and O/N Heterocycles, *Therapeutic Use of Medicinal Plants and their Extracts* 2, 165-309

Amin et al. [2009]. Oxidative markers, nitric oxide and homocysteine alteration in hypercholesterolimic rats: role of atorvastatine and cinnamon, *International Journal of Clinical and Experimental Medicine* 2, 254-265

Bakkali et al. [2008]. Biological effects of essential oils – A review, *Food and Chemical Toxicology* 46, 446

Bullerman [1997]. Inhibition of aflatoxin production by cinnamon, *Journal of Food Science* 39, 6, 1163-1165

Bumbudsanpharoke et al. [2015]. Applications of nanomaterials in food packaging, *Journal of Nanoscience and Nanotechnology* 15, 9, 6357-6372

Chao et al. [2008]. Cinnamaldehyde inhibits pro-inflammatory cytokines secretion from monocytes/macrophages through suppression of intracellular signaling, *Food and Chemical Toxicology* 46, 220-231

Fotland et al. [2011]. Risk assessment of coumarin using the bench mark dose (BMD) approach: Children in Norway which regularly eat oatmeal porridge with cinnamon may exceed the TDI for coumarin with several folds, *Food and Chemical Toxicology* 50, 3-4, 903-912

Gunawardena et al. [2014]. Anti-inflammatory properties of Cinnamon polyphenols and their monomeric precursors, in *Polyphenols in human health and disease*, Elsevier Inc., 409-425

Ho et al. [2013]. Inhibition of neuroinflammation by cinnamon and its main components, *Food Chemistry* 138, 4, 2275-2282

Iwata et al. [2016]. The Relation between Hepatotoxicity and the Total Coumarin Intake from Traditional Japanese Medicines Containing Cinnamon Bark, *Frontiers in Pharmacology* 7, Article 174

Janjarasskul & Suppakul [2018]. Active and intelligent packaging: The indication of quality and safety, *Critical Reviews in Food Science and Technology* 58, 5, 808-831

Hussein et al. [2015]. Perforation-mediated modified atmosphere packaging of fresh and minimally processed produce - A review, *Food Packaging and Shelf Life* 6, 7-20

Jain et al. [2017]. Effect of oral cinnamon intervention on metabolic profile and body composition of Asian Indians with metabolic syndrome: a randomized double-blind control trial, *Lipids in Health and Disease* 16, 113

Lv et al. [2012]. Phenolic composition and nutraceutical properties of organic and conventional cinnamon and peppermint, *Food Chemistry* 132, 3, 1442-1450

Manso et al. [2013]. Combined analytical and microbiological tools to study the effect on *Aspergillus flavus* of cinnamon essential oil contained in food packaging, *Food Control* 30, 370-378

Misra et al. [2014].Diabetes in South Asians, *Diabetic Medicine* 31, 1153–1162

Montero-Prado et al. [2011]. Active label-based packaging to extend the shelf life of "Calanda" peach fruit: Changes in fruit quality and enzymatic activity, *Postharvest Biology and Technology* 60, 211– 219

Paoletti et al. [2006]. Metabolic Syndrome, Inflammation and Atherosclerosis, *Vascular Health and Risk Management* 2, 2, 145–152

Popkin [2009]. *The World Is Fat: The Fads, Trends, Policies, and Products That Are Fattening the Human Race*, Pinguin Group (USA) inc., pp. 240

Ribeiro-Santos et al. [2017a]. Use of essential oils in active food packaging: Recent advances and future trends, *Trends in Food Science & Technology* 61, 132-140

Ribeiro-Santos et al. [2017b]. Revisiting an ancient spice with medicinal purposes: Cinnamon, *Trends in Food Science & Technology* 62, 154-169

Rideal & Walker [1903]. Standardization of Disinfectants, *Journal of the Royal Sanitary Institute* 24, 424

Saeed et al. [2018]. Phytochemistry and beneficial impacts of cinnamon (*Cinnamomum zeylanicum*) as a dietary supplement in poultry diets, *World's Poultry Science Journal* 74, 2, 331-346

Shikha & Alka [2018]. Cinnamon: an imperative spice for human health, *World Journal of Pharmacy and Pharmaceutical Sciences* 7, 3, 1078-1085

Tung et al. [2010]. Anti-inflammatory activities of essential oils and their constituents from different provenances of indigenous cinnamon

(Cinnamomum osmophloeum) leaves, *Pharmaceutical Biology* 48, 10, 1130-1136

Van Hul et al. [2017]. Reduced obesity, diabetes 1 and steatosis upon cinnamon and grape pomace 2 are associated with changes in gut microbiota and markers of gut barrier, *American Journal of Physiology – Endocrinology and Metabolism* 314, 4, E334-E352

Yldirim et al. [2018]. Active Packaging Applications for Food, *Comprehensive Reviews in Food Science and Food Safety* 17, 165-199

Zhu et al. [2011]. Short-term germ-killing effect of sugar-sweetened cinnamon chewing gum on salivary anaerobes associated with halitosis, *The Journal of Clinical Dentistry* 22, 1, 23-6

Plastic Attack

Campaigners call it an event to highlight "our absurd plastic culture"

Not that long ago, the "Plastic Attack" action received tremendous media coverage in Belgium. Newspaper articles and television news bulletins showed supermarket customers tearing off the packaging of the consumables and food products they had bought and dumping them into bins at the exit. Is the use of (food) packaging redundant? Will it soon be banned?

Admittedly, we face a problem – an old problem, one that emerged many years ago. The militant and committed artist, Clay Apenouvon, became fascinated by plastic and in 2010 he created his concept "Plastic Attack". This concept was meant to raise awareness worldwide of the environmental danger and harm caused by plastic. In his work, Apenouvon used a striking metaphor when he talked about the "Fatal beauty" of plastic [http://africanah.org/clay-apenouvon-togo/].

Packaging is the encasement of products in packages

Packaging includes protective wrappings and other external coverings that can provide protection, information, security and marketing benefits. Finding completely new materials or objects that achieve excellence in all four aspects will not be easy.

The basic benefit of packaging is to protect the packed goods – both, food and non-food items – prior to their sale. It prevents damage during transport and storage. Food packaging also significantly contributes to the hygienic transportation and storage of various foods and drinks.

Packaging reduces exposure to both chemical and microbiological contaminants, which can cause food poisoning or foodborne diseases[46]. Some packaging or packaging systems also actively prolong the shelf life of various foods and drinks, e.g. modified atmosphere packaging[47], active packaging[48], etc.

Packaging also provides information about the contents: mostly factual, legally mandatory or promotional information. And packaging is also in the front line when it comes to marketing. It provides a marketing opportunity by attracting customers to the product and by demonstrating the product's attributes. Through design and appropriate communication, packages can differentiate a product from similar products produced by competitors and help sell them. Well designed, impressive packaging can be very useful in promoting packed goods.

Packages are sometimes designed for containment: products (or objects) that contain multiple items use appropriate packaging to keep everything together before the items are displayed in the shop. Product containment can also allow a product to be sold in larger quantities. And product security depends on the packaging. Correct packaging procedures make items tamper-resistant, i.e. they can help reduce theft and prevent harm from dangerous products.

Packaging provides protection, information, security and marketing benefits. It is hard to imagine modern life without packaging. Shouting from the rooftops that packaging must be banned may be short-sighted,

---

46 Strictly speaking, the term "food poisoning" refers to consumption of foods that contain a toxin or poison. The key point is that the multiplication of bacteria to harmful levels takes place prior to consuming the contaminated food. In foodborne diseases, the food or water only acts as a vehicle for the disease to enter the body. The multiplication then takes place within the body where it spreads and remains for weeks or even months, potentially causing serious damage and even death.

47 Modified atmosphere packaging involves either actively or passively controlling or modifying the atmosphere surrounding the product within a package made of various types and/or combinations of films.

48 Active food contact materials absorb or release substances in order to improve the quality of packaged food or to extend its shelf life [European Food Safety Authority, https://www.efsa.europa.eu].

but it is nevertheless important to recognise that we face a complex and global packaging waste problem.

The message is: stop littering!

Consumer (food) packaging generates very large quantities of waste. Disposing of packaging introduces waste into the ecosystem, which produces a great many negative effects.

Litter is small waste that is left outside, either consciously or unconsciously, in places where it does not belong. Cigarette butts, chewing gum, food waste, wrappings, cans, bottles, drinking cups, tickets, umbrellas, handkerchiefs are all examples of litter. Even though the problem has been known for over a century – as early as 1870 Jules Verne (1828-1905) provided a graphic description of how floating debris accumulates in ocean gyres in the chapter on the Sargasso Sea of his famous novel *Twenty Thousand Leagues under the Sea* – the warnings have not been taken seriously. Did you know it takes some 75-80 years to degrade a discarded empty bag of crisps? And did you know that the complete breakdown of a polyethylene terephthalate bottle[49] takes ~500 years?

Littering is not only a soure of irritation; cleaning up the mess also costs a great deal of money. Rermoving the litter in Flanders costs over 60 million euros per year, which corresponds to almost 10 euros per inhabitant [https://www.vlaanderen.be/nl/natuur-en-milieu/afval/zwerfvuil-en-sluikstort]. And a lot of work remains to be done. Despite government efforts, there are still masses of waste on our streets and motorways. Generating awareness is the most important step in the fight against littering. All of us can play a role in protecting the environment by changing our behaviour as consumers, says Jan Verheyen, spokesman OVAM (Openbare Vlaamse Afvalstoffenmaatschappij, Public Waste Agency of Flanders).

The litter build-up is not so much a regional problem as a global problem. We have all seen the pictures of the Great Pacific garbage

---

49 Most soft drink bottles are made of polyethylene terephthalate (or PET).

patch (GPGP) or Pacific trash vortex, the gyre of marine debris particles in the central North Pacific Ocean that was discovered as long as ~30 years ago. The oceanic garbage build-up is a highly complex and very worrying unsolved problem. Lebreton et al. [2018] confirm that ocean plastic pollution within the GPGP is increasing exponentially and pollution build-up is occurring at a faster rate than in surrounding waters. Plastic debris accumulations were also observed much closer to home. The team of Andrés Cózar, an ecologist at the University of Cadiz in Spain, provided the first global map of the abundance of plastic debris in the open oceans. The map shows the existence of five areas of large-scale accumulation of floating plastic debris in the centres of the North Pacific, South Pacific, North Atlantic, South Atlantic and Indian Oceans. Moreover, the team measured plastic concentrations throughout the Mediterranean basin, from the Strait of Gibraltar to Cyprus, and found amounts of floating plastic debris comparable to those described for the five subtropical ocean gyres [Cózar et al. 2015].

Yet, garbage is both visible and invisible. It consists predominantly of small, suspended, often microscopic particles in the upper water column. Sometimes larger pieces of plastic float around in the water, and fish, sea birds, and sea mammals mistake them for food. When the animals eat the plastic, their bodies cannot digest it and the plastic provides the animal with a sensation of satiety. The animal then stops eating and soon dies of starvation - the fatal beauty of non-degradable plastic!

But what we cannot see is even worse. Micro- and nanoplastics are ubiquitous, in marine as well as in freshwater ecosystems, with microplastics found in places as far-flung as a Mongolian mountain lake [Horton et al. 2017] and in deep sea sediments [Courtene-Jones et al. 2017]. The major concern is that they are ingested by a number of aquatic biota, especially the filter feeders like molluscs, mussels, oysters, from where they enter the food chain, all of which could have physical and toxicological effects on aquatic organisms and on the final consumers, i.e. the oyster and mussel lovers.

That our seafood should be contaminated by microplastics is serious enough, but there is more, much more. Microplastics are everywhere: on land, but also in the air we breathe, in the water we drink and in all the food we eat. It is very disturbing to learn that the food we eat contains microplastics from distant sources as well as from the immediate environment and house dust [Catarino et al. 2018]. We are surrounded by invisible pieces of waste, and exposed to all kinds of unpleasant consequences. In the first study of its kind, Austrian researchers confirm they have found evidence of tiny plastic particles in the human gut. They analysed stool samples of people from different countries and found that all of them tested positive for microplastics. On average, 20 microplastic particles were found per 10 grams of stool [unpublished results].

Is it too late?

Every year, an estimated 8 million tons of plastic end up in the ocean, and the figure should rise to ~60 tons per minute (a doubling of the current supply) by 2050 if today's plastic use and lack of adequate waste management continue. The problem of ocean plastic waste is huge. Yet, despite everything, there is no reason to lose heart. I summarise the 8 essential steps that are required for efficient action. For more information I suggest you visit the World Economic Forum (WEF) website [Jensen 2018].

- We use too many single-use plastic items such as straws, plastic bags, cups, plates and cutlery, and must put an end to this practice.
- Leading fossil fuel based plastic manufacturers are planning to increase their production over the coming years. Instead, alternatives to non-degradable plastics should be developed. It is also recommended to target the industries responsible for major plastic waste with specific industry agreements and producer liability arrangements.
- Since fossil fuel based plastic is still cheaper to synthesise and buy than renewable plastic, governments should investigate the implementation of a tax on polluting plastic.
- The consumption of plastic is increasing faster than the capacity to handle its waste. An international aid programme should

therefore be established to develop waste management and recycling infrastructures.

- An international agreement with firm targets and time frames for implementation should be established, aiming at increased market responsibility to prevent new propagation and the strengthening of waste management.
- Efforts to map and monitor and research on adverse effects for health and environmental quality must be strengthened. This will cost money, but that money will be well spent. Who would dare to claim that public health and environmental quality are not the overriding priorities?
- Since a majority of the plastic in the ocean is thought to come from land-based activities and industry, everyone can and should contribute to the solution.
- To solve the plastic problem, we must ensure that action and clean-up operations are undertaken in areas where the problem is most acute. Much of the work, however, is hampered because of a lack of financial resources. The establishment of a global ocean fund, with waste management and the clean-up of marine areas high on the agenda, will be one step closer towards a plastic-poor future with no pollution of the world's oceans.

Plastic-poor in no way means plastic-free

The action *"Mei Plasticvrij* (a plastic-free month of May)" wanted to make the Flemish people aware of the ubiquitous presence of plastic waste. Its aim was to significantly reduce the production and use of plastic. A call to participate in the action appeared in all Flemish newspapers and magazines, and many joined the movement.

Since the dawn of the synthetic materials era, advances have been unparalleled in the history of materials. Chemists have discovered new catalysts and developed new synthesis routes to join small molecules into long polymer macromolecules with the appropriate properties for particular uses. Physicists and engineers have designed new processing methods and new technologies to enhance performances. Naturally, consumers are becoming increasingly more demanding. And, quite rightly, we expect products that will further enhance the quality of our lives and we want materials and technologies that are increasingly energy efficient, sustainable and capable of reducing global pollution. Our dream is an open and accessible world with a healthy living environment for all. It is also our challenge for the future.

The WEF published *"5 synthetic materials that will shape the future"*, a highly fascinating and relevant paper on important, but unexpected innovations and developments [https://www.weforum.org/]. Ignoring these opportunities would be very foolish. The WEF emphasised innovations of irrefutable importance.

Bioplastics are becoming steadily more important [Arikan & Oszoy 2017]. As we are all too often reminded, "common" plastics do not degrade and are a very visible source of environmental pollution. To complicate things even further, the raw materials of these polymers, which we call the monomers, are historically derived from crude oil, which is not renewable. But things are changing! Thanks to recent research and the development of improved enzyme and catalyst applications, it is becoming increasingly possible to convert renewable resources into the major building blocks needed for manufacturing plastics and synthetic rubbers. And when the reaction products are also biodegradable[50], they no longer constitute a huge problem for the environment. Currently, the global bioplastics market is thought to be growing at a rate of 20 % to 25 % per year. Their major advantages are a lower carbon footprint, independence, energy efficiency, and better eco-safety.

Plastic composites are reinforced by different types of fibre to make them stronger or more elastic. More recent high-performance developments within this field are nanocomposites, whereby plastics are reinforced using tiny particles of substances such as graphene[51]. These

---

50 Whether a plastic is biomass- or petroleum-based is a different question to whether it will biodegrade (a process by which microbes break down material if conditions are suitable). Technically, all materials are biodegradable, but for practical purposes, only those that degrade within a relatively short period of time are considered biodegradable.

51 The simplest way to describe graphene is that it is a single, thin layer of graphite —

have many potential uses [Chen et al. 2018], ranging from lightweight sensors on wind turbine blades to more powerful batteries and internal body scaffolds that speed up the healing process of broken bones.

No matter how carefully we select materials for engineering applications based on their ability to withstand mechanical stresses and environmental conditions, at a given time they will inevitably fail. Ageing, degradation and loss of mechanical integrity due to impact or fatigue are all contributing factors. Inspired by biological systems, new materials are now being developed which are able to heal in response to what would traditionally be considered irreversible damage. Polymers are not the only materials with the potential for self-healing, but they seem to be very good at it [Pang et al. 2018]. A series of novel techniques dedicated to polymerised products with features such as properties regulation, self-healing, reprocessing, solid state recycling, and controllable degradation are now being developed, heralding the opportunity of upgrading traditional polymer engineering. Although the exploration of this emerging topic is still in its infancy, the advances so far are encouraging and clearly directed to large scale applications.

Most polymers are insulators and therefore do not conduct electricity. However, a substantial upsurge in this field of polymer research emerged in 2000 after the award of a Nobel Prize to Alan MacDiarmid, Alan Heeger and Hideki Shirakawa for their contribution in discovering that a polymer named polyacetylene became conductive when impurities were introduced through a process known as doping. Not only does the same process make other similar polymers conductive, but some can even be converted into light-emitting diodes (better known as their acronym "LEDs"). This is an area where polymers still face considerable challenges since they are a class of exciting materials combining the advantages of both metals and plastics [Ouyang 2018].

Gels and synthetic rubbers can easily adjust their shape in response to external stimuli, which means they are able to respond to changes in

---

the soft, flaky material used in pencil lead. Graphite is an allotrope of the element carbon, meaning it possesses the same atoms, but they are arranged differently, which gives different properties to the material.

their surroundings. The external stimulus would usually be a change in temperature or acidity/alkalinity transition, but it could equally be light, ultrasound or chemical agents. This turns out to be incredibly useful in designing smart materials for sensors, drug delivery devices and many other applications, such as intelligent packaging[52]. Other possibilities for smart polymers include products like window coatings that can wash the windows when they are dirty, and medical stitches that disappear when an injury has healed.

Given this perspective, "plastic-free" is pure nonsense. I would have preferred "litter-free" or "waste-free". I would very much appreciate clean cities, clean motorways. And yes, I would love a natural, plastic-free, and productive ocean. Hopefully, consumers will no longer throw their rubbish on the streets. Hopefully, the industry will increasingly consider waste as a raw material. And, hopefully, decision makers will seriously and financially encourage the research we still need to warrant necessary innovations.

Yes, dear reader, I know, it is not always easy to be hopeful!

Make a feedstock out of waste

Looking beyond the current "take-make-dispose" extractive industrial model, circular economy aims to redefine growth, focusing on positive society-wide benefits. It entails gradually decoupling economic activity from the consumption of finite resources such as fossil fuel and designing waste out of the system [Ellen MacArthur Foundation 2017].

Europe could well take up a leading role in the transition to the plastics of the future. Its strategy [EC 2018] determines the foundations of a renewed plastics economy, where the design and production of

---

52 Intelligent packaging refers to systems that monitor the conditions of packaged foods; its concepts are based on the useful interaction between packaging environment and the packed food to provide active food protection. It is the newest technology within the food packaging field. Even though this technology is still growing and is not yet fully commercially viable, it has enormous potential to improve the safety, quality, and traceability of food products, as well as being very convenient for consumers [Biji et al. 2015; Ghaani et al. 2016].

plastics and plastic products focuses on reuse, repair and recycling needs, and where more sustainable materials are developed and promoted. This will deliver greater added value and prosperity in Europe and boost innovation as long as there is fair (governmental) funding. It will curb plastic pollution and its adverse impact on our environment and well-being. Yet, all stakeholders including the private sector, together with national and regional authorities, cities and citizens, will need to mobilise, since reuse and recycling of end-of-life plastics is still very low – much lower than for other materials such as paper, glass or metals. Still ~95 % of the value of plastic packaging materials, i.e. between 70 and 105 billion euros annually, is lost after a very short first-use cycle.

Rethinking and improving the way a complex value chain works requires effort and increased cooperation between all the key players, including the plastics producers and recyclers, the retailers and the consumers. It also calls for innovation and a shared vision to drive investment in the right direction. Increasing the sustainability of the plastics industry can generate new opportunities for innovation, competitiveness and job creation, in line with the objectives pursued by the European strategy [EC 2018].

Trashing excess packaging after purchase is no more than a drop in the ocean

Rethinking and improving, whereby bioplastics (and more particularly the biodegradable ones) can act as protagonists, will shape our future. At a time when there is so much talk about circular economy, we should now turn words into action and fatal beauty into a real opportunity.

Bibliography

Arikan & Oszoy [2015]. A Review: Investigation of Bioplastics, *Journal of Civil Engineering and Architecture* 9, 188-192

Biji et al. [2015]. Smart packaging systems for food applications: a review, *Journal of Food Science and Technology* 52, 10, 6125-6135

Catarino et al. [2018], Low levels of microplastics (MP) in wild mussels indicate that MP ingestion by humans is minimal compared to exposure via household fibres fallout during a meal, *Environmental Pollution* 237, 675-684

Chen et al. [2018]. A critical review on the development and performance of polymer/graphene nanocomposites, *Science and Engineering of Composite Materials*, published online

Courtene-Jones et al. [2017]. Microplastic pollution identified in deep-sea water and ingested by benthic invertebrates in the Rockall Trough, North Atlantic Ocean, *Environmental Pollution* 231, 1, 271-280

Cózar et al. [2015]. Plastic Accumulation in the Mediterranean Sea, *Plos ONE* 10, 4, pp. 12

Ellen MacArthur Foundation [2017]. *Towards the circular economy*, pp. 99

European Commission [2018], *A European Strategy for Plastics in a Circular Economy*, pp. 18

Ghaani et al. [2016]. An overview of the intelligent packaging technologies in the food sector, *Trends in Food Science & Technology* 51, 1-11

Horton et al. [2017], Microplastics in freshwater and terrestrial environments: Evaluating the current understanding to identify the knowledge gaps and future research priorities, *Science of the Total Environment* 586, 127-141

Jensen [2018]. *8 steps to solve the ocean's plastic problem*, https://www.weforum.org/agenda/2018/03/8-steps-to-solve-the-oceans-plastic-problem/

Lebreton et al. [2018], Evidence that the Great Pacific Garbage Patch is rapidly accumulating plastic, *Scientific Reports* 8, 4666, pp. 15

Ouyang [2018]. Recent Advances of Intrinsically Conductive Polymers, *Acta Physico-Chimica Sinica* 34, 11, 1211-1220

Pang et al. [2018]. Polymer engineering based on reversible covalent chemistry: A promising innovative pathway towards new materials and new functionalities, *Progress in Polymer Science* 80, 39-93

Astaxanthin from shrimp waste: a useful ingredient in shrimp packaging

You may have heard of beta-carotene and lycopene. Have any of you ever heard of astaxanthin?

It is a dark red pigment and a major carotenoid[53] – the carotenoid family comprises some 600 pigments – found in fruits and vegetables, in microalgae and aquatic animals such as krill, shrimp, and crayfish. It is responsible for the reddish coloration of crustaceans, shellfish, and the flesh of salmonoids. Astaxanthin, however, is much more than just a red pigment. It is primarily a powerful antioxidant. Its unique structure containing a keto and a hydroxyl group on each end of the molecule contributes to the exceptionally high capacity of astaxanthin to quench free radicals and reactive species of oxygen, and to inhibit lipid peroxidation[54]. It has many positive health effects, from diminishing wrinkles to upgrading our workout routine. Earlier research results showed that the standardized antioxidant activity is ~65–fold higher than vitamin C, ~54-fold more powerful than beta-carotene, and

---

53 Carotenoids are plant pigments responsible for bright red, yellow and orange hues in many food products; fruits that are high in carotenoids include squash, carrots, grapefruit, oranges and apricots [https://www.livescience.com/52487-carotenoids.html].

54 Lipid peroxidation is a process generated naturally in small amounts in the body, mainly by the effect of several reactive oxygen species such as hydroxyl radical, hydrogen peroxide, etc.

~14-fold higher than vitamin E [Biswal 2014]. Moreover, astaxanthin is by far much more potent than other carotenoids such as lutein and lycopene [Naguib 2000; Nishida et al. 2007].

Practically every cell in the human body can benefit from astaxanthin

Astaxanthin has potential health-promoting effects in the prevention and treatment of various diseases such as cancers, chronic inflammatory diseases, metabolic syndrome, diabetes, diabetic nephropathy, cardio-vascular diseases, gastrointestinal diseases, liver diseases, neuro-degenerative diseases, eye diseases, skin diseases, exercise-induced fatigue, male infertility, and mercury-induced acute renal failure [Yuan 2011].

Astaxanthin rejuvenates the human skin from within. Oral supplementation of antaxanthin-rich nutrients – the nutricosmetics, also known as "beauty pills" – is claimed to reduce wrinkles by resisting free radicals generated by solar radiation [Anunciato & da Rocha Filho 2012; Wakeman 2018]. Chew & Park [2004] have evidenced that astaxanthin helps balance the immune system by stimulating its infection and cancer fighting components. Moreover, it suppresses overactive immune responses that create needless allergic reactions, reduces immunopathology[55] and enhances longevity through an immune depressive effect [Dhinaut et al. 2017]. The beneficial effects of the enhanced intake of carotenoids such as astaxanthin typically lowers the risk of cancer. This has been supported by several epidemiological studies [Tanaka et al. 2012]. Also, the review paper by Zhang & Wang [2015] evidences that astaxanthin could have anticancer effects and may help prevent the proliferation and spread of cancer cells. Moreover, obese people develop dangerous fat accumulations in their livers, which predisposes them to cirrhosis and liver cancer, and astaxanthin supplements can reduce liver fats and triglyceride levels. Moreover,

---

55 Immunopathology corresponds to self-damage of the inflammatory response, resulting from oxidizing molecules produced when the immune system is activated.

astaxanthin supplementation slows the development of diabetic nephropathy [Manabe et al. 2008] and heals clouding of the eye lens (cataract) and diabetic retinopathy[56] [Sun et al. 2011]. Astaxanthin also has powerful antioxidant effects that can counter many cardiovascular complications. It helps normalize lipid profiles by reducing triglyceride and cholesterol levels while boosting beneficial high-density lipoprotein cholesterol (HDL-cholesterol, i.e. the good cholesterol). These effects reduce the risk of clot forming within the blood vessels [Yang et al. 2011]. According to the review by Fassett & Coombes [2009], there have been at least eight clinical studies measuring the effects of astaxanthin that have demonstrated that astaxanthin supplementation may lower markers of both inflammation and oxidative stress. Another review concludes that astaxanthin could protect against atherosclerosis, which is the build-up of plaque, which is caused by fat, cholesterol, calcium and other substances accumulating in the arteries [Kishimoto et al. 2016]. Astaxanthin also exerts beneficial effects in the brain by crossing the blood-brain barrier and penetrating the brain, eye, and central nervous system, which many antioxidants and even the well investigated carotenoid beta-carotene cannot do [Capelli & Cysewski 2013]. And finally, whether you are trying to kick up your workout routine or give your energy levels a boost at the gym, an extra dose of astaxanthin may also help. Animal studies, for instance, found that astaxanthin supplementation improved swimming endurance in mice [Ikeuchi et al. 2006] and illustrated that astaxanthin was able to help prevent exercise-induced muscle damage [Aoi et al. 2003]. Moreover, a study published some 8 years ago found that astaxanthin improved cycling time trial performance among 21 competitive cyclists [Earnest et al. 2011].

So it would seem that astaxanthin's unique "antioxidative artillery" provides for an impressive array of health benefits! In many ways it appears to be a panacea.

---

56 Diabetic retinopathy is a diabetes complication that affects eyes; it is caused by damage to the blood vessels of the light-sensitive tissue at the back of the eye.

Astaxanthin: a vital component of responsible nutritional supplementation programmes

Diets rich in seafood have long been recommended as a long-term nutritional intervention to preserve overall health and wellbeing. The association between the consumption of fish or seafood and beneficial effects on a variety of health outcomes has often been reported in epidemiologic studies and clinical trials. The recorded health benefits are mainly attributed to the omega-3 long-chain polyunsaturated fatty acids[57], which are abundant in fish and seafood. However, since fish has become a restricted food resource, there is now a growing interest in exploiting alternative sources such as antarctic krill[58]. Also, *in vivo* and clinical investigations using marine carotenoids, and more particularly krill oil, which is rich in astaxanthin, have shown promising results against free radical activity in different diseases [Sati & Bhatt 2018].

Given its truly impressive list of beneficial properties, it is not surprising that astaxanthin is widely used as a neutraceutical, a cosmetic, and even a colouring agent in aquaculture [Han et al. 2013]. Since microalgae can store high contents and are well known to accumulate it under stress conditions, unicellular green microalgae are suitable for the large scale production of astaxanthin (and some other chemical additives). The freshwater algal species *Haematococcus pluvialis* has often been grown because it can accumulate up to 4 % of the substance on a dry weight basis under stress conditions of enhanced salinity, nutrient

---

57 In omega-3 fatty acids the first double bond is between the third and fourth carbon atoms from the tail or methyl ($-CH_3$) end.

58 'Krill' is a general term used to describe about 85 species of free-swimming, open-ocean crustaceans known as euphausiids. Antarctic krill is one of the 85 species of krill that lives in the Southern Ocean. Antarctic krill are one of the most abundant and successful animal species on Earth. Scientists estimate there are about 500 million tonnes of Antarctic krill (*Euphausia superba*) in the Southern Ocean. The biomass of this one species may be the largest of any multi-cellular animal species on the planet. Most of the larger Antarctic animals, including seals, whales, seabirds, fish and squid, depend directly or indirectly on Antarctic krill [http://www.antarctica.gov.au/about-antarctica/wildlife/animals/krill].

deficiency, plant hormone treatment, and/or high light intensity [Ding et al. 2018; Galarza et al. 2018; Ho et al. 2018].

The necessary extraction, analysis, and storage procedures have been well optimized [Ambati et al. 2014; Dong et al. 2015].

Astaxanthin: a gateway to new and unexpected applications

A paper by Arancibia et al. [2014] concludes on a really fascinating note: ... *The incorporation of an astaxanthin-rich protein concentrate in a chitosan solution led to an increase in its antimicrobial capacity...* Packaging biofilms and coatings made from chitosan[59], obtained from the heads and carcasses of crustaceans, and enriched with astaxanthin, extracted from the shells of the same animals, can result in a significant improvement of the food's shelf life by delaying microbial spoilage.

In additional research [Arancibia et al. 2015], an active coating solution composed of chitosan and an astaxanthin-rich shrimp protein-lipid concentrate, both obtained from processing the discarded waste of Pacific white shrimp – *Litopenaeus vannamei*, a variety of prawn found in the eastern Pacific Ocean and commonly caught or farmed for food – was applied to preserving shrimp during chilled storage. The addition of protein-lipid concentrate increased the antioxidant capacity of the coating. It resulted in a lower-viscosity mixture that was still viscous enough to adhere to the shrimp while retaining its antioxidant capacity. Experimental shrimp storage trials have shown that the coatings, especially when enriched with protein-lipid concentrates, significantly delayed microbial growth. Also, the composite chitosan coating was imperceptible from a sensorial point of view and prevented blackspot[60] development.

---

59 Chitosan is a natural polycationic linear polysaccharide derived from chitin, a substance that develops in the hard outer shells of crustaceans such as crab, crayfish, shrimp and squid. Chitosan is recognized as a versatile biomaterial because of its non-toxicity, low allergenicity, biocompatibility and biodegradability [Cheung et al. 2015].

60 Blackspot or melanosis is a harmless, but objectionable discoloration or darkening in shrimp.

The authors of the paper concluded that chitosan and astaxanthin applications show great promise as a means of improving the quality of shrimp during cold storage.

This is quite obviously an important step forward

Finding a replacement for fossil fuel-based plastic food packaging is a matter of great urgency. Food containers and packaging – the majority of which are still made from synthetic polymers – make up a large share of the solid waste stream that clogs our landfills as well as our oceans, where macro and microplastics kill marine life. Furthermore, the chemical ingredients of plastic – most additives are not covalently bound and easily released from the polymer matrix – can be absorbed by fish, and eventually by humans who eat the fish. And like the petrol we put in our cars, synthetic plastic is totally unsustainable; it is made from fossil fuel, which is rapidly running out.

The quality of consumer goods is often associated with freshness, not with care. Long-term use is frequently undesirable, poorly resourceful. Yet humans continue to manufacture, use and dispose. There is however an alternative: the circular economy. It aims at turning goods that are at the end of their service lives into resources for others, closing the loops of industrial systems and minimizing waste. This approach can change the current economic logic because it replaces production with sufficiency: reuse what you can, recycle what cannot be reused, repair what is broken, remanufacture what cannot be repaired [Stahel 2016].

Packaging with shrimp waste is a wonderful idea! Farming shrimp for human consumption and packing it in materials made from discarded processing waste is a perfect example of sustainable approach.

Bibliography

Ambati et al. [2014]. Astaxanthin: Sources, Extraction, Stability, Biological Activities and Its Commercial Applications—A Review, *Marine Drugs* 12, 128-152

Anunciato & da Rocha Filho [2012]. Carotenoids and polyphenols in nutricosmetics, nutraceuticals, and cosmeceuticals, *Journal of Cosmetic Dermatology* 11, 1, 51-54

Aoi et al. [2003]. Astaxanthin limits exercise-induced skeletal and cardiac muscle damage in mice, Antioxidants & Redox Signaling 5, 1, 139-144

Arancibia et al. [2014]. Antimicrobial and antioxidant chitosan solutions enriched with active shrimp (*Litopenaeus vannamei*) waste materials, *Food Hydrocolloids* 35, 710-717

Arancibia et al. [2015]. Chitosan coatings enriched with active shrimp waste for shrimp preservation, *Food Control* 54, 259-266

Biswal [2014]. Oxidative stress and astaxanthin: the novel supernutrient carotenoid, *The International Journal of Health & Allied Sciences* 3, 147-53.

Capelli & Cysewski [2013]. *The World Best Kept Health Secret – Natural Astaxanthin*, Cyanotech Corporation, pp. 198

Cheung et al. [2015]. Chitosan: An Update on Potential Biomedical and Pharmaceutical Applications, *Marine Drugs* 13, 8, 5156-5186

Chew & Park [2004]. Carotenoid Action on the Immune Response, *The Journal of Nutrition* 134, 1, 257S-261S

Ding et al. [2018]. A strategy for boosting astaxanthin accumulation in green microalga *Haematococcus pluvialis* by using combined diethyl aminoethyl hexanoate and high light, *Journal of Applied Phycology* 30, pp. 11

Dhinaut et al. [2017]. A dietary carotenoid reduces immunopathology and enhances longevity through an immune depressive effect in an insect model, *Scientific Reports* 7, 12429, pp. 12

Dong et al. [2014]. Four Different Methods Comparison for Extraction of Astaxanthin from Green Alga *Haematococcus pluvialis*, *The Scientific World Journal*, pp. 7

Earnest et al. [2011]. Effect of astaxanthin on cycling time trial performance, *Sports Medicine* 32, 882-888

Fassett & Coombes [2009]. Astaxanthin, oxidative stress, inflammation and cardiovascular disease, *Future Cardiology* 5, 4, 333-342

Galarza et al. [2018]. Over-accumulation of astaxanthin in Haematococcus
    pluvialis through chloroplast genetic engineering, *Algal Research* 31,
    291-297

Han et al. [2013]. Astaxanthin in microalgae: pathways, functions and
    biotechnological implications, *Algae* 28, 2, 131-147

Ho et al. [2018]. Maximization of Astaxanthin Production from Green
    Microalga Haematococcus pluvialis Using Internally-Illuminated
    Photobioreactor, *Advances in Bioscience and Bioengineering* 6, 2, 10-22

Ikeuchi et al. [2006]. Effects of astaxanthin supplementation on exercise-
    induced fatigue in mice, *Biological and Pharmaceutical Bulletin* 29, 10,
    2106-2110

Kishimoto et al. [2016]. Potential Anti-Atherosclerotic Properties of
    Astaxanthin, *Marine Drugs* 14, 35, pp. 13

Manabe et al. [2008]. Astaxanthin protects mesangial cells from
    hyperglycemia-induced oxidative signaling, *Journal of Cellular
    Biochemistry* 103, 6, 1925-1937

Naguib [2000]. Journal of Agricultural and Food Chemistry 48, 4, 1150-1154

Nishida et al. [2007]. Quenching Activities of Common Hydrophilic and
    Lipophilic Antioxidants against Singlet Oxygen Using Chemiluminescence
    Detection System, *Carotenoid Science* 11, 16-20

Sati & Bhatt [2018]. Krill oil: the most powerful omega-3 known on earth,
    International Journal of Pharmaceutical Sciences and Research 9, 7,
    2693-2699

Stahel [2016]. Circular economy, *Nature* 531, 435-438

Sun et al. [2011]. Protective actions of microalgae against endogenous and
    exogenous advanced glycation endproducts (AGEs) in human retinal
    pigment epithelial cells, *Food and Function* 2, 5, 251-258

Tanaka et al. [2012]. Cancer Chemoprevention by Carotenoids, *Molecules* 17, 3,
    3202-3242

Wakeman [2018]. An open label pilot study to evaluate the effectiveness of
    a proprietary nutraceutical formulation on elements of skin function
    associated with aging, *International Journal of Scientifi Research* 7, 4,
    2277-2278

Yang et al. [2011]. Astaxanthin-Rich Extract from the Green Alga
    Haematococcus pluvialis Lowers Plasma Lipid Concentrations and
    Enhances Antioxidant Defense in Apolipoprotein E Knockout Mice[1-3], *The
    Journal of Nutrition* 141, 9, 1611-1617

Yuan [2011]. Potential health-promoting effects of astaxanthin: A high-value carotenoid mostly from microalgae, *Molecular Nutrition & Food Research* 55, 1, 150-165

Zhang & Wang [2015]. Multiple Mechanisms of Anti-Cancer Effects Exerted by Astaxanthin, *Marine Drugs* 13, 4310-4330

From exceptional delicacy to addiction

The indisputable explosion in sugar consumption cannot be ignored

In September 2011, the United Nations (UN) declared that for the first time in human history chronic non-communicable diseases such as heart disease, cancer, dementia and diabetes pose a greater health burden worldwide than infectious diseases, contributing to ~35 million deaths annually [Lustig et al. 2012]. In every country where people have adopted a diet dominated by low-cost, highly processed food, there have been rising rates of obesity and related diseases. The UN announcement targets tobacco, alcohol and diet as the predominant risk factors in non-communicable diseases.

Everyone knows that people today ingest far too much sugar. The sugar guideline of the World Health Organization (WHO) issued in March 2015 states that adults and children must restrict their sugar intake to less than 10 % of the total energy intake per day, which is the equivalent of ~12.5 teaspoons of sugar for adults, and suggests a further reduction to below 5 % of total energy intake per day [WHO 2015].

Why has the whole situation spiralled out of control? Sugar is the food nobody needs, but everybody craves. Human physiology evolved on a diet containing very little sugar and virtually no refined carbohydrates. It is quite possible that sugar entered our diets by accident. Probably sugarcane was primarily a fodder crop, used to fatten pigs, though humans may have chewed on the stalks from time to time. To bite the fibrous inner flesh, called bagasse, releases a sweet flavour. Crude sugar cane juice is reported to contain a sucrose[61] level between 12 and 15 %.

... The governor's wife died more than 300 years ago in colonial Maryland. Her coffin was made of expensive lead and her wrists were bound with silk ribbons. But one of the most telling signs of Anne Wolseley Calvert's wealth was the condition of her teeth. "She'd lost 20, and several others had decayed down to the root stubs," says Douglas Owsley, the head of physical anthropology at Smithsonian's National Museum of Natural History, whose team analyzed the remains. "One reason her mouth was in such poor condition was that she was affluent enough to afford sugar..." [Rothenberg Gritz 2017]. Today, sugar is accessible to everyone. As a result, there have been many unpleasant consequences. Sugar has become such a widespread commodity that lower-income people are those who now consume the most. Shoppers with no access to fresh produce end up consuming caloric sweeteners in everything they consume, from cereals to pasta sauce, from flavoured coffees to sports drinks.

The unsavoury history of sugar

Evidence from plant remains and DNA suggests that sugarcane was first grown in South East Asia [Denham & Haberle 2008]. Researchers are still trying to find (additional) early evidence of sugarcane cultivation at the Kuk Swamp in Papua New Guinea, where the domestication of related crops such as taro[62] and banana dates back to ~8000 BC [Fullagar et al. 2006]. The crop spread around the Eastern Pacific and Indian Oceans ~3500 years ago, carried by Austronesian and Polynesian seafarers.

The first chemically refined sugar appeared on the scene in India ~2500 years ago. From there, the technique spread east towards China

---

61 Sucrose is a disaccharide, composed of two monosaccharides: glucose (a hexagonal structure) and fructose (a pentagonal structure).

62 Taro (*Colocasia esculenta*) is probably native to southeastern Asia. It became a staple crop, cultivated for its large, starchy, spherical underground tubers, which are consumed as cooked vegetables, made into puddings and breads, and also made into the Polynesian poi, a thin, pasty, highly digestible mass of fermented taro starch [Encyclopaedia Britannica].

and west towards Persia and the early Islamic world, eventually reaching the Mediterranean in the 13th century. Cyprus and Sicily became important centres for sugar production. Throughout the Middle-Ages, sugar was considered a rare and expensive spice, rather than an everyday condiment. The first place to cultivate sugarcane explicitly for large scale refinement and trade was the island of Madeira, during the late 15th century. Then, the Portuguese realised that new and favourable conditions for sugar plantations existed in Brazil, where a slave-based plantation economy was established. The introduction of Brazilian sugarcane in the Caribbean in the 17th century led to the growth of an industry which was to feed the sugar craze of Western Europe.

By the late 16th century, São Tomé, the Portuguese island close to the equator, could not keep up with Brazil's rate of sugar production and started exporting slaves to Brazil and other New World islands to work on sugar plantations. It was a highly profitable business. Brazil out-produced all of the New World colonies as well as the Mediterranean countries. During the 1600s, coffee, tea, and chocolate also made their way to Europe and their arrival drastically increased the European sugar consumption. Increasing demand naturally triggered a greater reliance on slavery. The need for manual labour on the massive sugar plantations in Brazil and the Caribbean was met by the transatlantic slave trade, which resulted in ~12 million human beings being shipped from Africa to the Americas between 1500 and 1900. Mortality rates could reach up to 25 % on each voyage. Between 1 and 2 million dead must have been thrown overboard. In 1807, Thomas Jefferson (1743-1826), who was the principal author of the Declaration of Independence and later served as the third President of the United States (US), signed a bill that prohibited importing slaves to the US. Shortly after, the British House of Lords passed an act for the abolition of the slave trade. But despite these decisions, slavery remained a widespread practice until the end of the 19th century.

Andreas Sigismund Marggraf (1709-1782) discovered that sucrose can also be derived from beets and devised a method using alcohol to extract it [Marggraf 1747]. His student, Franz Carl Achard (1753-1821), later devised an economical industrial method to extract the sugar in its pure form. In 1801, with the support of King Friedrich Wilhelm III, Achard opened the first sugar beet refinery at Gut Kunern near Steinau, Silesia. In 1802, the refinery processed 400 tons of beets with a degree of efficiency of 4 %. Other refineries were soon built by his students. The beet sugar industry thrived in Europe throughout the Napoleonic Wars, though Napoleon was the subject of much ridicule for supporting the industry. When the wars ended, cheap Caribbean sugar was again exported to Europe, which severely damaged the sugar beet business. In 1837, Vilmorin[63], a French seed company, created the sugar beet, which has a high sucrose content and a structure designed for optimal sugar extraction [Gayon & Zallen 1998]. Moreover, slavery died out in the Caribbean, and European governments implemented policies to support their beet growers. With governmental support, the European beet sugar industry substantially expanded throughout the 20th century.

Is there a difference between cane sugar and beet sugar?

White table sugar comes from either cane or beets and is usually sold without its plant source identified. This is because chemically speaking the two products are identical. Refined table sugar is pure, crystallized sucrose. Sucrose is found naturally in honey, dates, and sugar maple sap, but it is most concentrated in sugarcane and sugar beets. The refining process renders the original plant irrelevant: the sucrose is completely extracted from the plant that produced it. However, in order to make sugarcane crystals purely white, they are processed with bone char or bone black. Beet sugar, on the other hand, does not require this step. This distinction is important to many vegans and vegetarians, who seek to minimize animal suffering.

Additionally, many bakers and pastry chefs claim there is a difference between brown sugars made from sugarcane and those made from sugar

---

63 The company Vilmorin has a long history in France, where it was family-controlled for almost two centuries, and which today is as a publicly traded company owned principally by the agro-industrial cooperative Groupe Limagrain, the largest plant breeding and seed company in the European Union.

beets. The molasses[64] that colours brown sugar comes from sugarcane processing; it is not a high-grade product of sugar beets. Brown sugar made from sugar beets has sugarcane molasses added.

In many ways, the story of sugar and tobacco are closely aligned

Both products were initially produced through slave labour. Tobacco became an important crop grown on the slave plantations in the 17th century. The southern states of America such as Virginia were the main areas growing tobacco, with small amounts grown on the Caribbean islands. Both products were also seen to be beneficial to health. In 1526, the Spanish writer Gonzalo Fernandez de Oviedo y Valdes (1478-1557) wrote that the enslaved Africans in the Americas say ... *that if they take tobacco when their day's work is over they forget their fatigue...* This shows that the enslaved Africans who were working on the plantations were also using tobacco. Reverend John Lindsay (1686-1768), a minister of the church in Jamaica, wrote about tobacco: ... *This Plant ... is pretty much planted by the Negroes for the use of the Pipe; to which the Negroes are greatly enslaved. Indeed, they allege that this alone is what makes their other slavery the more tolerable...* He was relaying the slaves' claim that the use of tobacco, which is a drug, made their lives easier to tolerate.

Although both sugar and tobacco have ancient origins, it was their sudden mass consumption from the mid-17th century onwards that created the health hazards and health risks[65] we associate with them today. The idea of "industrial epidemics" of non-communicable diseases being driven by the profit motives of major corporations applies to both. And while tobacco is widely acknowledged to be addictive, sugar can also drive behavioural responses that are indistinguishable from addiction. Before we know what is happening, the sugar addiction has taken hold.

---

64 Molasses are syrups that remain after the sugar is crystallized out of cane or beet juice.

65 A hazard is a potential source of harm or adverse health effect on a person or persons, whereas a risk is the likelihood that a person may be harmed or suffer adverse health effects if exposed to a hazard.

The sweet cravings will never leave you. A biscuit here, a sweetened drink there … we will not become obese overnight or rapidly develop a heart disease or lose bone density. Sugar addiction will produce its harmful effects only gradually, day after day, after day.

The forbidden fruit

In the 1970s, tobacco representatives told teens that smoking was not for young people. Smoking was like driving a car, drinking alcohol and having sex. So, why hinder the sale of "adult stimulants"? Young people grow up anyway and become adults. A very subtle form of advertising! Nobody smokes to look young. And young people want what is inaccessible to them, especially if it is strictly for adults. Teenagers do not like to be treated like children. This is something the tobacco companies obviously understood very well! Cigarette smoking has become a gargantuan reality: every year ~6000 trillion cigarettes are lit up, that is ~700 million per hour. We can understand why the tobacco industry will never do anything that might kill the goose that lays the golden eggs! Tragically, however, those smoking cigarettes are poisoning human lungs with tens of thoudands of tons of tar.

The tobacco industry is well known for having repeatedly refused to admit the dangers of smoking. It is infuriating to see how the industry targets teenagers and young adults, chemically manipulates nicotine and organizes fraud. The tobacco industry is a diabolical machine operated by institutions that are capable of infiltrating culture and science, subverting medicine and corrupting minds on a large scale. The famous internal memo *Doubt is our product* says much about Big Tobacco's approach and objectives [Proctor 2012].

Fear, uncertainty and doubt (FUD) is a strategy that has been widely used for a good half-century especially in sales and marketing, but also in public relations and even in political discourse. And tobacco companies have become masters in applying this strategy. All too often, policy makers bypass major problems rather than to confront them and prefer to address challenges separately rather than holistically. The FUD technique tries to influence others by spreading negative, often vague information or tries to inspire fear. It is painful to see how the chemical industry also makes frequent use of FUD in the production, processing, packaging and distribution as well as in the retailing and consumption of foodstuffs.

Tooth enemies

Here is a striking though little-known fact: Cristin Kearns, a researcher at the University of California in San Francisco, and her team dug through the archives of the sugar industry to discover another smoking gun. With the help of the man who "slaughtered" Big Tobacco, she arrived at the conclusion that Big Sugar intentionally prevented scientists from assessing the harmful effects of sugar ingredients [Kearns et al. 2015 & 2017].

The (American) sugar industry, unable to deny the role of sucrose in tooth decay, adopted a FUD strategy to pre-empt actions intended to reduce the negative effects of sugar consumption. This included, for example, the funding of research in close collaboration with the friendly and allied food industry on enzymes capable of breaking down dental plaque. There were moreover regular meetings with the National Institute of Dental Research (NIDR) management, and a report was also submitted to NIDR to serve as a basis for submitting projects for the National Caries Program. Any research that could possibly have harmed the interests of the sugar industry was omitted from the priorities. Not surprisingly, ~78 % of the sugar industry's submissions were incorporated into the NIDR call.

John Hickson, Vice President and Director of Research at the Sugar Research Foundation, made it very clear that several research results raised a number of questions: ... *Many labs of varying reputations state that sugar is a less desirable food source of calories than other carbohydrates, e.g. Yudkin...* Yudkin [1964] concluded that sugar consumption can be directly related to ischemic heart disease, whereas fat is only indirectly related. There is no doubt that Big Tobacco's FUD approach was an excellent source of inspiration. It is probably no coincidence that several hundred compounds, including sugars, are added to the tobacco to make the smoke less irritating and therefore more inhalable. Modifying tobacco to make smokers as addicted as possible: a cleverly concocted but highly unscrupulous approach!

Deceptive non-disclosure was yet another aspect of the strategy implemented by the sugar industry. It did not disclose evidence of damage revealed by laboratory investigations on animals. These results could have shown that the risk of coronary heart disease due to sucrose consumption exceeds that of starch consumption. In addition, it did not report the adverse results with respect to the association between dietary sugars and cancer, which could have led to further investigations of the carcinogenic character of sucrose [Kearns et al. 2017]. It is clear that the sugar industry has strongly reduced or even masked the existence of a link between the consumption of added carbohydrates and multiple health problems.

Why is obesity such a problem?

For the first time in history, more people are suffering from obesity than from starvation worldwide. According to the WHO, ~2.3 billion adults were overweight, and more than 700 million people obese in 2015. The number of obese persons increased considerably over the last decade and in all likelihood, there will be little or no change in the near future.

Today, no country is immune to this widespread health epidemic. Overweight and obesity[66] are major health issues in both the developed and the developing world. Clinically, obesity is an excess body fat accumulation that is detrimental to overall health [Ogden et al. 2007]. It is the result of a prolonged disproportion in the energy balance, with energy intake largely exceeding energy expenditure.

Weight gain is caused by various factors, including inherited biological traits, early life experiences, and behavioural, environmental and social factors that influence individual behaviour. Results from the Quebec family investigation have shown that high dietary restraint,

---

66 Overweight and obesity are defined by body mass index (BMI) measurements: BMI ≥25 means overweight, and ≥30 means obesity [Mei et al. 2002].

high disinhibition and susceptibility to hunger behaviours, in addition to short sleep duration, are all associated with excess adiposity[67] and/or obesity [Chaput et al. 2014]. People's energy intake has increased through the ready availability and low cost of energy dense, nutrient-poor food products and beverages, especially cereal-based foods such as cakes, biscuits, pies, pizza, etc. as well as confectionery and sugar-sweetened drinks. The omnipresence of cues promoting the intake of palatable food, coupled with the rewarding aspects of these heavily processed foods increases the motivation to eat to excess. Stress also affects food choice. People may increase the amount of high-fat and high-sugar food consumed in response to a stressor, making stress a risk factor for the development of obesity in vulnerable individuals.

In the 21st century, obesity should not only be viewed as a metabolic disorder, but rather as a multifactorial disease. Thus, strategies that focus on modulation of the reward system, reduction of stress reactivity and reverse compromised hippocampal function may be more effective than the currently available pharmacological approaches typically targeting appetite suppression. Overall, understanding the factors that increase the vulnerability of individuals to develop obesity is essential in developing more effective treatments [Morris et al. 2015].

And it goes without saying that providing education and support to individuals and populations within a strategy for promoting healthy food intake and appropriate physical activity are of critical importance in the prevention of obesity as well [Morris et al. 2015].

---

67 Adiposity: a condition of being severely overweight, or obese. The term "obesity" more frequently is used for this condition in the U.S. where obesity is usually defined by measuring a person's body mass index (BMI). There also is a measurement of body fat used by some researchers known as the body adiposity index (BAI). Unlike the BMI, weight is not taken to account in the BAI, which is based on a person's height and hip circumference.

Bibliography

Chaput et al. 2014. Findings from the Quebec family study on the etiology of obesity: genetics and environmental highlights, *Current Obesity Reports* 3, 54-66

Denham & Haberle [2008]. Agricultural emergence and transformation in the Upper Wahgi valley, Papua New Guinea, during the Holocene: theory, method and practice, *The Holocene* 18, 3, 481-496

Fullagar et al. [2006]. Early and mid Holocene tool-use and processing of taro (Colocasia esculenta), yam (Dioscorea sp.) and other plants at Kuk Swamp in the highlands of Papua New Guinea, *Journal of Archaeological Science* 33, 595-614

Gayon & Zallen [1998]. The Role of the Vilmorin Company in the Promotion and Diffusion of the Experimental Science of Heredity in France, 1840-1920, *Journal of the History of Biology* 31, 241-262

Kearns et al. [2015], Sugar Industry Influence on the Scientific Agenda of the National Institute of Dental Research's 1971 National Caries Program: A Historical Analysis of Internal Documents, *PLOS Medecine* 12, 3, pp. 22

Kearns et al. [2017], Sugar industry sponsorship of germ-free rodent studies linking sucrose to hyperlipidemia and cancer: An historical analysis of internal documents, *PLOS Biology* 15, 11, pp. 9

Lustig et al. [2012]. The toxic truth about sugar, *Nature* 482, 27-29

Marggraf [1747]. Experiences chimiques faites dans le dessein de tirer un veritable sucre de diverses plantes, qui croissent dans nos contrées» (Chemical experiments made with the intention of extracting real sugar from diverse plants that grow in our lands), *Histoire de l'académie royale des sciences et belles-lettres de Berlin*, 79-90

Mei et al. [2002]. Validity of body mass index compared with other body-composition screening indexes for the assessment of body fatness in children and adolescents, *The American Journal of Clinical Nutrition* 75, 978-985

Morris et al. [2015]. Why is obesity such a problem in the 21st century? The intersection of palatable food, cues and reward pathways, stress, and cognition, *Neuroscience & Biobehavioral Reviews* 58, 36-45

Ogden et al. [2007]. The epidemiology of obesity, *Gastroenterology* 132, 2087-2102

Proctor [2012]. *Golden Holocaust, Origins of the Cigarette Catastrophe and the case for Abolition*, University of California Press, Berkeley, California, pp. 774

Rothenberg Gritz [2017]. The Unsavory History of Sugar, the Insatiable American Craving, *Smithsonian magazine*, https://www.smithsonianmag.com/history/unsavory-history-sugar-american-craving-180962766/

WHO [2015]. *Guideline: Sugars intake for adults and children*, Geneva: World Health Organization, pp. 59

Yudkin [1964], Dietary fat and dietary sugar in relation to ischaemic heart-disease and diabetes, *The Lancet 2*, 4-5

Be ambitious, cut resource use, reduce waste and boost recycling!

Looking for a better relationship with our goods

Quality is all too often associated with newness, not with caring; long-term use is all too frequently undesirable, poorly resourceful. Yet, humans continue to make, use, and dispose. There is a valuable alternative though, i.e. the structural change from a linear (waste-based) economy to a circular (reuse) one [Ellen MacArthur Foundation 2003]. It aims at turning goods that are at the end of their service lives into resources for others, closing the loops of industrial systems and minimizing the generation of waste. This approach can change the current economic logic because it replaces production with sufficiency: reuse what you can, recycle what cannot be reused, repair what is broken, remanufacture what cannot be repaired [Stahel 2016]. Circular economy business models fall into two groups: one that fosters reuse and extends service life through repair, remanufacture, and upgrades and another that turns old goods into new resources by recycling the materials.

When it comes to circular economy, some people tend to think about nothing else than recycling materials. Yet, circular economy is much more than that. It is thinking beforehand of ways of maintaining the value of the product prior to recycling or recovering the materials. It is looking at options to recover the materials used in a product; recycling must be easy to achieve, without needing to expend when the products reach their end of their useful lives. Moreover, the products should be easy to break down and separate.

Since 2010, the Ellen MacArthur Foundation has been promoting this idea among academics, industry entrepreneurs and policymakers. A circular economy is restorative or regenerative by intention and design. It replaces the end-of-life concept with restoration, shifts towards the use of renewable energy, eliminates the use of toxic chemicals which impair reuse, and strives to eliminate waste through the superior design of materials, products, systems, as well as business models.

Such an economy is based on few simple principles. First of all, a circular economy aims to "design out" waste. Products are designed and optimised for a cycle of disassembly and reuse. This defines the circular economy and sets it apart from disposal and even recycling, whereby large amounts of embedded energy and labour are lost. Secondly, circularity introduces a strict differentiation between the consumable and durable components of a product. Unlike today, consumables in the circular economy will largely be made of biological ingredients or "nutrients" that are at least non-toxic and preferably even beneficial and can be safely returned to our biosphere. Durables[68] such as engines, computers, appliances, furniture, jewelry, consumer electronics, sporting goods, etc. are made of technical nutrients such as metals and many plastics that are unsuitable for the biosphere. These particular nutrients are designed from the start for reuse. Thirdly, the energy required to fuel this cycle should be renewable by nature, again to decrease resource dependence and increase system resilience [Ellen MacArthur Foundation 2013; Ghisellini et al. 2016; Rau & Oberhuber 2016; Ledsome et al. 2018; Wachs & Singh 2018]. We definitely need to be more proactive on the end-of-life question and its overall implications, and on how this relates to the management of the design process.

---

68 Durables are a category of consumer products that do not have to be purchased frequently because they are made to last a long time; they are also called durable goods or consumer durables [Merriam Webster].

It is well recognized fact that the markets for food and beverage packaging are large

Recycling food packaging waste into new food packaging presents unprecedented challenges, especially with regard to safety issues. The use of recycled food packaging not only increases the possible sources of contamination, but often also the numbers and levels of contaminants that can migrate[69] from the packaging into the packed foods and beverages. Migration potentially has adverse public health effects [Pivnenko et al. 2016; Muncke et al. 2017]. This also explains why governements are increasingly prepared to invest in monitoring.

The regulation for food packaging in Europe and the United States (US) requires the same level of safety for chemicals migrating into foods for all recycled and virgin materials alike [Muncke et al. 2017]. In the European Union (EU), the use of recycled plastics in food contact materials (FCM) is specifically regulated under the Commission Regulation (EC) N° 282/2008 on recycled plastic materials and articles intended to come into contact with foods. The US Food and Drug Administration considers recycling processes for plastic food contact articles on a case-by-case basis and invites recyclers of plastic to submit information on their processes for evaluation and comment. In the US, the use of recycled paper and board is regulated under 21 CFR 176.260 according to which waste paper shall not contain any poisonous or deleterious substance that is retained in the recovered pulp and migrates into packed food, except those specifically regulated under 21 USC 346 and 21 USC 348. In Europe, there is still no harmonized regulation for (recycled) paper and board FCM [Simoneau et al. 2016]. Some EU member states have introduced specific measures however and Switzerland has banned the use of recycled paper and board in direct contact with food.

---

69 The mass transfer of chemical contaminants from food packaging and contact materials into food is called migration; according to some scientists, contact materials are an underestimated source of chemical food contamination [https://www.foodpackagingforum.org/food-packaging-health/migration].

Paper and board have long been recovered and recycled into new fibre-based products

For successful recycling, separate collection systems for paper and board have been established to prevent contamination by food waste, for example. The production of recycled paper and board is comparable to the process for virgin fibres but requires additional steps. After separating the recovered paper and board into well-defined technical grades, they are mixed with water to produce a pulp. Next, non-fibrous parts such as staples, textiles, and tape are removed. Subsequently, the pulp is ground in a disperser, water is removed in drum filters or screw extractors, and the fibres are cleaned by chemical, thermal and/ or mechanical treatments. Optionally, bleaching and de-inking may be applied to enhance the appearance of the final product. The entangled fibres are then mixed with fresh fibres to achieve the required quality and processed on a paper (board) machine producing the final material [Geueke et al. 2018].

Chemical contaminants in waste paper [Van Bossuyt et al. 2016; Geueke et al. 2018] can include additives such as fillers, retention aids, sizing agents, coatings, biocides, and synthetic binders. Furthermore, since paper is commonly printed, dyed, glued, and labelled, printing inks, adhesives, photo-initiators, solvents, plasticizers, surfactants, and pigments are frequently detected in the waste paper. Contaminants may also be introduced during use and/or waste management, because paper and board are prone to absorbing chemicals. Geueke et al. [2018] emphasize the possible presence of 7 alarming chemical contaminant types that require our full attention: mineral oil hydrocarbons (MOH), bisphenols, phthalates, naphthalenes, photoinitiators, inorganic elements, and a few relatively rare substances such as 2-phenylphenol and phenantrene.

Nowadays, MOH contamination in food packaged with recycled paper and board receive plenty of attention and for that reason the entire next chapter "How to avoid mineral oil from getting into packaged food?" is devoted to the phenomenon of MOH migration into packed food.

Food contamination deserves all of our attention

Whatever we might think, the economy – whether linear or circular – should never pose public health risks. Known to have contaminated our packed foods for over 20 years [Droz & Grob 1997], MOH are now receiving a great deal of attention. Particular emphasis has been put on understanding and monitoring the migration of MOH from recycled paper and board. MOH generally consist of highly complex mixtures of mineral oil saturated hydrocarbons (MOSH) and mineral oil aromatic hydrocarbons (MOAH). In the absence of a functional barrier, MOH from printing inks and recycled fibres tend to migrate from the paper-based food packaging material through the gas phase into the dry food. The concentrations easily exceed the migration limit of 0.6 mg per kg food [Lorenzini et al. 2010] that is derived from the acceptable daily intake provided by the Joint FAO/WHO Expert Committee on Food Additives[70]. It was found that the maximum concentrations of MOSH in the packaging material could potentially contaminate the packed food at levels exceeding the migration limit by a factor of 100 and more [Lorenzini et al. 2010]. The recycling of newspapers printed with mineral oil based inks has been identified as the most significant source of MOH, but adhesives, waxes, processing aids, environmental as well as yet unidentified sources may further add to MOH contaminations in recycled paper and board [Biedermann & Grob 2012].

The finding that bisphenols are constantly and ubiquitously spread [Huang et al. 2018; Pahigian & Zuo 2018] through paper recycling has been supported by several studies showing their presence in waste paper as well as in recycled paper and board [Liao & Kannan 2011; Suciu et al. 2013; Goeyens 2014]. For example, an analysis of 15 types of paper from different fractions of household waste detected bisphenol A (BPA) and its structurally similar alternative bisphenol S in 100 and

---

70 JECFA is an international scientific expert committee administered jointly by the Food and Agriculture Organization of the United Nations (FAO) and WHO; it has been meeting since 1956, to evaluate the safety of food additives, contaminants, naturally occurring toxicants and residues of veterinary drugs in food [https://www.who.int/foodsafety/areas_work/chemical-risks/jecfa/en/].

73 % of the samples, respectively [Pivnenko et al. 2015]. BPA (and other bisphenols) possess oestrogenic, anti-androgenic, inflammatory and oxidative properties. Moreover, since bone responds to changes in sex hormones, inflammatory and oxidative status, BPA exposure can also adversely affect bone health in humans [Chin et al. 2018]. Unfortunately, everybody is exposed to BPA and its alternatives. We must remain on our guard: bisphenols are not harmless chemicals; they may cause many discomforts and illnesses [Rochester 2013; Huang et al. 2018].

Phthalates are a large group of chemicals used to soften and increase the flexibility of plastic and vinyl, but they are also used in many consumer products, including e.g. cosmetics and personal care products, plastic and vinyl toys, etc. Phthalates of all types have commonly been measured in food packaging from recycled paper and board. Typical sources in the recycled paper pulp are inks, lacquers and adhesives [Fierens et al. 2012] and they have quite often been identified and quantified in paper and board waste as well as in recycled paper. Their migration contributes significantly to the phthalate occurrence in packed food [Pivnenko et al. 2016; Geueke & Muncke 2017]. Phthalates potentially disrupt the hormonal pathways, which can lead to an association with birth defects in males, increased insulin resistance and obesity, decreased neurological development and associations with some cancers [Holland 2018].

In 1994, the migration of six diisopropylnaphthalenes (DIPN) isomers from recycled paper and board packaging was reported for the first time [Sturaro et al. 1994]. These last few years, further studies have demonstrated that DIPN migration from recycled paper and board packaging is still common [Sturaro et al. 2006; Lorenzini et al. 2013]. Mixtures of DIPN are applied as solvents in carbonless copy paper, substituting the previously used polychlorinated biphenyls [Barp et al. 2015]. Based on the results of animal studies, the U.S. Department of Health and Human Services concluded that naphthalene can reasonably be assumed to be a human carcinogen. The International Agency for Research on Cancer (IARC) concluded that naphthalene is possibly carcinogenic to humans, because there is enough evidence that naphthalene causes cancer in animals, but not enough evidence about such an effect in humans. The overall IARC evaluation is as follows: naphthalene is possibly carcinogenic to humans (Group 2B). Under the Environmental Protection Agency 1986 cancer guidelines, naphthalene was assigned to Group C, the group of possible human carcinogens.

The use of polymeric multifunctional photo-initiators is considered as a high quality solution for ultraviolet curing inks and varnishes for printing food packaging. They are characterized by higher molecular weight, fewer and lower volatility photodecomposition by-products, and a higher probability than conventional photo-initiators of being chemically bound into the cured polymer matrix. They are intended to disappear during the chemical reaction that dries the inks. However, residual levels often remain in the ink because of incomplete reaction. The migration of more than 20 different photo-initiator residues from food packaging has been reported by Aparicio and Elizalde [2015]. Of these, benzophenone and 4-methylbenzophenone have been identified most frequently in recycled paper and board [Vápenka et al. 2016]. Moreover, it was demonstrated that several of these photo-initiators react as endocrine disruptors [Peynenburg et al. 2010; Reitsma et al. 2013].

Paints and pigments have been identified as main sources of the inorganic contaminants in paper and board. Food packaging made from fresh fibres contained lower concentrations of aluminium, copper, molybdenum, barium, and lead than recycled paper and board [BMELV 2012]. Heavy metals such as lead, cadmium, zinc, and copper were present in recycled corrugated cardboard samples from the Turkish market [Mertoglu-Elmas 2017].

We need to urgently tackle the terrible ecological crisis

We have almost become used to seeing pictures of hurricanes, typhoons, devastating floods and severe droughts on our television screens. Last summer, the average temperature measured by the Royal Meteorological Institute in Brussels broke all previous records. We experienced the hottest summer since temperatures were first measured in 1901. Even so, the highly unusual climatic conditions tend to quickly recede into the background of our busy, superficial media world and soon, we stop thinking about them.

Extracting, making, using, and disposing generate a gigantic waste of raw materials and cause the loss of ecosystems, of biodiversity and the climate crisis we are experiencing today. Humanity now finds itself in a perilous situation. The system threatens people as well as most other living creatures on this planet. And we cannot repair this system through small-scale interventions and improvements. We need to fundamentally change the economy. We must realize that property goes together with responsibility. Today we are forced to own all kinds of items for which we cannot assume long-term responsibility. We cannot take care of all the raw materials that have been processed into our consumables. And what is more, we certainly are not able to reuse them. In fact, we do not even know which materials or chemicals have been used in the process, and neither are we familiar with their properties. The only solution is a circular economy approach.

Circular economy is a trilogy. Waste should become a starting material; consumables should be non-toxic and possibly even beneficial, whereas durables should be reused, recycled or re-manufactered; and energy sources should be sustainable, renewable by nature. This also applies to packaging and packaging materials. More than ever before we need quality packaging for food. Food packaging – much of it is single-use food wrapping – has created a tremendous waste problem that has now polluted almost every part of the world.

Both the manufacturers and the consumers have got us into this mess and it is now up to us to dig ourselves out of it! Merging ecology and economy is the only way of ensuring the success of circular economy.

Bibliography

Aparicio and Elizalde [2015]. Migration of Photoinitiators in Food Packaging: A Review, *Packaging Technology and Science* 28, 181-203

Barp et al [2015]. Migration of selected hydrocarbon contaminants into dry pasta packaged in direct contact with recycled paperboard, *Food Additives and Contaminants A* 32, 2, 271-283

Biedermann & Grob [2012]. On-line coupled high performance liquid chromatographyegas chromatography for the analysis of contamination by mineral oil. Part 2: migration from paperboard into dry foods: interpretation of chromatograms. *Journal of Chromatography A* 1255, 76-99

BMELV [2012]. Ausmaß der Migration unerwünschter Stoffe aus Verpackungsmaterialien aus Altpapier in Lebensmitteln, https://www.chm.tu-dresden

Droz & Grob [1997]. Determination of food contamination by mineral oil material from printed cardboard using on-line coupled LC-GC-FID, *Zeitschrift für Lebensmitteluntersuchung und -Forschung A* 205, 239-241

Chin et al. [2018]. A Review on the Effects of Bisphenol A and Its Derivatives on Skeletal Health, *International Journal of Medical Sciences* 15, 10, 1043-1050

Ellen MacArthur Foundation [2013]. *Towards the Circular Economy - Economic and business rationale for an accelerated transition*, pp. 99

Fierens et al. [2012]. Analysis of phthalates in food products and packaging materials sold on the Belgian market, *Food and Chemical Toxicology* 50, 7, 2575-2583

Geueke & Muncke [2017]. Substances of Very High Concern in food contact materials: migration and regulatory background, *Packaging Technology and Science*, DOI: 10.1002/pts.2288, pp. 13

Geueke et al. [2018]. Food packaging in the circular economy: Overview of chemical safety aspects for commonly used materials, *Journal of Cleaner Production* 193, 491-505

Ghisellini et al. [2016]. A review on circular economy: the expected transition to a balanced interplay of environmental and economic systems, *Journal of Cleaner Production* 114, 11-32

Goeyens [2014]. *Food and Packaging: a chemical spark*, ACCO, Leuven, pp. 147

Holland [2018]. Socio-economic assessment of phthalates, *OECD Environment Working Papers* 133, pp. 91

Huang et al. [2018]. Bisphenol A concentrations in human urine, human intakes across six continents, and annual trends of average intakes in adult and child populations worldwide: A thorough literature review, *Science of the Total Environment* 626, 971-981

Liao & Kannan [2011]. Widespread occurrence of bisphenol A in paper and paper products: implications for human exposure, *Environmental Science and Technology* 45, 21, 9372-9379

Ledsome et al. [2018]. Designing products for multiple lives, in *DS 93: Proceedings of the 20th International Conference on Engineering and Product Design Education*, Dyson School of Engineering, Imperial College, London, 616-621

Lorenzini et al. [2010]. Saturated and aromatic mineral oil hydrocarbons from paperboard food packaging: estimation of long-term migration from contents in the paperboard and data on boxes from the market, *Food Additives and Contaminants A* 27, 12, 1765-1774

Lorenzini et al. [2013]. Migration kinetics of mineral oil hydrocarbons from recycled paperboard to dry food: monitoring of two real cases, *Food Additives and Contaminants A* 30, 4, 760-770

Mertoglu-Elmas [2017]. The effect of colorants on the content of heavy metals in recycled corrugated board papers, *Bioresources* 12, 2, 2690-2698

Muncke et al. [2017]. Scientific Challenges in the Risk Assessment of Food Contact Materials, *Environmental Health Perspectives* 125, 9, 095001

Pahigian & Zuo [2018]. Occurrence, endocrine-related bioeffects and fate of bisphenol A chemical degradation intermediates and impurities: A review, *Chemosphere* 207, 469-480

Peynenburg et al. [2010]. AhR-agonistic, anti-androgenic, and anti-estrogenic potencies of 2-isopropylthioxanthone (ITX) as determined by in vitro bioassays and gene expression profiling, Toxicology in Vitro 24, 1619-1628

Pivnenko et al. [2015]. Waste paper for recycling: Overview and identification of potentially critical substances, *Waste Management* 45, 134-142

Pivnenko et al. [2016]. Quantification of chemical contaminants in the paper and board fractions of municipal solid waste, *Waste Management* 51, 43-54

Rau & Oberhuber [2016]. *Material Matters*, Bertram + de Leeuw Uitgevers, pp. 220

Reitsma et al. [2013]. Endocrine-Disrupting Effects of Thioxanthone Photoinitiators, *Toxicological Sciences* 132, 1, 64-74

Rochester [2013]. Bisphenol A and human health: A review of the literature, *Reproductive Toxicology* 42, 132-155

Simoneau et al. [2016]. *Non-harmonised Food Contact Materials in the EU: Regulatory and Market Situation*, EUR 28357 EN; doi:10.2788/234276

Stahel [2016]. Circular economy, *Nature* 531, 435-438

Sturaro et al. [1994]. Food contamination by diisopropylnaphthalenes from cardboard packages. Int. *Journal of Food Science and Technology* 29, 5, 593-603

Sturaro et al. [2006]. Contamination of dry foods with trimethyldiphenylmethanes by migration from recycled paper and board packaging, *Food Additives and Contaminants* 23, 4, 431-436

Suciu et al. [2013]. Recycled paper–paperboard for food contact materials: Contaminants suspected and migration into foods and food simulant, *Food Chemistry* 141, 4146-4151

Van Bossuyt et al. [2016]. Printed paper and board food contact materials as a potential source of food contamination, *Regulatory Toxicology and Pharmacology* 81, 10-19

Vápenka et al. [2016]. Contaminants in the paper-based food packaging materials used in the Czech Republic, *Journal of Food and Nutrition Research* 55, 4, 361-373

Wachs & Singh [2018]. A modular bottom-up approach for constructing physical input–output tables (PIOTs) based on process engineering models, *Journal of Economic Structures* 7, 1, pp. 26

How to avoid mineral oil from getting into packaged food?

What is the problem?

Mineral oil hydrocarbons (MOH) comprise a highly complex and diverse group of hydrocarbon mixtures containing thousands of chemical compounds of different molecular structure and size. They are mainly derived from crude oil, but are also synthetically produced from coal, natural gas and biomass. The chemical composition of most MOH mixtures is unknown; moreover, it seemingly varies from one batch to the other [EFSA, https://www.efsa.europa.eu/]. MOH can be intentionally added to foods after they have been refined, but they can also end up in food as contaminants. Contaminating MOH volatilise from the atmosphere, ocean environments, machinery used in food production and processing, as well as from food packaging and food contact materials [van de Ven et al. 2017] to be transferred to food products.

Rice, pasta, cereals, chocolate, etc.: many everyday food items can be contaminated with harmful MOH. Despite ubiquitous and frequent exposures little is known about the potential toxicological effects, particularly with regard to the aromatic[71] mineral oil fractions. Tarnow et al. [2016] tested mineral oils with various aromatic hydrocarbon contents using a battery of in vitro assays to address various hormonal (endocrine)

---

71 In organic chemistry, the term aromaticity is used to describe a cyclic or ring-shaped planar molecule with a ring of resonance bonds that exhibits more stability than other geometric or connective arrangements with the same set of atoms.

endpoints. In addition, these scientists also applied the comet assay[72] to test for genotoxicity[73]. Out of 15 mineral oils tested, 10 were found to potentially act as xenoestrogens[74]. For most of the oils, endocrine effects were triggered by constituents of the aromatic hydrocarbon fraction. Of 5 oils tested in the comet assay, 2 showed slight genotoxicity. Altogether it appears that mineral oils – e.g. the ones used in printing inks – are potential endocrine disruptors. It is therefore important to carefully assess the extent to which mineral oils possibly contribute to the total estrogenic burden in humans.

Currently, MOH are primarily separated into mineral oil saturated hydrocarbons (MOSH) and mineral oil aromatic hydrocarbons (MOAH), because their toxicological end points are different [Biedermann et al. 2009; Grob 2018a]. But even though the problem has been well known since the 1980s, the European Union (EU) has still to adopt regulations to prevent mineral oil contamination in foods.

So, why is it so difficult to set threshold values that may not be exceeded?

Some 30 to 40 years ago "white" or "well-purified" mineral oil was seen as suitable for nutritional use, meaning it could safely be consumed. White oils are largely (but not completely) free of MOAH. There is, however, little justification for the edibility of mineral oil. On the contrary, frequent granuloma[75] formation in human tissues has been ascribed to mineral oil [Dincsoy et al. 1982; Grob 2018b]. Since then, efforts have been undertaken to set acceptable daily intake values. Often

---

72 The comet assay (single-cell gel electrophoresis) is a simple method for measuring deoxyribonucleic acid (DNA) strand breaks in eukaryotic cells [Collins 2004].

73 Genotoxicity is defined as a destructive effect on a cell's genetic material (DNA, RNA) affecting its integrity [Shah 2012].

74 Xenoestrogens are defined as chemicals that mimic some structural parts of the physiological oestrogen compounds, therefore may act as oestrogens or could interfere with the actions of endogenous oestrogens [Słomczyńska 2008].

75 A granuloma is one of a number of forms of localized nodular inflammation found in tissues.

however the evaluations have been questioned [Grob 2018b]. The latest results emphasize that a far-reaching revision of the regulations is long overdue [Barp et al. 2017a & 2017b]. Independently of the conflicting scientific evaluations, there was also a change in public perception as white mineral oil became to be perceived no longer as a food-grade component, but as a contaminant of high concern.

Today the blame is often put on food packaging materials and more particularly, on recycled paper and board. The earliest findings however received little attention [Goeyens 2014]. Hazardous MOSH contaminations occurring in powdered baby milk and other dry foods packaged in cardboard boxes for several weeks were observed: the hydrocarbons contaminated the food at concentration levels between 10 and 150 mg per kg. The inks used for printing paper and cardboard are dispersions of synthetic organic pigments in a bonding agent system consisting essentially of resins, vegetable oils and high-boiling-point mineral oil products. The proportion of mineral oil material in the inks varies between 20 and 30 %. The more volatile mineral oil components slowly evaporate from the printed cardboard box and migrate into the food product. These observations date back as far as 22 years. They were published by Swiss scientists of the Official Food Control Authority of the Canton of Zurich [Droz & Grob 1997].

These and numerous recent measurement results [Grob 2018b, and references herein] raise serious concern among consumers, manufacturers and scientists. It is quite clear that new protective measures should have been taken sooner. In January 2017, however, the European Commission adopted Recommendation (EU) 2017/84 on the monitoring of MOH in food, and in materials and articles intended to come into contact with food. This non-binding recommendation comes after a petition by the non-profit organization Foodwatch[76] that called to act on MOH in food. It urges EU Member States to monitor MOH in many types of food and in food contact materials used to package food items.

---

76 Foodwatch is a non-profit campaigning organization that fights for safe, healthy and affordable food for all people [https://www.foodwatch.org/en/homepage/].

There are many different expected and/or unexpected contamination sources

Both jute and sisal bags are made of fibres that must be treated with a batching oil to improve spinning. These fibres are treated with some 5 to 7 % oil of which roughly half evaporates during subsequent airing to prevent a noticeable packed food off-flavour. Typically, bags of ~1.5 kg are used for packing 50 kg of food, which corresponds to ~45 g of oil in contact with the food. A hypothetical total MOH transfer would result in concentrations of ~900 mg per kg food. Merely one third of the MOH however volatilises to be transferred to the foods [Grob 2018b]: concentrations in hazelnuts for example mostly range between 10 and 50 mg per kg with a few outliers as high as ~500 mg per kg. Batching oil treatments of packaging bags can quite unexpectedly give rise to substantial MOH contaminations of foods such as hazelnuts, rice, cocoa, coffee and many other dry food products.

Commission Regulation (EU) No 10/2011 on plastic materials and articles intended to come into contact with food authorises the use of white mineral oils and waxes specified by an elevated molecular mass without a specific migration limit. In other words, only the overall migration limit of 10 mg per dm^2 food contact surface applies [Grob 2018b]. Nonetheless, several cases of MOH migration/contamination have been reported in the past. Castle et al. [1991] determined migration of MOH from polystyrene cups and beakers into beverages. Jickells et al. [1995] found low migration from cork lubricated with mineral hydrocarbons into wine as well as from paper jam cover discs. There are but few data on MOSH migration from polyolefins containing white mineral oil as an additive[77]. Migration into powdered formula for baby bottles was found to amount to ~5 mg per kg [Biedermann-Brem et al. 2012] and this demonstrated that the migration of virtually non-volatile

---

77 Additives play an important role both in the processability of plastic materials as well as in their applications; the incorporation of additives makes polymer materials suitable for multiple applications in the plastic market [Ambrogi et al. 2017].

substances into dry food may be significant when food particles are small [Eicher et al. 2015].

Today, it is recognized that recycled paperboard contains MOH [Biedermann & Grob 2010], largely from the printing inks (e.g. on newspapers and magazines). EU authorities face a dilemma. On the one hand, the recycling of paper and board is highly recommended for the sustainable use of materials to avoid or end imminent resource depletion. This is indeed provided for in the European Parliament and Council Directive 94/62/EC on packaging and packaging waste. On the other hand, it should never be accepted that the migration from recycled board exceeds by a factor of ~100 the level considered safe by the present official toxicological evaluation. Available MOH release results [Lorenzini et al. 2010, Vollmer et al. 2010; Biedermann et al. 2013, Lorenzini et al. 2013; Barp et al. 2015] seriously discredit the use of paperboard made from recycled fibres in food packaging if no suitable precautions to prevent migration are taken.

The largest amounts of recycled fibres are used in transport boxes. They not only contaminate foods in paperboard folding boxes, but also those in paper or plastic bags [Grob 2018b]. It was shown for pasta and rice that migration from transport boxes through plastic films and boxes of virgin fibre board was substantial. There were also some particular cases where pralines and chocolate candies registered contamination levels of ~30 mg MOH per kg.

Apart from food packaging, several other sources can lead to food contamination

Additives, processing aids and other food ingredients also contribute to the MOSH contaminations. The use of release agents in bakery ware and sugar products as well as the use of oils for the surface treatment of foods such as rice and confectionery are universally known [EFSA 2013, Grob 2018b]. Paraffin waxes are authorised for use in chewing gum: spruce sap chewing gum was first brought to the American market in the mid-1800s and later replaced by gum made using petroleum-derived paraffin wax. They are also used as coatings for fruits and vegetables, as well as in pesticide formulations [Fiorini et al. 2008; Teixeira et al. 2009]. Furthermore, MOH are used as de-foamers and anti-dusting agents for cereal grains [EFSA 2013].

Part of the contamination of food with MOH comes from the environment. As these MOH are largely in the particulate matter, they were analysed in dust sampled by filters. The molecular mass distribution corresponded to that found in the particulate matter from the exhaust of hot diesel engines, which also largely corresponded to that of engine lubricating oil [Brandenberger et al. 2005, Grob 2018b]. Handpicked sunflower seeds from the Zurich area were noticeably less contaminated than mechanically harvested seeds [Grob 2018b]. The machinery used for harvesting (e.g. diesel oil, lubricating oil) and for food processing (e.g. lubricating oils in pumps, syringe type dosing and other industrial installations) are possible food contamination sources just like the solvents consisting of individual alkanes or complex MOH mixtures that are used as cleaning agents. Other environmental contamination sources are debris from tyres and road bitumen.

MOH can also be used as binders for minor additives added as powder in feed formulas.

Food contamination must be avoided at all times

Meanwhile, it became obvious that high numbers of potentially migrating substances may be released in the packaged food. Grob et al. [2006] wrote ... *the number of substances migrating from food contact materials above the threshold of toxicological concern for genotoxic carcinogens is unknown, but might be about 100.000...* Many of the substances we ingest interfere with our hormonal system, meaning they can make people sick. How do we keep them out of our food? Ewender et al. [2012] investigated the permeation of mineral oil components from cardboard packaging materials. Although some possibilities exist to limit the migration, a functional barrier seems to be the best solution to stop permeation altogether.

Simply replacing recycled fibres for primary food packaging by virgin fibres may appear to be the safest and most elegant solution.

However, the production of fresh fibres is restricted by forest growth. The demand for paper and cardboard used for food packaging seems to exceed current forest renewal. Additionally, even if all primary food packaging were made of virgin fibres, mineral oil contamination would still be possible through evaporation off secondary packaging. In other words, the substitution of recycled by virgin fibres will reduce the risk of contamination but will not completely exclude it.

Since printing inks play a predominant role, it is worth trying to replace their mineral oil components by safer chemicals. There are however a number of technical limitations and it is obvious that a sensible and cautious approach would be to thoroughly assess possible substitutes for mineral oil components prior to their use. This would prevent having to face similar problems in the (near) future.

Decontamination during the paper and board recycling processes is a third option. An efficient removal of the mineral oil components would solve the problem. This option would involve more efficient cleaning processes so that recycled materials meet the official migration limits. It would also require a drastic reorganization and upgrading of current processes, which hardly seems feasible in the foreseeable future.

Finally, the application of good quality plastic barriers can significantly reduce the contamination of packed food products. Since all other measures require close cooperation up and down the supply chain, the introduction of barriers is now considered the most promising solution. Functional barriers[78] have been highly recommended to protect the foods against MOH in the packaging materials [German Federation of Food Law and Food Science 2017]. Per definition, behind a functional barrier, non-authorised substances may be used, provided their migration remains below a given detection limit. According to the Commission Regulation (EU) No 10/211, a maximum level of 0.01 mg per kg food is established for the migration of a non-authorised substance through the functional barrier. Substances that are mutagenic, carcinogenic or toxic to reproduction should not be used in food contact

---

78 Functional barriers are multilayer structures deemed to prevent migration of some chemicals released by food contact materials into food [Feigenbaum et al. 2005].

materials or articles without previous authorisation and are therefore not covered by the functional barrier concept.

Bibliography

Ambrogi et al. [2017]. Additives in polymers, in Jasso-Gastinel & Kenny (eds.) *Modification of Polymer Properties*, Elsevier, 87-108

Barp et al. [2015]. Migration of selected hydrocarbon contaminants into dry pasta packaged in direct contact with recycled paperboard, *Food Additives and Contaminants: Part A* 32, 2, 271-283

Barp et al. [2017a]. Accumulation of mineral oil saturated hydrocarbons (MOSH) in female Fischer 344 rats: Comparison with human data and consequences for risk assessment, *Science of The Total Environment* 575, 1263-1278

Barp et al. [2017b]. Mineral oil saturated hydrocarbons (MOSH) in female Fischer 344 rats; accumulation of wax components; implications for risk assessment, *Science of The Total Environment* 583, 319-333

Biedermann & Grob [2010]. Is recycled newspaper suitable for food contact materials? Technical grade mineral oils from printing inks, *European Food Research and Technology* 230, 5, 785-796

Biedermann et al. [2009]. Aromatic Hydrocarbons of Mineral Oil Origin in Foods: Method for Determining the Total Concentration and First Results, *Journal of agricultural and food chemistry* 57, 19, 8711-8721

Biedermann et al. [2013]. Migration of mineral oil, photoinitiators and plasticisers from recycled paperboard into dry foods: a study under controlled conditions, *Food Additives and Contaminants: Part A* 30, 5, 885-898

Biedermann-Brem et al. [2012]. Migration of polyolefin oligomeric saturated hydrocarbons (POSH) into food, *Food Additives and Contaminants: Part A* 29, 3, 449-460

Brandenberger et al. [2005]. Contribution of unburned lubricating oil and diesel fuel to particulate emission from passenger cars, *Atmospheric Environment* 39, 6985-6994

Castle et al. [1991]. Migration of mineral hydrocarbons into food. 1. Polystyrene container for hot and cold beverages, *Food Additives and Contaminants* 8, 6, 693-700

Collins [2004]. The comet assay for DNA damage and repair: principles, applications, and limitations, *Molecular Biotechnology* 26, 3, 249-261

Dincsoy et al. [1982]. Lipogranulomas in non-fatty human livers. A mineral oil induced environmental disease, *American Journal of Clinical Pathology* 78, 35-41

Droz & Grob [1997]. Determination of food contamination by mineral oil material from printed cardboard using on-line coupled LC-GC-FID, *Zeitschrift für Lebensmitteluntersuchung und -Forschung A* 205, 239-241

EFSA [2013]. Scientific Opinion on Mineral Oil Hydrocarbons in Food, *EFSA Journal* 10, 6, pp. 185

Eicher et al. [2015]. Migration by "direct" or "indirect" food contact? Dry or wetting foods? Some experimental data for paper and board. *Food Additives and Contaminants: Part A* 32, 1, 110-119

Ewender et al. [2012]. Permeation of Mineral Oil Components from Cardboard Packaging Materials through Polymer Films, *Packaging Technology and Science* 26, 7, 423-434

Feigenbaum et al. [2005]. Functional Barriers: properties and evaluation, *Food Additives and Contaminants* 22, 10, 956-967

German Federation of Food Law and Food Science [2017]. *Toolbox for Preventing the Transfer of Undesired Mineral Oil Hydrocarbons into Food*, Bund für Lebensmittelrecht und Lebensmittelkunde e. V., pp. 35

Goeyens [2014]. *Food and Packaging: a chemical spark*, ACCO, Leuven, pp. 147

Grob [2018a]. Toxicological Assessment of Mineral Hydrocarbons in Foods: State of Present Discussions, *Journal of agricultural and food chemistry* 66, 27, 6968-6974

Grob [2018b]. Mineral oil hydrocarbons in food: a review, *Food Additives and Contaminants: Part A* 35, 9, 1845-1860

Grob et al. [2006]. Food contamination with organic materials in perspective: packaging materials as the largest and least controlled source? A view focusing on the European situation, *Critical Reviews in Food Science and Nutrition* 46, 529-536

Lorenzini et al. [2010]. Saturated and aromatic mineral oil hydrocarbons from paperboard food packaging: estimation of long-term migration from contents in the paperboard and data on boxes from the market, *Food Additives and Contaminants: Part A* 27, 12, 1765-1774

Lorenzini et al. 2013. Migration kinetics of mineral oil hydrocarbons from recycled paperboard to dry food: monitoring of two real cases, *Food Additives and Contaminants: Part A* 30, 4, 760-770

Shah [2012]. Importance of Genotoxicity & S2A guidelines for genotoxicity testing for pharmaceuticals, *IOSR Journal of Pharmacy and Biological Sciences* 1, 2, 43-54

Słomczyńska [2008]. Xenoestrogens: mechanisms of action and some detection studies, *Polish Journal of Veterinary Sciences* 11, 3, 263-269

Tarnow et al. [2016]. Estrogenic Activity of Mineral Oil Aromatic Hydrocarbons Used in Printing Inks, *PLoS ONE* 11, 1, pp. 15

Teixeira et al. [2009]. Paraffin wax emulsion for increased rainfastness of insecticidal bait to control Rhagoletis pomonella (Diptera: Tephritidae), *Journal of Economic Entomology* 102, 3, 1108-1115

van de Ven et al. [2017]. *Mineral oils in food; a review of toxicological data and an assessment of the dietary exposure in the Netherlands*, RIVM Letter report 2017-0182, pp. 62

Vollmer et al. [2010]. Migration of mineral oil from printed paperboard into dry foods: survey of the German market, *European Food Research and Technology* 232, 1, 175-182

Humanity's "ancestral microbial heritage" must be preserved

The most extraordinary feature of life is its diversity

In the Anthropocene era [Crutzen 2006], i.e. the present era, during which human activities are exerting ever increasing impacts on the environment and in many ways outcompeting the natural processes, environmental sustainability has become one of our biggest issues. Because human activities have also grown to be significant geological forces, for instance through land use changes, deforestation and fossil fuel burning, it is justified to use the term "anthropocene" to define the current geological epoch. It is generally assumed that the Anthropocene started about two centuries ago, approximately coinciding with James Watt's first steam engine in 1784.

Increasing populations along with tremendous escalations in anthropogenic activities have raised questions about the sustainability of natural resources on the planet. Today, no part of the Earth is unaffected by the consequences of human activities. Global pollution is among the greatest threats to life and well-being that we have to face and will be facing in the future. Fast growing human populations and inherent increases in consumption per capita have put a great strain on natural resources. Additionally, urbanisation, industrialisation, and intensive agricultural practices have polluted the water resources, air and soil around the globe. Our natural resources are overexploited and, worse still, they have become contaminated with toxic chemicals that threaten the survival of future generations.

Animals and plants across the globe are being wiped out with ever increasing speed. According to recent estimates, the Earth is going through one of its most dramatic phases of biodiversity loss, the impact of which is unpredictable. The diversity of life on Earth is dramatically affected by human alterations of the ecosystems. Moreover, there is compelling evidence that the reverse is also true. Biodiversity in the broad sense[79] affects the properties of ecosystems and as a result, the assets that humans can obtain from them. Humans for example benefit from the diversity of organisms they have learned to use to produce medecines and food products.

Biodiversity has always been an integral part of human experience, which is why there are many moral reasons to preserve it for its own sake. Undeniably, what has been less recognised is that biodiversity also influences human well-being, including access to water and basic resources to be able to enjoy a satisfactory life and security in the face of global environmental change. Ecosystem processes are at the core of the Earth's most vital life support systems [Diaz et al. 2006]. And here is the problem: the human-caused rate of extinction of species of both plants as well as animals is currently hundreds of times higher than the past natural rate and if nothing changes the rate of extinction could be thousands of times higher in a not so distant future [Arora 2018].

Additionally, another tragic extinction crisis could be under way in the human guts and skins. Dominguez-Bello et al. [2018] warn that humanity faces a serious health crisis because many of the beneficial microbes that inhabit people's bodies are being eradicated. The overuse of antibiotics and widespread consumption of processed food products – typical ailments of our contemporary society – are dangerous habits.

---

79 Biodiversity in the broad sense is the number, abundance, composition, spatial distribution, and interactions of genotypes, populations, species, functional types and traits, and landscape units in a given system [Diaz et al. 2006].

Looking for the healthy microbiome

In 2008, a team of doctors and scientists ventured deep within the Venezuelan jungle and characterised the fecal, oral, and skin bacterial microbiome[80] and resistome[81] of members of an isolated Yanomami Amerindian village with no documented previous contact with Western people [Clemente et al. 2015] – a truly exceptional opportunity for Maria Gloria Dominguez-Bello, a microbiologist at the New York University department of Medicine. She was born in Venezuela and has been working in the Amazon for more than 20 years. Her research work focuses primarily on the human microbiome, i.e. the hundreds of trillions of bacteria and other microbes that colonise our bodies and outnumber our own cells by a factor of ~10.

Yes, the fact is we are not just single individuals walking about the planet; we are walking ecosystems.

The microbiome has emerged as one of the hottest areas of biomedical research. Dominguez-Bello's team investigates microbiome development from birth, and considers its functions for the host, impact by practices that reduce microbial transmission or disrupt the microbiota and strategies for restoration. They also study how Westernisation is changing environmental microbes and human exposures, integrating the fields of anthropology and architecture/urban studies into microbial ecology. A holistic understanding of the role of the Earth's microbial community and its genome – its microbiome – in the biosphere and in human health is key to meeting many of the challenges that face humanity in the 21st century [Dubilier et al. 2015].

---

80 Human bodies harbour a huge array of micro-organisms. While bacteria are the biggest players, they also host single-celled organisms known as archaea as well as fungi, viruses and other microbes. Together, these are dubbed the human microbiota. Our body's microbiome is all the genes these microbiota contain [Davis 2018].

81 The antibiotic resistome is the collection of all the antibiotic resistance genes, including those usually associated with pathogenic bacteria isolated in the clinics, non-pathogenic antibiotic producing bacteria and all other resistance genes [Wright 2007].

We know microorganisms digest the food we eat and provide us with valuable nutrients; we know that they prevent the growth of harmful microbes and regulate our immune systems, that they influence our risk of obesity and other health problems, and that they determine how effectively we process the medicines we take. If we are to truly understand our own health, we need to understand our microbes, especially since they come under assault from many of the foibles of our modern life. Fatty, calorific diets dramatically change the communities of microbes in our guts. Antibiotics kill them as readily as they kill harmful bugs. Then the question arises whether the current microbiome composition is still suitable for dealing with all the challenges. And if not, then it is vital to determine what the most appropriate microbiome composition should look like. That is why the Yanonami Amerindian people are so important. Investigating the natives of the Venezuelan jungle at least offers a glimpse of those microbiomes that are beyond the influence of mainstream civilisation. It comes as is no surprise that the results of the investigation [Clemente et al. 2015] suggested that westernisation has significantly affected human microbiome diversity.

These Yanomami harbour a microbiome with the highest diversity of bacteria and genetic functions ever reported in a human group. Despite their isolation, presumably for ~11000 years since their ancestors arrived in South America, and no known exposure to antibiotics, they harbour bacteria that carry functional antibiotic resistance (AR) genes, including those that confer resistance to synthetic antibiotics and are syntenic with mobilisation elements. These results suggest that westernisation significantly affects human microbiome diversity and that functional AR genes appear to be a feature of the human microbiome even in the absence of exposure to commercial antibiotics. AR genes are likely poised for mobilisation and enrichment upon exposure to pharmacological levels of antibiotics. The latter findings emphasise the need for an extensive characterisation of the functions of the microbiome and resistome in remote non-westernised populations before complete globalisation of modern practices affects potentially beneficial bacteria harboured in the human body.

It is logical that the science of microbiomes was born in the West

The developed world has the money, the science, the technology and the infrastructure. No wonder then that western research groups started studying the human (and animal) microbiota and microbiomes.

Only a handful of studies have looked beyond the western world. De Filippo et al. [2010] for example showed that children from a village in Burkina Faso have very different communities of gut microbes from children living in Florence, Italy. The authors emphasise the importance of preserving the treasure of microbial diversity present in ancient rural communities worldwide. Two years later, Yatsunenko et al. [2012] found similar results by comparing farmers from the Venezuelan Amazon and Malawian villages with U.S. city-dwellers. Their results confirm the need to consider the microbiome when evaluating human development, nutritional needs, physiological variations as well as the impact of westernisation.

The latter studies showed that the bacteria in the African and South American guts were dominated by plant digesting specialists, which are characterized by strongly activated genes for breaking down complex sugars and starches. By contrast, the American and European bacteria excelled at digesting the simple sugars found in processed food, together with the amino acids from a diet rich in animal protein. Both teams also found that the rural populations had more diverse communities of gut bacteria, while the urbanites were dominated by microbes that are linked to obesity. It is increasingly clear that the Western lifestyle has left us with a gentrified microbiome, in which only shadows of its former diversity (its former biodiversity) remained and which is dominated by completely different species. No one knows exactly why. It may be because our processed and sanitised foods, beverages and living areas deprive us of an influx of new microbes. It may also be that we select for species that are better at crowding others out.

Either way, researchers wonder what we have lost and whether this is related to the new epidemics of the modern cosmopolitan world.

An ambitious vision to deal with a problem of the same order of magnitude as climate change

The rates of occurrence of diseases such as diabetes, asthma and allergies have spiralled, and many researchers have suggested that the increase is due to significant losses in our microbiota. Human evolution and lifestyle changes, caused by both the agricultural and industrial revolutions, led to great advances in medicine and increased our average life expectancy. But at the same time the changes also greatly altered the ecological relationships and disease patterns of populations [Valle Gottlieb et al. 2017]. Studies involving populations that still enjoy a rural way of life and have traits similar to those that prevailed the Paleolithic period show that their gut microbiota are more robust, resistant and diverse in comparison to those of highly industrialised civilisations. The human diet has expanded and broadened to include the consumption of high-calorie foods, particularly from animal sources. For some time, researchers have strongly suspected that modern lifestyle and eating habits lead to reduced intake of beneficial bacteria. This suggests that non-pathogenic, beneficial bacteria are being eradicated by the currently predominant consumption of processed foods and frequent use of antibiotics.

Dominguez-Bello et al. [2018] delivered a very ambitious paper on how to solve the problem. They plan to capture and preserve the diversity of the human microbiota – they plan to build a Noah's Ark for the survival of germs – collected from people living in untouched, remote corners of the world who have not been impacted by modern society and/or processed foods.

In recent years, the human gut microbiota have emerged as a primary target area for health monitoring and modulation [Cho & Blaser 2012; Lozupone et al. 2012]. Alterations in the gut microbiota have been linked repeatedly to pathological states such as infections, auto-immune disorders, inflammatory bowel diseases and cancer. Researchers now believe that it will ultimately be possible to prevent diseases by reintroducing lost microbes [Vandeputte et al. 2017]. However, for this to happen, humanity's ancestral microbial heritage must be preserved.

Dominguez-Bello et al. [2018] suggest the best way to achieve this objective is to collect beneficial microbes from populations in remote Latin American and African areas. These microbes co-evolved with humans over tens or hundreds of millennia. They can help us digest our foods, strengthen our immune systems and protect us against invading germs, infections and allergic reactions.

Over a handful of generations, we have seen a staggering loss in microbial diversity and a simultaneous worldwide increase in immune and other disorders. For that matter, we observe that so-called bio-banking initiatives are springing up in research institutions around the world. So far, most of them have only focused on samples from industrialised, westernised regions. It is however of equal or even greater importance that the inhabitants of non-industrialized countries, especially in the extremely remote South American and African villages, be sampled also.

The international effort to preserve a greater diversity of microbiota will require enormous investments, but the rewards will certainly make the effort worthwile. Dominguez-Bello et al. [2018] conclude that we owe it to future generations to preserve the microbes that colonised our ancestors for ~200000 years of human evolution. And we must begin to preserve them before it is too late.

It is has become very urgent to improve the ecosystems in which we live. It is just as important to improve the ecosystems that live in us.

Bibliography

Arora [2018]. Environmental Sustainability—necessary for survival, Environmental Sustainability 1, 1-2

Cho & Blaser [2012]. The human microbiome: at the interface of health and disease, *Nature Reviews Genetics 13, 260-270*

Clemente et al. [2015]. The microbiome of uncontacted Amerindians, *Science advances* 1, 3, e1500183, pp. 12.

Crutzen [2006]. The "anthropocene", in Ehlers & Moss (eds.) *Earth system science in the anthropocene*, Springer, Berlin & Heidelberg, 13-18

Davis [2018]. The human microbiome: why our microbes could be key to our health, *The Guardian*, March 26, https://www.theguardian.com/news/2018/mar/26/the-human-microbiome-why-our-microbes-could-be-key-to-our-health

De Filippo [2010]. Impact of diet in shaping gut microbiota revealed by a comparative study in children from Europe and rural Africa, *Proceedings of the National Academy of Sciences* 107, 33, 14691-14696

Diaz et al. [2006]. Biodiversity Loss Threatens Human Well-Being, *PLoS Biology* 4, 8, e277, pp. 6

Dominguez-Bello et al. [2018]. Preserving microbial diversity, *Science* 362, 6410, 33-34

Dubilier et al. [2015]. Create a global microbiome effort, *Nature News* 526, 7575, 631-634

Lozupone et al. [2012]. Diversity, stability and resilience of the human gut microbiota, *Nature* 489, 220-230

Valle Gottlieb et al. [2017]. Impact of human aging and modern lifestyle on gut microbiota, *Critical Reviews in Food Science and Nutrition* 58, 9, 1557-1564

Vandeputte et al. [2017]. Practical considerations for large-scale gut microbiome studies, *FEMS Microbiology Reviews* 41, S154-S167

Wright [2007]. The antibiotic resistome: the nexus of chemical and genetic diversity, *Nature Reviews* 5, 175-186

Yatsunenko et al. [2012]. Human gut microbiome viewed across age and geography, *Nature* 486, 222-227

SHOULD WE BE THANKFUL FOR THE FOOD WE GET TO EAT?

A growing appetite for fast food

Rather slow than fast food!

The journalist and author Michael Wolff wrote in his riveting and explosive account of president Trump's administration [Wolff 2018]: *... Sometimes Trump would have a 6:30 p.m. meeting with former chief strategist Steve Bannon, but if not, more to his liking, he was in bed by that time with a cheeseburger, watching his three screens and making phone calls...* This may sound like a nice relaxing evening for Joe Average, but it is hardly the kind of behaviour you would expect from a President of the United States. Moreover, if all this is true, I have serious reservations about the eating habits of Donald Trump. Though fast food consumption is sometimes considered as "Liberty Hall", it is rather the opposite that is true. Recent scientific literature reinforces the link between fast food and bad cholesterol[82].

Never before have so many people watched so many entertaining cooking shows on television and read so much gastronomic writing. For years, cook books have scored best at Belgian book fairs, and I am personally very sorry that novels are far less appreciated. On the other hand, never before have so many people spent so little time cooking

---

82 Cholesterol travels through the blood on proteins called lipoproteins. Two types of lipoproteins carry cholesterol throughout the body. LDL (low-density lipoprotein), sometimes called "bad" cholesterol, makes up most of our body's cholesterol; high levels of LDL cholesterol raise our risk of suffering heart disease and stroke. HDL (high-density lipoprotein), or "good" cholesterol, absorbs cholesterol and carries it back to the liver. The liver then flushes it from the body. High levels of HDL cholesterol can lower our risk of heart disease and stroke [https://www.cdc.gov/cholesterol/ldl_hdl.htm].

food. Highly sophisticated kitchens do not necessarily encourage healthy cooking!

Fast food consumption has increased enormously during the last decades [Xue et al. 2016] and the increase is very likely to continue. Globally, fast food generates significantly higher revenues every year [Franchise Help 2018]. The economy of the United States (US), for example, has not risen by more than 3 % a year in the past 10 years. The burger business however is seriously booming. McDonald's, Burger King, and Wendy's reported a same-store sales jump of >3.2 % [Kramer 2017]. There are over 200 000 fast food restaurants in the US and it is estimated that 50 million Americans visit them every single day. Between 2013 and 2016, 36.6 % of American adults consumed fast food on a given day. The percentage of adults who consume fast food decreases with age: 44.9 % are aged 20-39, 37.7 % 40-59 and 24.1 % 60 and more. It is disappointing to note that this represents approximately between one fifth and one third of the population. Moreover, among those who consumed fast food, men were more likely than women to eat fast food at lunch, but women were more likely to report eating fast food as a snack [Fryar et al. 2018].

This obviously increasing trend is not without its consequences: ... *Out-of-home foods (takeaway, take-out and fast foods) have become increasingly popular in recent decades and are thought to be a key driver in increasing levels of overweight and obesity due to their unfavourable nutritional content...* the study by Janssen et al. [2017] concludes. Residential fast food outlet availability is increasingly considered a contributing factor to elevated obesity prevalence by researchers as well as policymakers [Foresight 2007]. Obesity has become endemic in many countries of the world and it is suggested that diets commonly contain an overabundance of energy-dense food products. Most notably, obese people adopt modern, "westernized" diets and lifestyles. The pace of the technological revolution is outstripping human evolution and for an increasing number of people weight gain is the inevitable – but largely involuntary – consequence of exposure to a modern lifestyle. Adolescent obesity is indeed one of the major global health challenges of the 21st century. This is not to eliminate personal responsibility altogether, but we must remember that the forces that drive obesity are for many people simply overwhelming.

There is however no single reason why people eat out-of-home foods. The Janssen et al. [2017] study presents several key factors that influence fast food consumption. Many of them are intertwined. Economic weakness and financial instability of the consumer appear to be strong determinants of access to out-of-home foods and consequent consumption. Additionally, the biological and psychological drives combined with a culture where overweight and obesity is becoming the norm [Foresight 2007; Popkin 2009] have made it "fashionable" to consume out-of-home food.

Yet, reactions weren't long in coming. Slow Food is an international association committed to bringing back the real value of food and respect for food producers, who work in harmony with the environment and ecosystems [Pussemier & Goeyens 2017]. The association strongly believes in the importance of food education for young generations. It moves towards a multidisciplinary approach that recognises strong connections between people, plate, and planet [Centre for Alternative Technology 2014]. While we are over-consuming high impact food, the planet's resources remain finite and the impact is felt on the world's terrestrial and aquatic ecosystems. If we are to build a future where people and nature thrive, we need to reconsider the food we eat and how it is produced.

Regular fast food consumption means more calories and fewer nutrients

The investigation by Donin et al. [2017] emphasises that children aged 9 to 10 who eat more than one takeaway meal per week (~28 % of the subjects) have higher body fat mass and greater skinfold thickness than those who never or seldom consume them (~26 %). They also have higher total energy intake, higher percentage energy intake from both total and saturated fat and higher energy density[83] from food intake. Regular fast

---

83 Energy density is the amount of energy stored in a given food mass.

food consumers also have lower protein, starch and micronutrient (e.g. vitamin C, folate and iron) intakes, suggesting a dietary pattern rich in calories, but poor in nutrients. These unhealthy dietary patterns and their subsequent risk markers for coronary heart disease, type 2 diabetes and obesity in children could have undesirable health consequences if continued into later life, the scientists warn [Donin et al. 2017].

Obesity and its high numbers of serious co-morbidities[84] exact a heavy toll in both human health and economic terms and this situation is deteriorating every year [Apovian 2013].

The epidemic of obesity is associated with elevated risk of type 2 diabetes mellitus, hypertension, obstructive sleep apnea, coronary heart disease and stroke [Barnett & Kumar 2009; Costa et al. 2018]. Types of dyslipidemia[85] include elevated LDL cholesterol, decreased HDL cholesterol, and elevated triglycerides. Results from a German study of 7124 adults, representing a nationally representative sample, similarly found significantly increased risks among obese compared with non-obese subjects for cardiovascular diseases, cardiometabolic risk factors, osteoarthritis[86] and, among women, diabetes and gallbladder disease [Schienkiewitz et al. 2012].

In addition to being associated with several cardiovascular risk factors, obesity is also associated with an increased risk of all-cause mortality. A meta-analysis, carried out by Guh et al. [2009] also observed an increased risk of several types of cancer among obese patients. Worldwide, the burden of cancer attributable to obesity expressed as population attributable fraction is 11.9 % in men and 13.1 % in women. There is convincing evidence that excess body weight is associated with an increased risk of cancer at as many as 13 anatomic sites, including

---

84 Co-morbidity is associated with worse health outcomes, more complex clinical management, and increased health care costs [Valderas et al. 2009].

85 Dyslipidemia is defined as having blood lipid levels that are too high or low; blood lipids are fatty substances, such as triglycerides and cholesterol [Medical News Today - https://www.medicalnewstoday.com/articles/321844.php].

86 Sometimes called degenerative joint disease or "wear and tear" arthritis, osteoarthritis is the most common chronic condition of the joints. It occurs when the cartilage or cushion between joints breaks down leading to pain, stiffness and swelling [Arthritis Foundation - https://www.arthritis.org/about-arthritis/types/osteoarthritis/].

endometrial, esophageal, renal and pancreatic adenocarcinomas; hepatocellular carcinoma; gastric cardia cancer; meningioma; multiple myeloma; colorectal, postmenopausal breast, ovarian, gallbladder and thyroid cancers [Avgerinos et al. 2019].

A systematic review of the overall body of evidence also confirms that advancing age, male sex, and higher body mass index increase obstructive sleep apnea (OSA) prevalence. OSA is a condition characterized by repeated episodes of partial or complete obstruction of the respiratory passages during the sleep. The body's response to obstructed breathing leads to arousal of the brain, sympathetic activation, and oxygen desaturation in the blood. Repeated episodes of upper airway obstruction during sleep may result in sleep fragmentation and non-restorative sleep. Those who suffer from OSA may complain of tiredness, excessive day-time sleepiness, insomnia, or morning headaches, but the condition is often asymptomatic. Weight loss has been accompanied by a substantial improvement in characteristics related not only to obesity, but also to OSA, suggesting that weight loss might be a cornerstone treatment of both conditions [Romero-Corall et al. 2010].

So far, relatively little is known about the associations between takeaway meal consumption and chronic disease risk markers in children. Yet, our governments should seriously start considering health protection initiatives to reverse the current trends in takeaway meal consumption and to improve childhood diet and nutrition both at home and school. So why wait any longer?

Overall, there is strong demand for further research on the out-of-home food phenomenon

To understand the complex interplay between biological, psychological, cultural and other determinants, it is essential to improve our understanding of the factors responsible for out-of-home food consumption, to investigate the major differences between countries and to support the building up of a coherent body of evidence as well as the development of the effective measures we desperately need.

And if the health risks associated with the regular consumption of out-of-home food products do not put you off, then perhaps the environmental consequences will. Not only do fast food products affect our health; they are also bad for the environment. High rates of obesity in richer countries cause up to ~1 billion extra tonnes of greenhouse gas (GHG) emissions every year, compared with countries with leaner populations, according to a study that assesses the additional food and fuel requirements of overweight. This finding is particularly worrying, say Roberts & Edwards [2010], because obesity is dramatically on the rise in many rich nations. The authors also assert that the recent increasing prevalence of obesity in the developed world is an inevitable consequence of wholesale shifts of the frequency distributions of body mass index of whole populations, not just more "rogue" obese individuals. In their model, they compared a population of 1 billion lean people, with weight distributions equivalent to a country such as Vietnam, with 1 billion people from richer countries, such as the US, where about 40 % of the population is classified obese. It appeared the fatter population needed 19 % more food energy for its energy requirements. The authors also factored in greater car use by the overweight. ... *The heavier our bodies become the harder it is to move about in them and the more dependent we become on cars...* they wrote.

The whole chain of fast food production has a considerably adverse influence on our environment [Pussemier & Goeyens 2017]. First, fast food stores sell huge quantities of meat. Most, if not all, of this meat is produced at factory farms (intensive cattle farming) that significantly contribute to GHG emissions and global warming. Second, most of these products are transported over long distances, thereby further increasing the impact on air quality. They also have a negative effect on water quality, because pathogens, hormones, drugs and the fertilizers they use for the cultivation of feed crops tend to seep into surrounding groundwater, potentially causing outbreaks of waterborne illness, fish kills, and other hazards. And finally, fast food restaurants also tend to use too much packaging. The overuse of wrappers, straws, bags, boxes, and plastic as well as paper ware is one of the biggest sources of urban litter and waterway and ocean contamination.

Just the once will not hurt

The occasional cheeseburger can do no harm. The same cannot be said about the daily cheeseburger in bed. The obesity epidemic shows no sign of abating, and that is bad news for public health. There is a very urgent need to resist the environmental forces that trigger gradual weight gain, obesity and related diseases in the population.

Consumers must learn to adjust to sustainable food production and healthy food consumption. They must accept to pay slightly higher prices for better food products. It is a well-known fact that eating too much meat is not good for your health. But then, vegetarianism is good for your health only when diets are well-balanced, when vegetarian dishes contain enough vitamins and essential amino acids. And we should all prefer unrefined and unprocessed food products [Satija et al. 2017] over ingredient-rich ready-made dishes and delicatessen.

We should prefer healthy food, which local and short supply chains can easily provide. A first move to slightly more expensive, but higher quality foods could be a giant step in the right direction in our pursuit of healthy food and sustainable food production. No doubt that even a small improvement of our eating habits would be good for us and good for the planet.

It is no coincidence that many years ago the father of modern nutrition, the American chemist Wilbur Olin Atwater (1844-1907), noted that: ... *the general impression of hygienists (is) that our diet is one-sided and that we eat too much ... fat, starch and sugar. This is due partly to our large consumption of sugar and partly to our use of such large quantities of fat meats ... How much harm is done to health by our onesided and excessive diet no one can say. Physicians tell us that is very great...* [Pojman et al. 2017].

How much harm has been done to our health by one-sided diets?

Bibliography

Apovian [2013]. The Clinical and Economic Consequences of Obesity, *American Journal of Managed Care* 19(11 suppl), S219-S228

Avgerinos et al. [2019]. Obesity and Cancer Risk: Emerging biological mechanisms and perspectives, *Metabolism*, in press

Barnett & Kumar [2009]. *Obesity and Diabetes*, John Wiley & Sons Inc., The Atrium, Southern Gate, Chichester, pp. 314

Centre for Alternative Technology [2014]. *People, Plate and Planet - The impact of dietary choices on health, greenhouse gas emissions and land use*, pp. 46

Costa et al. [2018]. The Relationship between Obesity, Insulin Resistance and Aldosterone Levels, *Current Research in Diabetes & Obesity Journal* 6, 1, pp. 3

Donin et al. [2017]. Takeaway meal consumption and risk markers for coronary heart disease, type 2 diabetes and obesity in children aged 9–10 years: a cross-sectional study, *Archives of Disease in Childhood* 0, 1-6

Foresight [2007]. *Tackling Obesities: Future Choices – Project Report*, Government Office for Science ondon), pp. 164

Franchise Help [2018]. Fast Food Industry Analysis 2018 - Cost & Trends, https://www.franchisehelp.com/industry-reports/fast-food-industry-analysis-2018-cost-trends/

Fryar et al. [2018]. *Fast Food Consumption Among Adults in the United States, 2013–2016*, NCHS Data Brief 322, pp. 6

Guh et al. [2009]. The incidence of co-morbidities related to obesity and overweight: A systematic review and meta-analysis, *BMC Public Health* 9, 88, pp. 20

Janssen et al. [2017]. Determinants of takeaway and fast food consumption: A narrative review, *Nutrition Research Reviews*, https://doi.org/10.1017/S0954422417000178, published online

Kramer [2017]. Burger sales are booming, http://www.foodandwine.com/news/fast-food-industry-growing-us-economy

Pojman et al. [2017]. *Environmental Ethics: Readings in Theory and Application, 7th Edition*, Cengage Learning, pp. 833

Popkin [2009]. *The World is Fat*, Avery, pp. 240

Pussemier & Goeyens [2017]. *AgricultureS & Enjeux de société*, Les presses agronomiques de Gembloux, pp. 112

Roberts & Edwards [2010]. *The Energy Glut: The Politics of Fatness in an Overheating World*, Zed Books Ltd, pp. 192

Romero-Corall et al. [2010]. Interactions Between Obesity and Obstructive Sleep Apnea - Implications for Treatment, *Chest* 137, 3, 711-719

Satija et al. [2017]. Healthful and Unhealthful Plant-Based Diets and the Risk of Coronary Heart Disease in US Adults, *Journal of the American College of Cardiology* 70, 4, 411-422

Schienkiewitz et al. [2012]. Comorbidity of overweight and obesity in a nationally representative sample of German adults aged 18-79 years, *BMC Public Health* 12, 658, pp. 11

Valderas et al. [2009]. Defining Comorbidity: Implications for Understanding Health and Health Services, *Annals of Family Medicine* 7, 4, 357-363

Wolff [2018]. *Fire and Fury: Inside the Trump White House*, Henry Holt and Company, pp. 336

Xue et al. [2016]. Time Trends in Fast Food Consumption and Its Association with Obesity among Children in China, *PLoS ONE* 11, 3, pp. 14

Love hormone oxytocin's boozy characteristics

Avoir l'esprit ouvert n'est pas l'avoir béant à toutes les sottises [Rostand 1967]. To have an open mind is not to have it gaping at all nonsense.

How much can I trust information on the internet?

Information on the internet ranges from truth to fiction to intentional misinformation. It is always important to develop a critical eye towards everything one reads, not least towards the praise and compliments for the "miraculous" molecule, oxytocin (OT). Throughout history, business and marketing experts have tried to be creative in how they inform the public about their products. There are always new hearts to be conquered.

Creativity works and some companies will always be able to talk anyone into anything: *How can you reduce stress naturally? Buy OT Hormone in a Convenient OT Nasal Spray* [https://www.OTfactor.co/] *... OT hormone, the love hormone, calms and soothes for natural stress relief ... Researchers have demonstrated how this wonder substance can reduce stress and anxiety ... When participants used a nasal spray with the love hormone, they lowered their stress levels and felt more relaxed, with a more positive outlook on life ... Some people buy OT nasal spray to enhance the bonding between themselves and their sexual partner ... OT spray could also increase feelings of trust and increase the maintenance of monogamy ... High levels of the hormone can help stimulate childbirth, and afterwards, it helps to stimulate the production of breast milk ... The love hormone could help children and adults with autism develop better* *social skills ... Scientific studies showed how using this spray helped groups work together...*

Trying to understand what is at stake should be done without interference or pressure from the outside and without being influenced by dogmas or ready-made ideas. So, I went and looked into the peer reviewed scientific literature and found there is more than a little truth in internet advertising.

The way puppies look at you is irresistible; puppies will make your heart melt!

Researchers in Japan have described several experiments that suggest people and their four-legged best friends have mutually developed an instinctive bonding mechanism in the several thousand years since dogs were first domesticated [Nagasawa et al. 2015]. As part of the experiment dogs were put into a room with their owners and the scientists studied their interaction by measuring OT levels in urine samples. People whose dogs had the most eye contact with their masters – a mutual gaze – registered the largest increases in OT levels. Moreover, the dogs had an OT peak that correlated with that of their owners. In a similar experiment with wolves – the not domesticated, close relatives of dogs – no such result was recorded despite the fact that the wolves involved in the experiment had been raised by people. This OT study shows that there is an inter-species OT-mediated positive loop, facilitated and modulated by gazing. A similar rise in OT occurs when human mothers and infants look at each other. This suggests that early dogs may have hijacked this response to better bond with their new "human families".

Moreover, based on previous results, Petersson et al. [2017] expected touch and forms of behaviour related to calm and anti-stress to be positively related to OT levels in both dogs and owners, whereas behaviour related to activation or stress would be associated with cortisol[87] levels. The authors found that OT as well as cortisol levels,

---

87 Cortisol is a steroid hormone that regulates a wide range of processes throughout the body, including metabolism and immune responses; it also has a very important role in helping the body respond to stress.

in both dogs and their owners, are associated with the way the owners interact with their dogs and also with forms of behaviour caused by the interactions.

The attachment relationship between a dog owner and his dog can be regarded as functionally similar to the relationship that prevails between a parent and a child. Several studies demonstrated that this type of relationship is characterized by behavioural and neuroendocrine similarities close to the ones described for mothers and infants [Stoeckel et al. 2014; Nagasawa et al. 2015].

Will Cupid's arrows assume the form of a nasal OT spray?

Several new studies show that OT makes us more sympathetic, supportive and open with our feelings [Gravotta 2013]. Wudarczyk et al. [2013] even outlined a proposal for the use of OT in the therapeutic neuro-enhancement of contemporary romantic relationships. The authors argue that an intranasal dose of OT in conjunction with marriage counselling can improve closeness between married partners.

OT has good and bad effects, however, that may be different for different individuals and couples depending on a range of personal, interpersonal as well as contextual factors. And the authors of the publication warn against careless OT-based treatment plans: … *Yet while the existence of negative effects in early trials may simply point to the need to develop complementary administration paradigms that could moderate or even reverse these bad effects in applied settings, the importance of pre-screening and the close involvement of a trained professional in any therapeutic program cannot be overstated…*

The first piece of evidence that indicates that OT is nature's "love glue" or "cuddle chemical" comes from researchers who measured OT levels in couples. For years, Psychology Professor Ruth Feldman at Bar-Ilan University (Israel) focused on the role of OT in mother–child bonding [Feldman et al. 2007]. More recently, she decided to investigate romantic bonds by comparing OT levels in new lovers and single persons. The increase in OT during the period of falling in love was the highest ever found [Schneiderman et al. 2012]. New lovers had twice the amount usually seen in pregnant women. Moreover, OT was also correlated with the longevity of a relationship. The couples with the highest levels were the ones who were still together six months later.

One way to clarify the question whether OT is responsible for the stability of a couple's bond or whether disconnected couples fail to trigger their OT release system is to administer OT rather than simply measure naturally occurring levels. The research team of couple therapist and Professor Beate Ditzen at the University of Zurich (Switzerland) recruited adult couples who received OT or placebo intra-nasally before engaging in a conflict discussion in the laboratory. OT increased positive communication behaviour and reduced salivary cortisol – meaning it reduced stress levels – compared to placebo [Ditzen et al. 2009]. The team believes OT might help to enhance the effects of a standard treatment, such as cognitive behavioural therapy, by possibly making the benefits of social interaction more accessible to the individual. But OT administration will probably never replace the standard treatments. The authors emphasize that the study does not show that OT should be used as the actual treatment.

OT in women also reduced the levels of salivary alpha-amylase, whereas in men it increased these levels [Ditzen et al. 2012]. The release of salivary alpha-amylase was reported to react to physiological and psychological stressors. Several studies showed increased levels of alpha-amylase before and after psychological stress. Since salivary alpha-amylase does not seem to be closely related to other biological stress markers such as catecholamines and cortisol, it may be a useful additional parameter for the measurement of stress. Interestingly, men under OT were faster to detect the valence of positive stimuli, conceptually associated with sexuality, bonding, and social relationships [Unkelbach et al. 2008].

It may well be that oxytocin improves the welfare of humans and other animals

Duncan and Olsson [2001] were among the first scientists to distinguish the state of suffering from the pleasurable state. States of suffering evolved to motivate behaviour in "need situations", which require immediate action. States of pleasure, on the other hand, evolved to motivate behaviour in "opportunity situations" where there is a long-term benefit associated with performing the behaviour, but no need to act immediately.

Studies on animal welfare are now gradually moving from methods focusing on reduction of stress to methods increasing pleasure and stress tolerance in the animals' lifetime [Chen & Sato 2017] and consequently, assessments of good welfare are becoming increasingly important. Affiliative behaviour and positive social interaction are being used as good welfare indicators.

Chen & Sato [2017] investigated how OT relates to positive social behaviour, pleasure and stress tolerance as well as which management factors stimulate OT release. They focus on how OT, as a good welfare indicator, is affecting the welfare of farm animals and what kind of animal management increases OT concentrations. The release of OT is related to the performance of positive normal behaviour and enrichment such as (daily) brushing [Grandin & Shivley 2015], which can further accelerate OT secretion. Further studies on farm animal welfare should pay more attention to management practices that induce OT and hence improve the comfort and stress tolerance of the animals. Merely focusing on how to control stress in farm animals, e.g. by administering tranquillizers, beta-blockers etc. is notably insufficient.

... There were groups of cattle being driven in the chutes, which were roadways about fifteen feet wide, raised high above the pens. In these chutes the stream of animals was continuous, it was quite uncanny to watch them, pressing on to their fate, all unsuspicious – a very river of death... [Sinclair 2015]. The realisation that the comfort and stress tolerance of farm animals must be improved has come quite late, I believe. More than 100 years after it was first published, *The Jungle* has lost none of its same emotional power. Upton Sinclair's novel remains a must read.

Scientists were struck by the incredible similarities between oxytocin and alcohol

OT generates trust and generosity but it can also fuel aggression. Mitchell et al. [2015] at the University of Birmingham in the UK have noted the striking similarity in the socio-cognitive effects that can be induced by OT and the effects of excessive alcohol consumption. Research revealed that although OT and alcohol target different receptors in the brain, they cause common action on transmissions in the prefrontal cortex[88] and the limbic structures[89], i.e. in the brain structures that control how we perceive stress and anxiety. The result is lowered inhibition especially in stressful situations like a job interview or asking someone out on a date. "Taking compounds such as OT or alcohol can make these situations seem less daunting," Mitchell said.

While OT is associated with positive feelings, its close similarity with alcohol means that we cannot ignore its potential danger. Like alcohol, OT can also facilitate increased aggression and envy, boastfulness, and selfish behaviour. Also, like alcohol, OT's ability to lower social inhibition can have dangerous effects. Both substances can enhance our perception of trustworthiness – a side effect with potentially dangerous consequences.

Though many of us would like to believe in the effectiveness and utility of the intranasal OT spray, the substance needs to be regarded with scepticism and rigour [Leng & Ludwig 2016]. The possible effects of intranasal OT definitely justify additional, proper dose-response studies. Will the OT nasal spray ever be used as an alternative to alcohol? This to me seems hardly likely. But understanding exactly how OT suppresses

---

88 The gray matter of the anterior part of the frontal lobe that is highly developed in humans and plays a role in the regulation of complex cognitive, emotional, and behavioural functioning [Merriam Webster].

89 The limbic system is the part of the brain involved in our behavioural and emotional responses, especially when it comes to forms of behaviour we need for survival: feeding, reproduction and caring for our young, and fight or flight responses [Queensland Brain Institute, https://qbi.uq.edu.au/brain/brain-anatomy/limbic-system].

certain modes of action and alters our behaviour could provide real benefits for a great many people.

Hopefully, ongoing and future investigations will shed new light on the bright and dark sides of the love hormone and will open up avenues that have not so far been considered [Mitchell et al. 2015].

Another quote by Jean Rostand: ... *la vérité que je révère, c'est la modeste vérité de la science, la vérité relative, fragmentaire, provisoire, toujours sujette à retouche, à correction, à repentir* [Rostand 1963]. The truth that I revere is the modest truth of science, the relative, fragmentary, and provisional truth that is always subject to improvement, correction, and repentance.

Similar effects and yet, a cure; could research also lead to a "sobriety" pill?

In 2014 the World Health Organisation called on governments to do more to prevent alcohol-related deaths and diseases. Each year over three million people die due to alcohol-related causes. Alcohol consumption cannot only lead to dependence, but also increases people's risk of developing more than 200 diseases, including liver cirrhosis and some cancers. In addition, compulsive drinking can lead to violence and injuries. A new scientific study concludes there is no safe level of drinking alcohol. The study, published by GBD 2016 Alcohol Collaborators [2018], shows that in 2016 nearly three million deaths globally were attributed to alcohol use, including 12 per cent of deaths in males between 15 and 49. Imagine, then, if problem drinkers could be given a "miracle" pill that would make them less likely to drink, less intoxicated if they drunk and more capable of enduring the potentially life-threatening alcohol withdrawal syndrome. Research exploring the interactions between the love hormone OT and alcohol gives some grounds for hope that such a pill might one day exist.

OT causes both immediate and long-lasting inhibition of alcohol consumption in rodents [Bowen et al. 2011]. The authors suggest that exogenous OT administered during adolescence can have subtle, yet enduring effects on anxiety, sociability and the motivation to consume alcohol. Such effects may reflect the inherent neuroplasticity[90] of brain OT systems and a feed-forward effect whereby exogenous OT up-regulates endogenous OT systems. Furthermore, repeated exposure to OT promotes addiction-resistant behaviour characterised by reduced anxiety, higher sociability and greater activity of the natural OT system [McGregor & Bowen 2012].

Later research published by Bowen et al. [2015] provides perhaps one of the most striking demonstrations of OT's interaction with alcohol. OT was infused into the brains of rats that were afterwards given an intoxicating dose of alcohol. The OT completely prevented the discoordination caused by the alcohol in the rat equivalent to a field sobriety test. Rats given OT behaved just like sober rats. The scientists went on to demonstrate that OT prevents alcohol from acting at specific sites in the brain involved in alcohol intoxication, sites known as delta subunit-containing GABA-A receptors[91]. This was a particularly striking discovery inasmuch as OT is normally thought to bind primarily to its own OT receptors and a population of receptors for the closely related peptide vasopressin.

So, at least in rodents, OT reduces both the short- and long-term alcohol consumption. It also prevents alcohol-induced intoxication, reduces the severity of alcohol withdrawal and promotes resistance to addiction and relapse. Faehrmann et al. [2018] are now reviewing the neurobiological mechanisms of OT effects on stress-related pathways and are discussing the potential use of OT in the treatment of alcohol addiction. Their investigations show that OT exerts substantial anxiolytic effects and facilitates pro-social behaviour. OT can be safely applied as intranasal preparation. Yet, the authors conclude that the research strongly suggests that application of OT may beneficially influence the mechanisms of relapse and craving by reducing anxiety, stress

---

90 Neuroplasticity can be defined as the brain's ability to change, remodel and reorganize for purpose of better ability to adapt to new situations by forming new neural connections throughout life.

91 The GABA-A receptors are the major inhibitory neurotransmitter receptors in mammalian brain [Sigel & Steinmann 2014].

vulnerability and social withdrawal in abstinent alcohol-dependent patients.

Early days yet

The more we learn about how OT causes such a wide range of positive effects on alcohol-induced behaviour, the closer we may be getting to a "sobriety" pill being science rather than science fiction.

Sobriety and love: can we kill two birds with one stone? Hopefully we can, but there is still so much more we need to know.

Bibliography

Bowen et al. [2011]. Adolescent Oxytocin Exposure Causes Persistent Reductions in Anxiety and Alcohol Consumption and Enhances Sociability in Rats, *PLoS ONE* 6, 11, e27237

Bowen et al. [2015]. Oxytocin prevents ethanol actions at δ subunitcontaining GABA-A receptors and attenuates ethanolinduced motor impairment in rats, *Proceedings of the National Academy of Sciences* 112 , 10, 3104-3109

Chen & Sato [2017]. Role of oxytocin in improving the welfare of farm animals – A review, *Asian-Australasian Journal of Animal Sciences* 30, 4, 449-454

Ditzen et al. [2009]. Intranasal Oxytocin Increases Positive Communication and Reduces Cortisol Levels During Couple Conflict, *Biological Psychiatry*. 65, 9, 728-731

Ditzen et al. [2012]. Sex-specific effects of intranasal oxytocin on autonomic nervous system and emotional responses to couple conflict, *Biological Psychiatry* 72, 3, e3–e4

Duncan & Olsson [2001]. Environmental enrichment: from flawed concept to pseudo-science, in *Proceedings of 35th International Congress of the ISAE*, University of Natural Resources and Applied Life Sciences, Vienna, pp. 73

Faehrmann et al. [2018]. Oxytocin und die suchterhaltenden Mechanismen der Alkoholabhängigkeit, Neuropsychiatrie 32, 1-8

Feldman et al. [2007]. Evidence for a Neuroendocrinological Foundation of Human Affiliation - Plasma Oxytocin Levels Across Pregnancy and the Postpartum Period Predict Mother-Infant Bonding, *Psychological Science* 18, 11, 965-970

GBD 2016 Alcohol Collaborators [2018]. Alcohol use and burden for 195 countries and territories, 1990–2016: a systematic analysis for the Global Burden of Disease Study 2016, *The Lancet* 392, 1015-1035

Grandin & Shivley [2015]. How Farm Animals React and Perceive Stressful Situations Such As Handling, Restraint, and Transport, *Animals* 5, 1233-1251

Gravotta [2013]. Be Mine Forever: Oxytocin May Help Build Long-Lasting Love, *Scientific American*, February 13

Leng & Ludwig [2016]. Intranasal Oxytocin: Myths and Delusions *Biological Psychiatry* 79, 3, 243-250

McGregor & Bowen [2012]. Breaking the loop: Oxytocin as a potential treatment for drug addiction, *Hormones and Behavior* 61, 331-339

Mitchell et al. [2015]. Similar effects of intranasal oxytocin administration and acute alcohol consumption on socio-cognitions, emotions and behaviour: Implications for the mechanisms of action, *Neuroscience and Biobehavioral Reviews* 55, 98-106

Nagasawa et al. [2015]. Oxytocin-gaze positive loop and the coevolution of human-dog bonds, *Science* 348, 6232, 333-336

Petersson et al. [2017]. Oxytocin and Cortisol Levels in Dog Owners and Their Dogs Are Associated with Behavioral Patterns: An Exploratory Study, Frontiers in psychology 18, article 1796, pp. 8

Rostand [1963]. *Le droit d'être naturaliste*, Éditions Stock, Paris, pp. 216

Rostand [1967]. *Inquiétudes d'un biologiste*, Éditions Stock, Paris, pp. 154

Schneiderman et al. [2012]. Oxytocin during the initial stages of romantic attachment: Relations to couples' interactive reciprocity, *Psychoneuroendocrinology* 37, 8, 1277-1285

Sigel & Steinmann [2014]. Structure, Function, and Modulation of GABA-A Receptors, *Journal of Biological Chemistry* 287, 48, 40224-40231

Sinclair [2015]. *The Jungle (first edition 1906)*, Signet Classics, Penguin Group, New York, pp. 400

Stoeckel et al. [2014]. Patterns of Brain Activation when Mothers View Their Own Child and Dog: An fMRI Study, *PLoS ONE* 9, 10, pp. 12

Unkelbach et al. [2008]. Oxytocin Selectively Facilitates Recognition of Positive Sex and Relationship Words, *Psychological Science* 19, 1092-1094.

Wudarczyk et al. [2013]. Could intranasal oxytocin be used to enhance relationships? Research imperatives, clinical policy, and ethical considerations, *Current Opinion in Psychiatry* 26, 5, 474-484

Grubs can be eaten raw and when they are cooked they taste like roasted almonds – or so they say!

… A distinguished novelist has said that to watch flies trying to tug their legs off the paper one after another 'til they are twice their natural length is one of his favorite amusements. I have never found any difficulty in believing it of him. It is an odd fact that considerateness, if not actually kindness, to flies has been made one of the tests of gentleness in popular speech. How often has one heard it said in praise of a dead man: "He wouldn't have hurt a fly!" As for those who do hurt flies, we pillory them in history. We have never forgotten the cruelty of Domitian. "At the beginning of his reign," Suetonius tells us "he used to spend hours in seclusion every day, doing nothing but catch flies and stab them with a keenly sharpened stylus. Consequently, when someone once asked whether anyone was in there with Cæsar, Vibius Crispus made the witty reply: 'Not even a fly.'" … One of the most agonising of the minor dilemmas in which a too sensitive humanitarian ever finds himself is whether he should destroy a spider's web, and so, perhaps, starve the spider to death, or whether he should leave the web, and so connive at the death of a multitude of flies. I have long been content to leave Nature to her own ways in such matters … The ladybird, the butterfly, and the bee – who would put chains upon such creatures? These are insects that must have been in Eden before the snake. Beelzebub, the god of the other insects, had not yet any engendering power on the earth in those days, when all the flowers were as strange as insects and all the insects were as beautiful as flowers… [Lynd 1921].

No unscrupulous swatting!

Whether they are insects right here in Europe or in one of the planet's most exotic locales, many insect species are a true delight to watch. But then of course they can also be slimy, cringe-inducing creatures, often swatted by humans or ruthlessly eliminated with insecticides. Moreover, many of us fail to recognize that beetles, wasps, moths, caterpillars, grasshoppers, etc. are unexplored nutrition sources that can help reduce global food insecurity [van Huis et al. 2013].

This might suggest that insects are there for the taking, but nothing is further from the truth. The feature article in The New York Times Magazine recently published by Brooke Jarvis [2018] discusses the drastic drop-off in the insect populations. The author makes a terrifying report: all over the world species are disappearing and among those who survive the number of individuals has plummeted. This loss of biodiversity is part of what is known as the sixth mass extinction: it is the sixth time in the history of the world that a large number of species are disappearing in unprecedented fast succession – a phenomenon caused this time not by asteroids or ice ages but by humans. And it is nothing but a huge disaster, because insects play an invaluable role in pollination, soil decomposition and plant growth. They actively participate in the equilibrium of our planet's ecosystems, and their absence could trigger chain reactions for plants as well as for animal species including men. The New York Times Magazine insists: ... *Nature's resilient, but we're pushing her to such extremes that eventually it will cause a collapse of the system...* Is the apocalypse close for insects? And what does this decline mean for the rest of life on Earth? Scientists sincerely hope that insects will have a chance to embody nature's resilience.

So, if we ever want to eat insects, it is time we fine-tune our technologies.

Why do we have such an aversion in the West towards eating insects?

Human beings often consider insects as a nuisance, as nothing more than pests intent on destroying our crops and tormenting humans and other animals. Nothing could be further away from the truth. Insects can provide food at low environmental cost and positively contribute to livelihoods. They play a fundamental role in nature.

Yet, many westerners continue to ignore these benefits. Contrary to popular belief, insects are not merely "famine foods" eaten in times of food scarcity. Even though they do not belong to our gastronomic tradition in the West, many Asians, Africans and Latin Americans actually choose to eat insects, mainly because of their palatability and their established place in local food cultures.

Of the ~1 million known insect species, a reported ~2000 different insect species [Jongema 2017] are already eaten in various countries across the globe and are actually an integral part of the diet of >2 billion people worldwide [van Huis et al. 2013]. Most consumed insects include beetles, caterpillars, bees, wasps, ants, termites, grasshoppers, locusts and crickets [Holland 2013]. The concept of utilising insects for food (as well as for feed) is appealing because of their high nutritional content, with a lot of media hype around their desirable protein content. Insects have a high reproductive rate and feed conversion efficiency, making them ideal for farming purposes. Their feed conversion ratio is highly efficient becaus they are poikilothermic[92]. Additionally, insects are supposed to be environmentally friendly: they can recycle waste matter, require little space, food and water to grow and reproduce, and they are amenable to vertical farming.

---

92 A poikilotherm is an animal whose internal temperature varies considerably; it is the opposite of a homeotherm or animal which maintains thermal homeostasis. Poikilothermic animals include types of vertebrate animals, specifically some fish, amphibians, and reptiles, as well as a large number of invertebrate animals [Wikipedia].

As man evolved, the hunter-gatherers collected much more than edible plants

Early humans probably hunted for insects too. Insects could be found everywhere and many animals ate them. So why would they not have been eaten buy humans? Early humans took their cue from insectivorous animals to decide which insects were edible and tasty.

Years later, Romans and Greeks would dine on beetle larvae and locusts. The Greek scientist and philosopher Aristotle even wrote about harvesting tasty cicadas. In the Old Testament book of Leviticus (11, 20-23), the authors stated: ... *All flying insects that walk on all fours are to be regarded as unclean by you. There are, however, some flying insects that walk on all fours that you may eat: those that have jointed legs for hopping on the ground. Of these you may eat any kind of locust, katydid, cricket, or grasshopper. But all other flying insects that have four legs you are to regard as unclean...* This "green light" was obviously bad news for locusts and grasshoppers. John the Baptist lived in the desert for months on a diet of locusts and honeycomb!

Locusts were also a nutritious, cheap and plentiful source of food for the ancient Algerians. They prepared the insects by boiling them in salt water and drying them in the sun. And the Australian Aborigines made meals of moths. After cooking them in sand, they burned off the wings and legs and sifted the moths through a net to remove their heads, leaving nothing but delectable moth meat. The Aborigines were and continue to be entomophagists[93]. They eat honeypot ants[94] and witchetty grubs, the large, white, wood-eating larvae of several species of moths.

---

93 Entomophagy is the human consumption of insects and arachnids in the form of eggs, larvae, pupea and adults. Arachnids (class Arachnida) are any member of the arthropod group that includes spiders, daddy longlegs, scorpions, and (in the subclass Acari) the mites and ticks, as well as lesser-known subgroups [Encyclopaedia Britannica].

94 They carry their community's emergency food supply on their backs: they develop swelled abdomens, filled with food by other worker ants.

Insects are good for us

The protein, fat, amino acid, fatty acid and mineral content of many edible insects often compares favourably with that of beef, pork and chicken. Using the nutrient value score as a measure of comparison, it appears that commercially available insects have a nutritional value that is either comparable to or higher than that of chicken and beef. Scientists, decision makers, and business managers are increasingly aware of the importance of new protein sources, which is why it is recommended to consume insects as environmentally sustainable and nutritious alternatives to conventional livestock products [Payne et al. 2016a & 2016b].

The proteins found within most insect species are high quality proteins [Bukkens 1997] since they contain the essential amino acids that correspond to the reference standards set out by the Food and Agricultural Organisation and the World Health Organisation (WHO). The WHO released a report containing the daily requirements of essential amino acids for the average healthy adult as well as for children and infants [Yi et al. 2017]. And when comparing the required amino acid profile for a healthy adult with the amino acid profile of edible insect species, it is observed that most insects contain all the essential amino acids for growth. This could be of great benefit to more deprived communities, where deficiencies in essential amino acids are quite common.

Compared to other livestock animals, moreover, insects seem to contain more polyunsaturated fatty acids[95] and higher levels of minerals, such as iron and zinc, and more vitamins B1, B2, and B3 [van Huis et al. 2013].

Asiatic rhinoceros beetles (*Oryctes rhinoceros* L.) and winged termites (*Macrotermes nigeriensis* S.) constitute real live, crawling and flying stocks of nutrients and minerals [Omosoto et al. 2015]. Both insects

---

95 Polyunsaturated fatty acids (PUFA) are fatty acids that contain more than one double bond in their backbone; this class includes many important compounds, such as essential fatty acids [Wikipedia]

are rich sources of proteins, minerals, fibre and fat. Their levels of anti-nutrient and/or secondary metabolites are lower, when compared to other food sources. Also, these two insects are rich in antioxidants. They can be used to substitute animal proteins like beef and mutton. The inclusion of these insects in the human diet tends to enrich the body with mineral salts.

Yet another example is that of Manipur – a state in north-eastern India, with the city of Imphal as its capital [Wikipedia]. The people of many ethnic origins who live there capture and consume different insect species living in puddles, ponds, lakes, and rivers. In the valley region of the Manipur state, there are many inland freshwater lakes that act as ideal habitats for aquatic edible insects. They are highly valued and sought after by Malipur locals because of their taste and enhanced availability. The existence of an insect consumption culture in Manipur ensures that the nutritional needs of the indigenous people are met.

Although the consumption of edible insects has sometimes been trivialized, entomophagy can play a predominant role in food security, public health, environmental quality management, as well as being a source of income [Ayieko et al. 2010; Shantibala et al. 2014]. For the communities living in the Lake Victoria district (Africa), for example, insect consumption could well be a major step towards the commercialisation of insects. Making people aware of the need to protect the sources of insects and encouraging them to protect the insect fauna may become much easier. Entomophagy is no longer merely a survival strategy for the poor; it is becoming a food habit for healthconscious individuals; a food for the future.

Entomophagy is most certainly something to be reckoned with in the future. Insect consumption deserves to be scrutinized and evaluated. It is by no means exceptional and can only grow in importance over the coming years.

There are still not enough regulations to ensure the microbiological safety of edible insects

The Dutch Food and Consumer Product Safety Authority has released a preliminary report on micro-organisms relevant to insects and the threshold limits of each micro-organism considered safe to be consumed [https://www.nvwa.nl/]. The list of micro-organisms relevant to insects is largely based on EU safety regulations for meat and seafood products. As insects move from novel foods to commercial food ingredients, however, governments will need to re-evaluate their legislation to incorporate insects as a recognised food ingredient. And they had better begin straight away.

As you would expect with food sources containing protein, there are reports of immunoglobulin-mediated allergic reactions occurring from consuming insects [Srinroch et al. 2015]. Carmine dye, a popular red colorant derived from female cochineal insects, has been reported to cause severe allergic reactions in patients. And in China, where the consumption of insects is considered a delicacy, there are reported cases of allergic reactions caused by silkworm pupae, ranging from mild reactions to more serious cases of anaphylactic[96] shock [Ji et al. 2008].

The allergic reactions induced by entomophagy are comparable to the allergies due to the consumption of arthropod species such as crustaceans. It is suggested that patient sensitivity is a result of previous exposure to insect allergens (inhalation, contact or accidental consumption) or cross-reactivity between the insect allergen and a potential crustacean allergen [Srinroch et al. 2015].

The perceived safety of consuming insects is an important factor in securing consumer acceptance. It is therefore imperative to further investigate and understand the safety of eating insects before advocating their consumption [van Huis et al. 2017]. Hence, it is suggested to use commonly known edible insect species reared on pollutant-free feed in controlled farming environments to reduce the potential risks associated with eating insects.

---

96 Anaphylaxis is a severe allergic reaction that requires immediate treatment.

Bugs as drugs

Insects also provide ingredients that have been a staple of traditional medicine for centuries. Many of these ingredients have not been evaluated experimentally, though preliminary trials have shown many have beneficial properties [Cherniak 2010].

Several varieties of ants are also consumed as food in countries like China, Thailand, India and some African countries [van Huis 2013]. The Chinese black ant (*Polyrhachis dives*) for example has been a traditional edible insect in China for centuries and in addition to its nutritional value the insect has been used in traditional medicine for the treatment of rheumatoid and osteoarthritis, inflammatory diseases, and diabetes [Huang & Xiao 2003]. Tang et al. [2015] have also confirmed that other parasites constitutes a promising field of research. Chinese black ants contain chemicals with anti-inflammatory, immunosuppressive, and renoprotective activities.

The best-studied medical application of insects is the use made of the maggots of the blow fly (Calliphoridae) that feed on necrotic tissue. In 1931, John Hopkins physician William Stevenson Baer (1872-1931) published the first truly scientific study of the maggots' effectiveness in wound care [Baer 1931 & 2011]. He first observed maggots in action during his service as a battle field surgeon in World War I. After the war he pursued his investigations on selected patients from 1919 until completion of his pioneering research in 1929. In his most compelling clinical trial, Baer introduced maggots into the open wounds of 21 patients and observed rapid debridement – doctor-speak for rapid removal of dead tissue. Moreover, it turned out that the maggots also removed pathogens from the wound sites. Within two months, all 21 of Baer's patients had been completely healed and released from hospital. Fly larvae aid in wound healing via several mechanisms [Cherniak 2010 and references herein]. Larval secretions break the larger molecules into smaller fragments; this gives rise to fibroplast aggregation and tissue repair. Moreover, the maggots feed on necrotic tissue that would otherwise form a breeding place for infections and produce antibacterial substances.

The review paper by Testa et al. [2017] also refers to the possible beneficial pharmacological effects of edible insect consumption. Several research teams have studied the possible use of edible antlions[97] and edible moths. In developing countries, the number of diabetic patients related to insulin resistance is very high. The main reason for this is that nutrient consumption patterns have shifted from a healthy traditional high-fibre, low-fat, low-calorie diet towards the consumption of calorie-rich foods, containing refined carbohydrates, fats, red meats, and low fibre. Mujahid et al. [2013] decided to study the hypoglycemic activity of the combination of bitter gourd or bitter melon (*Momordica charantia*) extract and antlion larvae (*Myrmeleon sp.*) extract in insulin-induced type 2 Diabetes Mellitus. Based on the results obtained in laboratory rat experiments, the authors concluded that the combination of bitter gourd and antlion extracts strongly reduced blood glucose levels.

Clanis bilineata is an edible and, incidentally, very beautiful moth whose larvae are widely consumed in China. In a study by Xia et al. [2013], chitooligosaccharides[98] from larvae skins were prepared and their hypolipidemic activity determined in rat experiments. The results of this study clearly indicated that chitooligosaccharides could provide suitable alterative hypolipidemic sources for humans.

Another recent study highlights the potential of the desert locust, *Schistocerca gregaria*, as an unconventional source of dietary and therapeutic sterols[99] [Cheseto et al. 2015].

Enghoff et al. [2014] suggest that the defensive secretions of millipedes act as potent insect repellents. Whether millipedes will ever become a

---

97 The antlions are a group of about 2,000 species of insect in the family Myrmeleontidae, known for the fiercely predatory habits of their larvae, which in many species dig pits to trap passing ants or other prey [Wikipedia].

98 Oligosaccharides are polymers containing a small number (~10) of simple sugars or monosaccharides; chitooligosaccharides are derived from chitin, a primary component of the exoskeletons of arthropods, such as crabs, lobsters and shrimps [Wikipedia].

99 Sterols or steroid alcohols occur naturally in plants, animals, and fungi, with the most familiar type of animal sterol being cholesterol. Cholesterol is vital to animal cell membrane structure and functions as a precursor to fat-soluble vitamins and steroid hormones [Wikipedia].

major human food remains to be seen. Nevertheless, millipedes have been shown to constitute a valuable food source for an evergrowing human population, especially in rural Africa. Additionally, millipede chemicals such as cyanide and benzoquinones for deterring (malaria transmitting) mosquitoes and for influencing *Plasmodium* and other parasites constitute a promising field of research. Tang et al. [2015] also confirmed that Chinese black ants contain chemicals that display anti-inflammatory, immunosuppressive, and renoprotective activities.

There is a buzz in the air and it is all about the human practice of eating insects

Western governments are showing an interest as there is huge potential for feeding growing numbers of humans and their livestock and for doing so in a sustainable way. We are even beginning to see restaurants with insects on the menu.

We should not ignore the expansion of the world population, neither should we be blind to the benefits of entomophagy. The conventional livestock production is land and water thirsty and this comes at a dramatic cost to our environment [Pussemier & Goeyens 2017]. Additional or alternative protein sources with lower environmental impacts should be considered good news. We still have a great deal to learn, however. Many authors have already noted the need for ad hoc studies to determine the roles of anti-nutrients and their possible implications for animal health, and one of the most interesting findings is the use of insects as starting points for developing drugs. Potential hypocholesterolemic and hypoglycemic agents, derived from some insects, will definitely require additional efforts to determine their possible uses for human health. Likewise, the antioxidant characteristic exhibited by some insects requires in-depth research before their use can be standardised in many therapies.

The review by Testa et al. [2017] shows that the use of insects as food and feed appears to have many positive aspects from the economic, environmental and nutritional points of view – a real challenge therefore as well as an opportunity for the 21st century. It is always a good time to invest in the future. It is always a good time to make a significant contribution to sustainability, to environmental quality, and to public health.

Hopefully, the financing agencies will understand these concerns. Deafness and short-sightedness are no recipes for the future. A generous and open-minded attitude is what is needed to stimulate new developments. And we must realise that eradicating insects is a move in the wrong direction!

Bibliography

Ayieko et al. [2010]. Processed products of termitesand lake flies: Improving entomophagy for food security Within the Lake Victoria region, *African Journal of Food Agriculture Nutrition and Development* 10, 2, 2085-2098

Baer [1931]. The Treatment of Chronic Osteomyelitis With the Maggot (Larva of the Blow Fly), *Journal of Bone and Joint Surgery* 13, 3, 438-475

Baer [2011]. The Classic: The Treatment of Chronic Osteomyelitis With the Maggot (Larva of the Blow Fly), *Clinical Orthopaedics and Related Research* 469, 4, 920-944

Bukkens [1997]. The nutritional value of edible insects, *Ecology of Food and Nutrition* 36, 2-4, 287-319

Cherniak [2010]. Bugs and drugs, Part 1: Insects. The "New" Alternative Medicine for the 21 st Century, *Alternative Medicine review* 15, 2, 124-135

Cheseto et al. [2015]. Potential of the Desert Locust *Schistocerca gregaria* (Orthoptera: Acrididae) as an Unconventional Source of Dietary and Therapeutic Sterols, *PLoS ONE* 10, 5, e0127171

Enghoff et al. [2014]. Millipedes as Food for Humans: Their Nutritional and Possible Antimalarial Value — A First Report, *Evidence-Based Complementary and Alternative Medicine* 2014

Holland [2013]. U.N. Urges Eating Insects; 8 Popular Bugs to Try, *National Geographic* May 14

Huang & Xiao [2003]. Study on Polyrhachis vicina, *Research and Practice of Chiness Medecines* 17, 60-62

Jarvis [2018]. The Insect Apocalypse Is Here, *The New York Times Magazine*, November 27

Ji et al. [2008]. Anaphylactic shock caused by silkworm pupa consumption in China, *Allergy* 63, 1407-1408

Jongema [2017]. *Worldwide list of recorded edible insects*, https://www.wur.nl/en/news-wur.htm

Lynd [1921]. Why we hate insects, in *The Pleasures of Ignorance*, Dossier Press, 57-63

Mujahid et al. [2013]. A combination of bitter gourd ethanolic extract with ant lion larvae aqueous extract for a blood glucose-lowering agent, *International Food Research Journal* 20, 2, 851-855

Omosoto et al. [2015]. Nutrient Composition, Mineral Analysis and Anti-nutrient Factors of Oryctes rhinoceros L. (Scarabaeidae: Coleoptera) and Winged Termites, Marcrotermes nigeriensis Sjostedt. (Termitidae: Isoptera), *British Journal of Applied Science and Technology* 8, 1, 97-106

Payne et al. [2016 A]. Are edible insects more or less 'healthy' than commonly consumed meats? A comparison using two nutrient profiling models developed to combat over- and undernutrition, *European Journal of Clinical Nutrition* 70, 285-291

Payne et al. [2016 B]. A systematic review of nutrient composition data available for twelve commercially available edible insects, and comparison with reference values, *Trends in Food Science & Technology* 47, 69-77

Pussemier & Goeyens [2017]. *AgricultureS et Enjeux de Société*, Presses Universitaires de Liège, pp. 112

Shantibala et al. [2014]. Nutritional and antinutritional composition of the five species of aquatic edible insects consumed in Manipur, India, *Journal of Insect Science* 14, 14, pp. 10

Srinroch et al. [2015]. Identification of novel allergen in edible insect, *Gryllus bimaculatus* and its cross-reactivity with *Macrobrachium* spp. Allergens, *Food Chemistry* 184, 160-166

Tang et al. [2015]. Constituents from the edible Chinese black ants (Polyrhachis dives) showing protective effect on rat mesangial cells and anti-inflammatory activity, *Food Research International* 67, 163-168

Testa et al. [2017]. Ugly but tasty: A systematic review of possible human and animal health risks related to entomophagy, *Critical Reviews in Food Science and Nutrition* 57, 17, 3747-3759

Van Huis et al. [2013]. *Edible insects: future prospects for food and feed security*, Food and Agriculture Organization of the United Nations, Rome

Xia et al. [2013]. Hypolipidemic activity of the chitooligosaccharides from Clanis bilineata (Lepidoptera), an edible insect, *International journal of biological macromolecules* 59, 96-98

Yi et al. [2017]. Extracting Tenebrio molitor protein while preventing browning: effect of pH and NaCl on protein yield, *Journal of Insects as Food and Feed* 3, 1, 21-31

Gourmet products from the sea affected by plastic debris

... Fry breadcrumbs in butter until crisp and golden. Sprinkle the breadcrumbs, black pepper, chives and parsley over the oysters. Grill under a preheated grill for 2 minutes. Serve with lemon wedges and brown bread and butter... Delicious!

The ocean is choking

Oceanic plastic pollution is a recent, anthropogenic and worldwide catastrophe. It is persistent, pervasive and pernicious. Once the plastic gets into the estuaries, shallow seas and deep oceans it causes harm to the seawater ecosystems and organisms, damages coastal economies, perturbs leisure activities, and ultimately affects human health [Plastic Oceans - http://www.plasticoceans.net]. The Great Pacific Garbage Patch for instance is a gyre of debris particles in the North and Central Pacific Ocean, west of the Californian beaches. Vast amounts of pelagic plastics and chemical sludge are caught up in oceanic currents. The garbage patch is an oceanic desert, filled with microscopic pieces of plastic, some tiny phytoplankton, and very few big fish or mammals. Fishermen and sailors seldom travel through the area, because of the scarcity of large fish and the gentle breezes. The United Nations Environment Programme report [2006], Ecosystems and Biodiversity in Deep Waters and High Seas, argues that well over 60 % of the marine world and its rich biodiversity is vulnerable and increasingly at risk. In the epipelagic upper layer[100] of the Central Pacific Ocean, there are up to 6 kilos of marine litter to every kilo of plankton.

The first scientific papers on oceanic plastic pollution appeared in the literature in the early seventies. Now, over 40 years later, Jambeck et al. [2015] have estimated that 275 million metric tons of plastic waste were generated in 192 coastal countries in 2010, with 4.8 to 12.7 million metric tons entering the ocean. The distribution and abundance of plastic debris in the world's oceans are still largely unknown; what we do know for sure is that it affects all organisms, small invertebrates as well as billfish, sharks and tunas, cetaceans and whales, and seabirds [Cózar et al. 2014].

The small size of weathered plastic debris renders it untraceable to its source and extremely difficult to remove from open ocean environments. Moreover, given the ubiquitous occurrence of micro-particles, their ingestion by marine organisms and subsequent impact on marine life is a growing cause for concern. The suspension filter-feeding species are particularly at risk. I was very unpleasantly surprised by the striking and alarming title: "Tiny bits of plastic in ocean are hurting oyster reproduction" [Monahan 2016 - http://www.sciencemag.org/news].

Bad news for lovers of highly prized crustaceans and shellfish! And yet, the internet is replete with tips on how to prepare oysters, and tasty serving suggestions.

An oyster's life is pretty simple

Eating, for example, means the oysters suck up the water, keep in the tasty plankton, and spit out the water. Unfortunately, the major drawback of their particular "eating habit" is that the oysters feed abundantly on unpalatable, tiny pieces of plastic, which happen to be the same size as their favourite unicellular plankton.

---

100 The surface layer of the ocean is known as the epipelagic zone and extends from the surface to ~200 meters. It is also known as the sunlight zone because this is where most of the visible light exists. With the light comes heat and this heat is responsible for the wide range of temperatures that occur in this zone [http://www.seasky.org/deep-sea/ocean-layers.html].

And how do oysters reproduce when they spend their adult life attached to a hard surface and are unable to move? When the water gets warmer during summer, male oysters release sperm balls that disintegrate and release the sperm upon contact with the seawater. Other male oysters, sensing this, soon follow suit and also release their sperm balls into the water. A male oyster releases hundreds of thousands of sperm balls, each containing approximately 2000 sperm. Females then bring the sperm into their shells through respiratory action and fertilize their eggs internally. The fertilized eggs develop inside the female for about 10 days before they are released into the water. The larvae then become part of the planktonic community, the community of all the small organisms that live in the water column but are incapable of swimming against a current. After approximately one month, the larvae metamorphose to their juvenile form and are ready to settle on hard surfaces. Attached baby oysters that are lucky enough to survive predation and sedimentation, will grow and eventually produce the next oyster generation.

Microplastics are the collusive bad guys

Recent research has shown that experimental micro-polystyrene exposure affects the feeding and absorption efficiency of oysters as well as their gamete quality and fecundity. Also, it impacts the growth of the offspring.

Sussarellu et al. [2016] have shown that in laboratory conditions microplastics are largely ingested by oysters. The particles end up in the oysters' guts, as a result of which the animals invest less energy in reproduction, either by disrupting their digestion or their hormone systems. Female oysters exposed to microplastics produce fewer eggs and males significantly slower sperm. Additionally, the oysters have fewer offspring that achieve maturity more slowly: strong negative effects were shown on broodstock fecundity and offspring growth at larval stages. The two explanatory hypotheses discussed in the paper, a fall in energy allocated to reproduction via interference in digestive processes and endocrine disruption, are not mutually exclusive. It is believed that, considering the strength of the impact on reproductive health indices, both forms of disruption may have occurred. The authors conclude that further investigations are still necessary: first, to provide full environmental data on small microplastics <10 μm, requiring fundamental analytical developments and second, to compare our experimental results with in situ and experimental studies that closely mimic in situ conditions.

High demand has led to a huge boost in oyster farming

The benefits of this delicacy extend well beyond their palatability. Ever since Giacomo Girolamo Casanova, the fabled 18th century playboy, is said to have eaten fifty of them every day for breakfast, these succulent bivalve molluscs have gained a reputation as aphrodisiacs. Recently, Mirza et al. [2005] discovered there may be some truth in this. Oyster flesh contains D-aspartic acid and N-methyl-D-aspartate. When fed to male and female laboratory animals, these compounds induce higher levels of the sex hormones testosterone and progesterone. On the occasion of an American Chemical Society conference, the authors concluded that the presence of D-aspartic acid and N-methyl-D-aspartate in oysters could correlate with their aphrodisiac properties.

Oysters are the darlings of a sustainable seafood movement and for good reason. When it comes to choosing sustainably farmed seafood, the oyster is pretty hard to beat. Oyster farmers have no need to use pesticides or antibiotics to keep their oysters healthy neither do the oysters need to be given feed. And above all, oysters are tasty and trendy. Worldwide, aquaculture accounts for 97 % of total oyster production. China is by far the largest producer, with 80 % of total world production, followed by Korea, Japan, the USA and the EU. The EU is self-sufficient as regards oysters and trade flows with third countries are insignificant. Intra-EU trade is also quite limited and is concentrated on flows from France to Italy. The French market is the largest for oysters in the EU.

Raw oysters: a real but dangerous delicacy

Raw oysters are considered a delicacy in many parts of the world and in many world cultures. It is however important to understand that consuming raw oysters can lead to serious illness if insufficient care is taken in making wise decisions.

The most common bacterium that causes food-borne illness associated with the consumption of raw oysters is *Vibrio vulnificus*. Infection caused by this organism can be seriously life-threatening. This is especially the case if the person who has become infected suffers from a liver disease, a weakened immune system, or diabetes.

Raw oyster consumption is associated with many persisting myths and misconceptions. These include thinking that hot sauce will kill any bacteria present in the oyster when in fact only prolonged exposure to heat and the appropriate cooking procedure will have that effect. Another common misconception is that consuming raw oysters with quantities of alcohol will help you avoid infection should bacteria be present. Still other people are convinced that only oysters that come from polluted waters can cause food poisoning. Actually, *Vibrio vulnificus* infection is not caused by pollution, but has everything to do with the type of waters in which oysters are grown, live, and thrive.

As a matter of fact, there is no infallibly safe way of consuming raw oysters. As is the case with other seafood options, it is important that oysters be thoroughly cooked or undergo commercial freezing if harmful, disease-causing bacteria are to be eliminated.

Under no circumstances should the elderly, very young children, and pregnant women consume raw oysters because of the high risk they run of developing complications due to food poisoning.

Oysters as well as many other bivalves are now in big trouble

It is high time to clean up the sea. Only then will oysters be able to live and grow in clean, healthy, plastic-free conditions.

… Fry breadcrumbs in butter until crisp and golden. Sprinkle the breadcrumbs, black pepper, chives and parsley over the microplastics.

Grill under a preheated grill for 2 minutes. Serve with lemon wedges and brown bread and butter... Delicious? Really?

Bibliography

Cózar et al. [2014]. Plastic debris in the open ocean, *Proceedings of the National Academy of Sciences* 111, 28, 10239-10244

Jambeck et al. [2015]. Plastic waste inputs from land into the ocean, *Science* 347, 6223, 768-771

Mirza et al. [2005]. *Do marine mollusks possess aphrodisiacal properties?*, presented at the 229th ACS National Meeting, in San Diego, CA, USA

Sussarellu et al. [2016]. Oyster reproduction is affected by exposure to polystyrene microplastics, *Proceedings of the National Academy of Sciences* 113, 9, 2430-2435

UNEP [2006]. Ecosystems and Biodiversity in Deep Waters and High Seas

Which is worse: a policy that costs jobs or lives?

Endocrine disrupting chemicals are simply everywhere

Endocrine disrupting chemicals (EDC) – sometimes referred to as hormonally active agents or hormone disruptors – have been identified in consumer products, electronics, furniture, personal care products, clothes, and food. Recent research has revealed that they have been detected in human blood and urine at levels known to pose health risks. EDC have been associated with an array of adverse health effects, including obesity and diabetes, female and male reproduction impairment, hormone-sensitive cancers in females, prostate cancer, thyroid disruption, and neurodevelopment and neuroendocrine effects [Gore et al. 2015].

In 2008, the Endocrine Society convened a group of experts to review the state of the science on endocrinological effects of environmental EDC. This led to a landmark Scientific Statement [Diamanti-Kandarakis et al. 2009]. EDC have been defined as the many hundreds of exogenous chemicals and mixtures of chemicals that interfere with any aspect of hormone action [Zoeller et al. 2012]. Today, there is far more conclusive evidence about whether, when, and how EDC perturb endocrine systems, including in humans [Gore et al. 2015]. For this reason, we urgently need to minimise further exposures, identify new EDC as they emerge and understand the specific underlying reaction mechanisms in order to develop methods that enable interventions whenever EDC-associated diseases occur. This is without any doubt a global challenge for the 21st century. It is especially important because new chemicals may otherwise be released on to the market without the appropriate prior safety testing. Yet, action on EDC lags behind controls on hazards such as carcinogens.

Among the known EDC, some are being closely monitored

This includes bisphenol A and its alternatives, all kinds of phthalates, parabens found in cosmetics and food materials, perfluorinated chemicals among others used in non-stick cookware, herbicides, pesticides such as the well-known atrazine and 1,1'-(2,2,2-trichloroethane-1,1-diyl) bis(4-chlorobenzene) or DDT, as well as the industrial polychlorinated biphenyls and polybrominated diethyl ethers, and their inherent impurities such as halogenated dibenzo-p-dioxins and dibenzofurans. We are exposed to a harmful chemical cocktail every single day!

Atrazine as well as DDT are banned in Europe. In the United States (US), on the other hand, if any of the community drinking water systems in the Atrazine Monitoring Program meets or exceeds the trigger value 2.6 ppb[101] for finished water or 12.5 ppb for raw water over a 90-day rolling average for 2 out of 5 consecutive years, atrazine use is banned in the water system's watershed. The DDT success story started in the 1940s, but not without some slight reservations: ... *DDT is an insecticide. It kills "bugs" of all sorts. In fact it seems destined already to take a place as the best weapon yet discovered in man's ages-long war with a hitherto unconquerable enemy, the insects. It is not a panacea; it will not kill all insects but it will kill more of them than anything else so far known. It has been rather badly presented to the public as a "miracle" insect killer and entangled with all the sentimental appeal naturally clinging to something that saved soldiers' lives and health and hastened the day of victory. That is perhaps why the public may expect too much of it now. It will undoubtedly do a great deal, but it is not a miracle; it is a chemical fact. It will kill not only insects but other cold-blooded and warm-blooded forms of life, because it is a powerful chemical. The only element of the story that smacks of the miraculous is the fact that it came along just when we needed it – and badly – to help win the war...* [Leary et al. 1946]. Strong opposition

---

101   1 ppb (parts per billion) corresponds to 1 microgram per litre.

to DDT was focused by the publication of Silent Spring [Carson 1962]. Its publication was a seminal event for the environmental movement and resulted in a large public outcry that led to a ban on the use of DDT in agriculture in the US in 1972. A worldwide ban on its agricultural use was formalised under the Stockholm Convention on Persistent Organic Pollutants [http://www.pops.int/]. Despite the clear prohibition of DDT applications, a Belgian study on organic contaminants evidenced some alarmingly high concentrations in eggs from free-range hens [Van Overmeire et al. 2006 & 2009]. The government showed very little interest. And yet, DDT is obviously persisting in the environment and is detectable in body fluids such as breast milk. Since DDT and its derivatives are present in the environment in every part of the world, in all living organisms, in the food we consume, and in our bodies where these contaminants lie dormant, every effort should be made to clean up the hot spots and to inform all the people that even minute exposures to DDT can have negative health effects.

These and many other unidentified EDC have one property in common: they are ubiquitous. EDC even build up in our bodies, where they have a negative impact on multiple endocrine endpoints and act through a huge number of different mechanisms. Furthermore, EDC often have multiple congeners and metabolites that can affect the body through various mechanisms.

A wide range of issues are thought to be crucial for improving our understanding of EDC mechanisms. Like "real" endogenous hormones[102], hormone disruptors can act at extremely low concentrations. What is more, they exhibit complex dose-response curves [Calabrese 2008; Zoeller & Vandenberg 2015]. It should also be noted that hormone levels, receptors, and physiological responses change dramatically during the life cycle. Exposures to proper levels of hormones are necessary for normal ontogenic processes[103] to occur during foetal and infant development. Too much or too little of a hormone may result in

---

102 An endogenous hormone is produced or synthesized within the organism or system [Merriam-Webster].

103 Ontogeny is the development or developmental history of an individual organism.

neurological impairments (e.g. thyroid hormone deficiency), sexual development disorders (e.g. abnormal androgen or oestrogen levels) and even death. Depending on when an individual is exposed and on the nature and concentration of the EDC, an adverse outcome may be evident either at birth or at a later stage in life [Gore et al. 2015].

Unlike endogenous hormones, EDC are not natural ligands and do not interact with hormone receptors with the same specificity and affinity. They can however interfere with the natural systems. Part of the complexity is due to exogenous chemicals being added in addition to the endogenous hormonal level. Hence, complex mixtures, dose additivity, and synergism are the norm. Even "weak" oestrogens can significantly alter hormonal action and obviously, there is no effect threshold. It is essential we stop thinking of those chemicals as acting singly. EDC act in mixtures, which in turn dramatically complicates experimental designs.

EDC also act on enzymes involved in steroidogenesis[104], steroid metabolism, and protein/peptide synthesis. They affect intracellular signalling processes and cell proliferation, growth, and death. There is convincing evidence that EDC exposures affect the expression of genes and proteins in different cells, tissues, and organs. Recent research suggests that some EDC may cause molecular epigenetic[105] changes including in the germline[106]. This latter point is extremely important because it suggests that the legacy of EDC exposures may go beyond the individual and can last even if there is no further exposure [Fowler

---

104 Steroid hormones are derivatives of cholesterol that are synthesised by a variety of tissues, most prominently the adrenal gland and gonads.

105 Conrad Waddington introduced the term *epigenetics* in the early 1940s. He defined epigenetics as "the branch of biology which studies the causal interactions between genes and their products which bring the phenotype into being." In the original sense of this definition, epigenetics referred to all molecular pathways modulating the expression of a genotype into a particular phenotype. Over the years, with the rapid growth of genetics, the meaning of the word has gradually narrowed. Epigenetics has been defined and today it is generally accepted to be "the study of changes in gene function that are mitotically and/or meiotically heritable and that do not entail a change in DNA sequence [Dupont et al. 2009].

106 The germline is the cellular lineage of a sexually reproducing organism from which eggs and sperm are derived [Merriam-Webster].

et al. 2012]. It really is worrying to think that exposed parents may be unknowingly compromising their children's and grandchildren's health.

In response to scientific evidence lobbyists have done their best to manufacture a level of doubt

Scientists who deny endocrine disruption and dismiss expert reviews are responsible for scientific inaccuracies and misrepresentations. Critics dismiss low-dose, nonlinear and non-monotonic[107] exposure–response relationships for EDC, even though the latter are well documented [Trasande 2016]. It is imperative that decision makers use science-based criteria to protect human health. It is high time they stop donning lab coats and leave the science to the scientists. EDC criteria should acknowledge the growing weight of evidence of how a chemical can disrupt hormones and generate adverse outcomes.

Yet the policy in Belgium is simply inadequate. Dr. Peter Piot, director of the prestigious London School of Hygiene and Tropical Medicine, could not understand why the federal Minister of Public Health refused to restrict the sale of alcohol and tobacco to minors. The minister's argument was that limiting sales costs jobs. "It does not cost jobs, it costs lives" says Dr. Piot in an interview with the Flemish weekly journal Knack [Vandersmissen 2016].

Alcohol is a psychoactive substance with dependence-producing properties that has been widely used in many cultures for centuries. However, as is the case for EDC and tobacco, the improper use of alcohol causes disease on a large scale, and constitutes a social and economic burden for society [WHO 2014]. Europe is facing an epidemic of liver cirrhosis among 35 to 45-year-olds – the result no doubt of a great deal of binge drinking! Alcohol-related harm is determined by the volume of alcohol consumed, by the pattern of drinking, and by the quality of the alcohol consumed. In the laboratory, alcohol is known to be a strong extraction solvent: for example, it extracts the flavour-

---

107 A monotonic function is a function which is either entirely non-increasing or non-decreasing.

lending essential oils from the slice of lemon we eagerly add to our gin tonic. Unfortunately, it also extracts the pesticides and plenty of other environmental contaminants, says Professor Jan Tytgat, toxicologist and pharmacologist at the Katholieke Universiteit Leuven.

A large number of pesticides is still used without restrictions and end up as residues in our food. So people are exposed to them on a daily basis. This is of great concern considering that low EDC doses may disrupt the normal function of the hormonal system – particularly that of young people – and ultimately lead to serious adverse effects and diseases later in life. A future mother eating a fresh fruit salad from conventional agriculture may think she is providing healthy vitamins to her future baby, but in fact she might be exposing it to a cocktail of EDC. What is more, pesticides are not the only chemicals we are exposed to in our daily lives – neither are they the only EDC. In its 2017 annual report, the European Food Safety Authority (EFSA) proudly announced that food residues in European food products were below the Maximum Residues Level, the highest level of a pesticide residue that is legally tolerated in our food [EFSA 2017]. However, EFSA failed to report that almost half the European food contains residues from at least one pesticide and about a third contains multiple pesticide residues. What EFSA did not say was that the evaluation of pesticide safety does not consider the effects of pesticide cocktails, neither does it consider the endocrine disruption potential of individual pesticides or mixtures [Matisová & Hrouzková 2012]. And no one will be held accountable if EFSA concludes that the safe levels are not so safe after all, even if this puts the human population at risk. Chemical risks are traditionally and far too often evaluated molecule by molecule, which is certainly not a good idea [Goscinny 2017].

Another frightening fact: ... *The number of substances migrating from food contact materials above the threshold of toxicological concern for genotoxic carcinogens is unknown, but might be about 100.000, i.e. the large majority has not been listed as officially approved...* [Grob et al. 2006]. The number should be given serious consideration. A great deal of attention has already been paid to food contamination by chemicals migrating from packaging materials such as mineral oil [Grob 2018], ink curing agents [Van Den Houwe et al. 2017], bisphenol A and its alternatives [Rosenmai et al. 2014; Huang et al, 2018; Hwang et al. 2018], all kinds of phthalates [Birnbaum & Schug 2013; Kim et al. 2018; Weiss et al. 2018], etc. [Muncke et al. 2017]. But what is worse is that in addition to many known chemicals, the impurities that occur in the raw materials as well as the multifold unidentified reaction products also contaminate our diet [Nerin et al. 2013]. The need to consume healthy food has never been greater!

It is abundantly clear that exposure to ubiquitous phthalates triggers unavoidable harmful consequences for the population. Two alarming conclusions were published during the preparation of this book. Phthalates have been considered obesogens and contribute to overweight and obesity in children. This was why Xia et al. [2018] evaluated the changes in urine metabolites in response to environmental phthalate exposure among overweight or obese children and investigated the metabolic mechanisms involved in the obesogenic effect of phthalates on children at puberty. They concluded that disrupted arginine and proline metabolism[108] associated with phthalate exposure might contribute to the development of overweight and obesity in school-age children. On the other hand, a systematic review of the epidemiology literature evidenced that phthalate exposure at levels seen in human populations may have male reproductive effects, more particularly exposures to bis(2-ethylhexyl) phthalate (DEHP) and dibutyl phthalate (DBP). The latter conclusion was primarily based on studies of anogenital distance, semen parameters and testosterone for DEHP and semen parameters and time to pregnancy for DBP [Radke et al. 2018].

Overall, the epidemiological literature suggests that phthalate exposure during gestation may contribute to reduced anogenital distance and neurobehavioral effects in male infants or children. Several other studies also suggest that adult phthalate exposure may be associated with poor sperm quality. In fact, these phthalate effects were

---

108   The central pathways for the biosynthesis of the amino acids arginine and proline from glutamate.

already announced by Birnbaum [2013], Birnbaum & Schug [2013], and Gennings et al. [2014].

It is no exaggeration to say that our food and beverages include some rather unexpected sources of exposure such as coffee and even drinking water for example. The production and delivery of ready-to-use consumer food require adequate packaging – often plastic containers that can withstand high temperature used for cooking. Single serve coffee containers have simplified the making of authentic Italian espresso coffee with the added benefit of reducing time and maintaining a consistent flavour for each serving. Coffee capsules can be made from different materials and are specifically designed to be used in specific brewing devices: the brewing process produces a concentrated brew generally known as coffee surrogate. Although the use of these containers has been declared to be safe by manufacturers, the actual release of contaminants in food, and in particular of EDC, deserves serious attention. De Toni et al. [2017] detected small amounts of phthalates in all the coffees; more specifically, DEHP and diisobutyl phthalate were ubiquitously present despite the high variability among the samples, whereas diethyl phthalate and di-n-butylphthalate were detected, but to a lesser extent.

In its background document for the development of World Health Organization (WHO) Guidelines for Drinking water Quality, reference is made to contaminating DEHP, i.e. the main plasticizer used in many flexible polyvinyl chloride products and in vinyl chloride co-polymer resins: ... *IARC has concluded that DEHP is possibly carcinogenic to humans (Group 2B). Induction of liver tumours in rodents by DEHP was observed at high dietary dose levels. A relationship between the occurrence of hepatocellular carcinoma and prolonged induction of peroxisomal proliferation in the liver was suggested, although the mechanism of action is still unknown. On the basis of toxicity data in experimental animals, the induction of peroxisomal proliferation in the liver seems to be the most sensitive effect of DEHP, and the rat appears to be the most sensitive species ... In 1988, JECFA evaluated DEHP and recommended that human exposure to this compound in food be reduced to the lowest level attainable. The Committee considered that this might be achieved by using alternative plasticizers or alternatives to plastic material containing*

DEHP ... Consequently, the TDI is 25 µg/kg of body weight. This yields a
guideline value of 8 µg/litre (rounded figure), allocating 1% of the TDI to
drinking-water [WHO 2003].

This puts EDC once more at the centre of our health concerns

Over the past decades there have been significant advances in our
understanding of EDC: their numbers, mechanisms of action, biological
effects, and impacts on human and wildlife health [Birnbaum 2013].
The convergence of wildlife, laboratory animal, and epidemiology data
suggests that EDC are a major cause of all kinds of diseases. Additionally,
it is now accepted that the development phase (in utero and during the
first years of life) is a very sensitive time for EDC-induced health effects.
Nevertheless, many questions remain unanswered and identifying
chemicals with endocrine activity has become a major challenge. We are
probably assessing only the "tip of the iceberg": we know that EDC are
not uniform, that they have different properties, sources, and trajectories
in the environment.

Organic chemicals are a major part of everyday life in the modern
world [Carpenter 2013]. Without any doubt, chemicals have made our
lives much easier. But, at the same time, it is important to recognise that
there have been downsides to the chemical revolution. We eat foods
that are often produced a long way from home; foods that depend on
fossil fuel to bring them to our supermarkets. Because we all like our
fruit and vegetables to look perfect, they must be treated with pesticides
and fungicides, and with herbicides to keep the weeds under control.
Since foods deteriorate over time, many fresh foods are treated with
preservatives to make them look fresh even if they are not. Food
additives are in almost every prepared product to reduce spoilage rates
and to improve colour and flavour. It is not just fruit and vegetables that
now contain chemicals that never used to be there. Nowadays, our meat
comes from animals treated with antibiotics and growth hormones. Our
fish come from waters contaminated with persistent organic pollutants
(POP). And many of the fish come from fish farms, where fish are caged
and fed food that is contaminated with chemicals. But even the wild fish

contain lipophilic POP. The same contaminants will be found in our meat, eggs and dairy products as a result of the contemporary practice of adding waste animal fats and products into the feed we give to our domestic farm animals. Moreover, whereas canned foods used to come in bare aluminium cans, the cans are now lined with bisphenol derivatives to avoid metal taste; we assume the bisphenols stay on the inside of the can, which is not the case. When we freeze our foods, we place them in plastic containers and bags. We drink from plastic bottles and cups and assume that the plasticisers – e.g. all kinds of phthalates – do not leach into the food and beverages, which again is not the case.

Even before our food reaches the kitchen, it contains many chemicals that reflect what the animals ate or were treated with. Moreover, there are chemicals on the fruits and vegetables that are only partially removed by washing. In conclusion, there is a huge variety of chemicals in the food we eat or drink, which we could call the cocktail of contaminants.

Various governmental actions are intended to prevent organic chemicals from being produced and used before they can be guaranteed not to escape into the environment, not to lead to exposure to organisms and pose significant health hazards. Such actions are however difficult and costly to put in place. Tests often consider acute lethality in animal models or study animal as well as human cells in cultures. To investigate the subtle effects on the nervous and/or immune systems and the delayed risk of developing cancer is much more difficult to achieve and there is no absolute certainty that humans will respond exactly like laboratory animals do. In a way we have all become guinea pigs.

Another major problem is that most of the testing and trying to understand the hazardous effects of chemicals in animal and cellular models focus on one chemical at a time. But in the real world we are exposed to mixtures of contaminants, to cocktails of contaminants. And to make things even more complex, most approaches assume that one chemical has only one site of action. DDT for example kills insects by blocking the action potential in insect nerves and causing paralysis. In humans, on the other hand, DDT increases the risk of a great variety of diseases, including cancer, cardiovascular disease, diabetes, nervous system effects and changes in immune system function. It is therefore highly improbable that the effects on the different organs are mediated by the same mechanism.

Today our knowledge of the development of adverse health effects through the consumption of food EDC is incomplete and much more research is required. But disregarding the current science-based criteria would be a major error. And you know what they say about an ounce of prevention being worth a ton of cure...

Bibliography

Birnbaum [2013]. State of the Science of Endocrine Disruptors, *Environmental Health Perspectives* 121, 4, A107

Birnbaum & Schug [2013]. Phthalates in our food, *Endocrine disruptors* 1, 1, e25078, pp. 6

Calabrese [2008]. Hormesis: why it is important to toxicology and toxicologists, *Environmental Toxicology and Chemistry* 27, 7, 1451-1474

Carpenter [2013]. *Effects of Persistent and Bioactive Organic Pollutants on Human Health*, Wiley & Sons, Inc., Hoboken, New Jersey, pp. 598

Carson [1962]. *Silent Spring*, Houghton Mifflin Harcourt, Boston, pp.

Diamanti-Kandarakis et al. [2009]. Endocrine-disrupting chemicals: an Endocrine Society scientific statement, *Endocrine Reviews* 30, 293-342

Dupont et al. [2009]. Epigenetics: Definition, Mechanisms and Clinical Perspective, *Seminars in Reproductive Medicine* 27, 5, 351-357

EFSA [2017]. The 2015 European Union report on pesticide residues in food, *EFSA Journal,* 15, 4, pp. 134

Fowler et al. [2012]. Impact of endocrine-disrupting compounds (EDC) on female reproductive health, *Molecular and Cellular Endocrinology* 355, 231-239

Gennings et al. [2014]. *Report to the U.S. Consumer Product Safety Commission by the Chronic Hazard Advisory Panel on Phthalates and Phthalate Alternatives*, pp. 597

Gore et al. [2015]. EDC-2: The Endocrine Society's Second Scientific Statement on Endocrine-Disrupting Chemicals, *Endocrine Reviews* 36, 6, E1-E150

Goscinny [2017]. *Enhanced screening methods for pesticides in food based on travelling-wave ion-mobility-high-resolution mass spectrometry*, PhD thesis, University of Liège, pp. 157

Grob et al. [2006]. Food contamination with organic materials in perspective: packaging materials as the largest and least controlled source? A view focusing on the European situation, *Critical Reviews in Food Science and Nutrition* 46, 529-536

Grob [2018]. Mineral oil hydrocarbons in food: a review, *Food Additives & Contaminants Part A* 35, 9, 1845-1860

Huang et al. [2018]. Bisphenol A concentrations in human urine, human intakes across six continents, and annual trends of average intakes in adult and child populations worldwide: A thorough literature review, *Science of the Total Environment* 626, 971-981

Hwang et al. [2018]. Simultaneous analysis and exposure assessment of migrated bisphenol analogues, phenol, and p-tert-butylphenol from food contact materials, *Food Additives & Contaminants Part A* 35, 11, 2270-2278

Kim et al. [2018]. Risk assessment for phthalate exposures in the elderly: A repeated biomonitoring study, *Science of The Total Environment* 618, 690-696

Leary et al. [1946]. *DDT and the Insect Problem*, McGraw-Hill Book Company Inc., New York, pp. 182

Matisová & Hrouzková [2012]. Analysis of Endocrine Disrupting Pesticides by Capillary GC with Mass Spectrometric Detection, *International Journal of Environmental Research and Public Health* 9, 3166-3196

Muncke et al. [2017]. Scientific challenges in the risk assessment of food contact materials, *Environmental health perspectives* 125, pp. 9

Nerin et al. [2013]. The challenge of identifying non-intentionally added substances from food packaging materials: A review, *Analytica Chimica Acta* 775, 14-24

Radke et al. [2018]. Phthalate exposure and male reproductive outcomes: A systematic review of the human epidemiological evidence, *Environment International* 121, 1, 764-793

Rosenmai et al. [2014]. Are structural analogues to bisphenol a safe alternatives?, *Toxicological sciences* 139, 1, 35-47

Trasande et al. [2016]. Peer-reviewed and unbiased research, rather than 'sound science', should be used to evaluate endocrine-disrupting chemicals, *Journal of Epidemiology & Community Health* 70, 11, 1051-1056

Van Den Houwe et al. [2017]. Migration of 17 Photoinitiators from Printing Inks and Cardboard into Packaged Food – Results of a Belgian Market Survey, *Packaging Technology and Science* 29, 2, 121-131

Vandersmissen [2016]. Peter Piot: 'Alcoholbeleid van Maggie De Block kost mensenlevens', *Knack* 13.12.16

Van Overmeire et al. [2006]. Chemical contamination of free-range eggs from Belgium, *Food Additives and Contaminants* 23, 11, 1109-1122

Van Overmeire et al. [2009]. Assessment of the chemical contamination in home-produced eggs in Belgium: General overview of the CONTEGG study, *Science of the Total Environment* 407, 4403-4410

Weiss et al. [2018]. Daily intake of phthalates, MEHP, and DINCH by ingestion and inhalation, *Chemosphere* 208, 40-49

WHO [2003]. *Di(2-ethylhexyl)phthalate in Drinking-water*, Background document for development of WHO Guidelines for Drinking-water Quality, pp. 13

WHO [2014]. *Global status report on alcohol and health*, pp. 376

Xia et al. [2018]. Phthalate exposure and childhood overweight and obesity: Urinary metabolomic evidence, *Environment International* 121, 1, 159-168

Zoeller et al. [2012]. Endocrine-disrupting chemicals and public health protection: a statement of principles from The Endocrine Society, *Endocrinology* 153, 4097-4110

Zoeller & Vandenberg [2016]. Assessing dose-response relationships for endocrine disrupting chemicals (EDC): a focus on non-monotonicity, *Environmental Health* 14, 42, pp. 5

If you want less packaging waste, swallow the package !

Adding thyme and/or basil to your next salad dressing will enhance its flavour

And, more importantly, it will ensure the safety of the produce. Washing lettuce in a solution containing either basil (*Ocimum basilicum*) or thyme (genus *Thymus* with ~350 species) essential oil (EO), at a concentration of 1 %, resulted in the number of *Shigella* bacteria dropping below their detection level [Bagamboula et al. 2004]. *Shigella* is the causative agent of human shigellosis. It is one of the leading bacterial causes of diarrhea worldwide and may cause significant intestinal damage. EO, the concentrated hydrophobic liquids containing volatile plant aroma compounds, as well as some of their individual components are known to exhibit antibacterial activity against foodborne pathogens [Burt 2004; Calo et al. 2015]. EO are not really oils as such since they do not contain the fatty acids that constitute what would otherwise be considered an actual oil.

Kavanaugh & Ribbeck [2012] have evidenced that thyme EO is very effective in eradicating *Pseudomonas* and *Staphylococcus aureus* biofilms, and we have just heard that recent designs and developments of EO-based, antimicrobial edible films and coatings boost meat shelf life [Kassem et al. 2011; Sánchez-Ortega et al. 2014]. Historically, culinary spices and herbs have been used for their health-enhancing properties and as food preservatives. Papyri from Ancient Egypt identified coriander, fennel, juniper, cumin, garlic and thyme as health promoting spices. Moreover, spices and herbs also played an important role in ancient Greek medical science. Hippocrates (460-377 BC) wrote about spices and herbs, including thyme. And the ancient Romans were extravagant users of spices and herbs as well.

Thyme was also a symbol of courage. The ancient Greek term for the "vital root" is *thymos* – a Homeric word meaning vitality, courage, or spirit. The phrase "the smell of thyme" became an expression of stylish praise. Thyme's association with bravery continued throughout medieval times, when it was a ritual for women to give their knights a scarf that had a sprig of thyme placed over an embroidered bee. Since the 16th century, thyme oil has been recommended for its antiseptic properties, as a mouthwash as well as for its topical application.

The antimicrobial properties of basil oil against a wide range of foodborne bacteria, yeasts and mould have long been known. Researchers successfully applied basil-based EO against several strains of pathogens [Lang & Buchbauer 2011 and references herein]. Moreover, basil EO is used as a digestive tonic. Originally, basil was native to India, Asia and Africa. It features prominently in different cuisines throughout the world, including Italian, Thai, Vietnamese and Laotian.

The name "basil" is derived from the old Greek word *basilikon*, meaning "royal", which illustrates the ancient culture's attitude towards a herb considered very noble and sacred. Traditional reverence for basil has continued in other cultures. In India, basil was cherished as an icon of hospitality, while in Italy it was a symbol of love.

In addition to their antimicrobial properties, EO are well known to retard oxidative degradation. Amiri [2012] reported that EO and some methanol extracts showed almost similar antioxidant activities when compared to butylated hydroxytoluene (BHT). BHT is a synthetic standard antioxidant, primarily used as an antioxidant food additive. Given the current worldwide interest in finding new and safe antioxidants from natural sources to prevent oxidative deterioration of foods and to minimise oxidative damage of living cells, researchers have been investigating new components, including phenolic diterpenes, phenolic carboxylic acids, biphenyls, and flavonoids extracted from rosemary, sage, oregano, and thyme [Amorati et al. 2013]. The addition of EO to edible products, either by mixing them directly or incorporating them into active packaging and edible coatings, represents an alternative to delay and prevent autoxidation.

Essential oils are complex chemical mixtures

They are usually extracted from different plant parts by steam distillation. This involves heating flowers, leaves and/or roots with steam until the oil vaporizes. Other extraction methods include water distillation, and maceration. Several factors affect both the quality and composition of the extracts, more particularly the soil composition, plant organ, vegetative cycle phase and climate. EO compositions comprise a main group which has terpene and terpenoid origin and a second consisting of aromatic and aliphatic components.

Three consulted scientific publications [Grigore et al. 2010; Boruga et al. 2014; Zengin & Baysal 2015] emphasise that all thyme-EO samples contained the monoterpene hydrocarbon, p-cymene as well as the terpenoidic phenol, thymol. The concentrations of these components always exceeded 5 %, with maximal values of 31 % for p-cymene and 48 % for thymol, respectively. The following components were identified in two of the studies: γ-terpinene, linalool, borneol, carvacrol and caryophyllene. The concentrations of the latter never exceeded 5 %.

The composition of basil EO is significantly different from that of thyme. Three studies on its chemical composition [Politeo et al. 2007; Koba et al. 2009; Joshi 2014] confirm the predominance of linalool, bergamotene, and 1,8-cineole. Two of the studies indicate the importance of eugenol. The concentrations of these components are highly variable, with highest values of 41 % being reported for linalool.

As recently as the 1960s, edible films had very little commercial use

One was familiar with the wax layers on fruit, used to prevent moisture loss and create a shiny fruit surface for aesthetic purposes. These practices were accepted long before the underlying chemistry was correctly understood and they continue today.

Why do we need edible films? Plenty of our foods come directly from nature; they can often be eaten immediately from the tree or vine, or picked up off the ground. Present-day transportation and storage requirements, however, and the advent of ever larger supermarkets and warehouse stores means that foods are usually not consumed in the orchard, field, or close to processing facilities. And it takes a great deal of time before a food product reaches the consumer's table. As the products are handled, transported and stored, they start to dehydrate, deteriorate, and lose their appearance, flavour and nutritional value. If no special measures are taken, damage can occur within days or even hours.

Any type of material used for enrobing a food product that may be eaten without further removal is considered an edible film or coating. It replaces or strengthens natural layers to prevent moisture losses, while selectively allowing for controlled exchange of important gases, such as oxygen, carbon dioxide, and ethylene, all of which are involved in the respiration and ripening processes of the plant. Films and coatings can also provide surface sterility and prevent loss of components with important nutritional value. Coating and wrapping the food items ultimately extend their shelf life. Generally, their thickness does not exceed 0.3 mm.

Essential oils included in edible coatings as the natural preservation method of oilseed kernels!

With this title the authors of the paper [Riveros et al. 2016] drew my attention to a remarkable, new area of application. The enrichment of an edible carboxymethyl cellulose (CMC) coating [Debeaufort et al. 1998] with thyme and basil EO improves the sensory stability of roasted sunflower seeds during storage. Moreover, thyme EO increases chemical stability. Sunflower seeds are very susceptible to rancidity and off-flavours developing through lipid oxidation. The purpose of the Riveros et al. study was to evaluate the combined effect of a CMC-based, edible coating – CMC is often used in food preparations under E 466 as a viscosity modifier or thickener and to stabilize emulsions – with thyme and basil EO to preserve the chemical and sensory quality parameters of roasted sunflower seeds during storage.

According to the study results, the use of CMC edible coatings improves the sensory and chemical stability of roasted sunflower seeds by hindering the lipid oxidation and subsequent development of rancid flavours. The addition of thyme or basil EO to the coating improves the sensory stability of roasted sunflower seeds during storage. And thyme EO could very well constitute an effective natural antioxidant for this food product.

It could also be used for other foods with similar physical and chemical characteristics. Hopefully, these promising results will open new vistas for additional research in related fields, and the research will gain momentum and hasten the process of change. We trust the pace of discoveries will be faster than the evolution of bacteria.

Perhaps EO will progress from being rather traditional food additives and curative agents and become widely used, efficient chemicals in food technology as well as in modern medical domains.

Can I eat some water, please?

Common plastic bottles roughly take 500-1000 years to degrade. Obviously, there is a complete mismatch between how long they are used for and how long the environment takes to decompose them. Transparent plastic bottles made from polyethylene terephthalate (PET) are recycled into new bottles, plastic containers for fruits and vegetables, textile fibres, carpets and stuffing for mattresses, jackets and sleeping bags [https://www.fostplus.be/en][109]. Tons of empty bottles however are dumped all over the country every year and many of them ultimately end up in the ocean where their disappearance is much slower than the supply of new bottles. The giant accumulation of plastic called the Great Pacific Garbage Patch contains at least 79000 tons of discarded plastic,

---

109 Fost Plus is responsible for promoting, coordinating and financing the selective collecting, sorting and recycling of household packaging waste in Belgium. On its website the cooperation claims it recycles ~680000 tonnes of packaging, or almost 90 % of all packaging that finds its way onto the Belgian market.

covering an area of ~1.6 million square km [https://abcnews.go.com/]. Of course, there is more than water bottles in the garbage patch, but they occupy much of the space. And when the fossil fuel and energy required to produce plastic bottles are factored in, it becomes clear that a sustainable solution is needed to stop or at least significantly reduce the damage to our environment. I am simply referring to what is floating around in the ocean without even speaking about tidying up the mess. Has a sustainable and satisfactory solution already been found? What about edible packaging?

"... I've slurped water. I've guzzled it. I've sipped it. But I've never eaten it. That changed when I tried my first Ooho. Ooho – or edible water – is the brainchild of Pierre Paslier and Rodrigo Garcia Gonzalez, who wanted to create an alternative to plastic bottles, the ones many of us buy every day and toss away. Their ingenious solution is an edible, seaweed-based membrane that holds water..."

This was the introduction of a striking article published by Julia Platt Leonard on April 17, 2017. Ooho is a blob-like, edible water capsule that stores a big sip of water within a biodegradable, tasteless membrane chiefly made from calcium chloride and a seaweed derivative called sodium alginate [http://www.oohowater.com/]. Alginate is a biomaterial that has numerous applications in biomedical science and engineering because of favourable highly desirable properties including biocompatibility and ease of gelation. To date, alginate hydrogels are particularly attractive in wound healing, drug delivery, and tissue engineering applications [Lee & Mooney 2012].

The water inside the membrane quenches the thirst while the membrane itself can either be swallowed or spat out. It will hardly cause any unwanted effects: it is both easily digestible and biodegradable. The inventors believe that Ooho can be the global solution to water and other "on-the-go" drinks. Much less energy (and much less CO_2 emission) is required to produce Ooho compared with PET bottles. This makes it a far more sustainable alternative to synthetic plastic bottles. Oohos are also much cheaper to manufacture compared to plastic bottles. Also, their green credentials are likely to resonate with sustainability-conscious audiences.

Paslier and Gonzalez found inspiration in a very unusual place. Their exploration began by looking at fake caviar. Oh yes, caviar is supposed to be a delicacy of salt-cured roe from wild sturgeons. Some people will do anything for a quick profit however, including producing and selling fake caviar. Fraudsters replace the real delicacy with small fish balls basically made of alginate, which is an extract from brown seaweed. Simply google "fake caviar" and you will find how to make small caviar-like balls. This of course is not meant as an invitation to set up a fake seafood business!

Drinks in edible, easily digestible membranes: it may sound futuristic, but it isn't

Edible packaging and coatings are time-honoured practices. As early as the twelfth century, citrus fruits from Southern China were preserved for the Emperor's table by placing them in boxes, pouring molten wax over them, and sending them by caravan to the North [Hardenburg 1967, Pavlath & Orts 2009]. While their quality would not have been acceptable to our modern society, the method was quite effective for its time and was used for centuries for lack of more efficient solutions.

Another example with a long history also has its roots in Asia: yuba, a very famous delicacy in some places. Soybeans are somehow connected to most Japanese delicacies, including the versatile and nutritious tofu skin, known as yuba in Japan. Yuba is the by-product of boiled soy milk. Just like the natural process we all have observed when heating cow's milk, a film (yuba) forms on the surface of boiling soy milk. While most people will discard the "icky" skins from cow's milk, the Japanese keep the yuba. They love it mainly because of its nutritional value: it contains ~55 % protein and ~25 % vegetable oil on a dry weight basis, and it is low in cholesterol [Shurtleff & Aoyagi 2012]. But yuba has also a delicate form and an easily adaptable natural flavour. Japanese people eat it from breakfast to dessert. Yuba films have been traditionally utilized for wrapping meats and/or vegetables. The good oxygen barrier capacity of soy protein isolate (SPI) films can be utilized in the manufacture of multilayer packaging, with the protein films functioning as the oxygen barrier part. SPI coatings on pre-cooked meat products offer a good protection against lipid oxidation as well as moisture loss. Moreover, incorporating additives such as antioxidants, flavouring agents, etc. can improve the overall quality of the packed food products [Buffo & Han 2005]. Also, SPI films may find applications such as micro-encapsulating agents of flavours and pharmaceuticals or in coatings of fruits, vegetables and cheese [Petersen et al. 1999]. And SPI coatings can be used on certain food products such as meat pies and cakes, which require films that are highly permeable to water vapour [Gennadios et al. 1993].

These are but a few examples of the wide range of applications. Often, we are so familiar with edible films and coatings that we do no longer think about them. Did you notice that the fruits in the bowl were treated? Did you think about the coating when you bit into the apple you were eating?

Some 25 years ago, the use of edible films and coatings as carriers of active substances was already suggested as a promising application of food packaging [Cuq et al. 1995]. They are now commonly used.

Edible packaging is not completely without its critics

Some people feel that the edible nature of the packaging defeats its main objective, which is to protect the food from dirt, chemical contaminants and germs and to improve its shelf life. And there is a psychological barrier that people need to overcome when ingesting soluble polymers (or in other words "soluble plastic"), even when they are biopolymers and were given a special flavour.

The Ooho company wants to gain its place on the market as an alternative for single-serve water bottles, generally bought in food and drink outlets. Moreover, large-scale outdoor events such as festivals, major sporting events, etc. might also be an access route to the market. But then, is water really the number one drink at the big festivals?

There are however quite significant challenges that the company must overcome before it can diffuse into the mass market. While Ooho capsules are suitable in single-serve settings, their practicality outside this particular area appears to be somewhat questionable. Unlike bottles, Oohos have a short shelf life of a few days, carry a potential choking hazard and only offer single-gulp consumption. Moreover, the fragility of the product's membrane means they are less suitable for long-distance transportation and use throughout the day, or throughout a few days (at most).

Hygiene is another problem that must be addressed since, without packaging, the membrane is exposed to chemical and microbiological contamination, which can be harmful when ingested. Food safety regulators will be concerned about the number of hands and surfaces food and beverages wrapped in edible packaging are likely to get in contact with on their way to a shop shelf and ultimately to a consumer. The company may need to provide Oohos with some protective packaging, which of course would go against their packaging-free mission. To decide that the edible packaging must be protected by additional packaging might prove self-defeating.

Ooho is an innovative product idea and will serve as an excellent, sustainable alternative to packaged water products in single-serve, on-the-go settings, especially at mass events. Outside this channel, however, the functionality of the product becomes somewhat restricted. In all likelihood, further innovation will be required if Ooho is to replace plastic water bottles on all consumption occasions.

Is edible packaging a crazy idea or a promising development?

The production of edible films is still mainly at the laboratory scale. It is also considered to be expensive compared with synthetic plastic films. Research on cost reduction and production on larger scales are necessary to promote the feasibility of commercialized edible packaging. The feasibility of commercialized systems depends on the complexity of the production process, size of investment for film production or coating equipment, potential conflicts with conventional food packaging systems, and manufacturer resistance to the use of new materials [Han & Gennadios 2005].

Additionally, food manufacturer demand is for long shelf life for products in interstate as well as international commerce. Edible packaging materials are themselves inherently susceptible to biodegradation and their protective functions are therefore stable for shorter durations than is the case for conventional packaging. The stability and safety of edible packaging under the intended storage and use conditions will therefore require further investigation.

We are well on the way to developing a new packaging concept, but more progress is needed. Scientists, industrial partners and public authorities must join forces.

Bibliography

Amiri [2012]. Essential Oils Composition and Antioxidant Properties of Three Thymus Species, *Evidence-Based Complementary and Alternative Medicine*, Article ID 728065, 8 pages

Amorati et al. [2013]. Antioxidant Activity of Essential Oils, *Journal of Agricultural and Food Chemistry* 61, 46, 10835-10847

Bagamboula et al. [2004]. Inhibitory effect of thyme and basil essential oils, carvacrol, thymol, estragol, linalool and p-cymene towards Shigella sonnei and S. flexneri, *Food Microbiology* 21, 1, 33-42

Borugă et al. [2014]. Thymus vulgaris essential oil: chemical composition and antimicrobial activity, *Journal of Medicine and Life* 7, 3, 56-60

Buffo & Han [2005]. Edible films and coatings from plant origin proteins, in Han (ed.) *Innovations in Food Packaging*, Elsevier Ltd, 277-300

Burt [2004]. Essential oils: their antibacterial properties and potential applications in foods—a review, *International Journal of Food Microbiology* 94, 223-253

Calo et al. [2015]. Essential oils as antimicrobials in food systems e A review, *Food Control* 54, 111-119

Cuq et al. [1995]. Edible films and coatings as active layers, in Rooney (ed.) *Active Food Packaging*, Springer, 111-142

Debeaufort et al. [1998]. Edible Films and Coatings: Tomorrow's Packagings: A Review, *Critical Reviews in Food Science and Nutrition* 38, 4, 299-313

Gennadios et al. [1993]. Temperature Effect on Oxygen Permeability of Edible Protein-based Films, *Journal of Food Science* 58, 212-214

Grigore et al. [2010]. Chemical composition and antioxidant activity of Thymus vulgaris L. volatile oil obtained by two different methods, *Romanian Biotechnological Letters* 15, 4, 5436-5443

Han & Gennadios [2005]. Edible films and coatings: a review, in Han (ed.) *Innovations in Food Packaging*, Elsevier Ltd, 239-262

Hardenburg [1967]. Wax related coatings for horticultural products; in *Agricultural Research Service ARS 51-15*, Washington D.C., pp. 26

Joshi [2014]. Chemical composition and antimicrobial activity of the essential oil of Ocimum basilicum L. (sweet basil) from Western Ghats of North West Karnataka, India, *Ancient Science of Life* 33, 3, 151-156

Kassem et al. [2011]. Improving the quality of beef burger by adding thyme essential oil and jojoba oil, *Archivos de zootecnia* 60, 787-795

Kavanaugh & Ribbeck [2012]. Selected Antimicrobial Essential Oils Eradicate Pseudomonas spp. And Staphylococcus aureus Biofilms, *Applied and Environmental Microbiology* 78, 11, 4057-4061

Koba et al. [2009]. Chemical composition and antimicrobial properties of different basil essential oils chemotypes from Togo, *Bangladesh Journal of Pharmacology* 4, 1-8

Lang & Buchbauer [2011]. A review on recent research results (2008–2010) on essential oils as antimicrobials and antifungals. A review, *Flavour and Fragrance Journal* 27, 13-39

Lee & Mooney [2012]. Alginate: properties and biomedical applications, *Progress in Polymer Science* 37, 1, 106-126

Leonard [2017]. *Edible water: how eating little balls of H2O could be the answer to the world's plastic pollution*, Independent, https://www.independent.co.uk/life-style/food-and-drink/edible-water-eating-ooho-skipping-rocks-lab-no-packaging-plastic-pollution-world-h20-a7682711.html

Pavlath & Orts [2009]. Edible Films and Coatings: Why, What, and How?, in Embuscado & Huber (eds.), *Edible Films and Coatings for Food Applications*, Springer, 1-23

Petersen et al. [1999]. Potential of biobased materials for food packaging, *Trends in Food Science & Technology* 10, 2, 52-68

Politeo et al. [2007]. Chemical composition and antioxidant capacity of free volatile aglycones from basil (Ocimum basilicum L.) compared with its essential oil, *Food Chemistry* 101, 379-385

Sánchez-Ortega et al. [2014]. Antimicrobial Edible Films and Coatings for Meat and Meat Products Preservation, *The Scientific World Journal*, Article ID 248935, 18 pages

Shurtleff & Aoyagi [2012]. *History of Yuba – The film that forms atop heated soymilk*, Soyinfo Center, pp.418

Zengin & Baysal [2015]. Antioxidnant and Antimicrobial Activities of Thyme and Clove Essential Oils and Application in Minced Beef, *Journal of Food Processing and Preservation* 39, 1261-1271

Are food manufacturers always fair about their products?

In several of its documents and reports the World Health Organization has recognized food contamination as a global challenge. Access to sufficient safe food is a basic necessity for human health. Ensuring food safety and security[110] in our highly globalised world represents increasingly difficult and often under-appreciated challenges for governments, commercial organizations and individuals [Fukuda 2015]. The effect of globalisation are clearly acknowledged in this statement: *… food contamination that occurs in one place may affect the health of consumers living on the other side of the planet[111]*. In fact, a vast majority of people experience a foodborne or waterborne disease at some point in their lives.

This makes the consumption of contaminated food a very serious issue. There must be enough food to meet the requirement of all human beings. And the quality of the food must be excellent for bad diets are the cause of many illnesses and may kill.

---

110 Food security has been defined by the Food and Agriculture Organization (FAO) of the United Nations (UN) as: *Food security exists when all people, at all times, have physical, social and economic access to sufficient, safe and nutritious food which meets their dietary needs and food preferences for an active and healthy life. Household food security is the application of this concept to the family level, with individuals within households as the focus of concern* [FAO 2003]. Food safety is an umbrella term that encompasses many facets of handling, preparation and storage of food to prevent illness and injury. Included under the umbrella are chemical, microphysical and microbiological aspects of food safety.

111 10 facts on food safety available on line at https://www.who.int/features/factfiles/food_safety/en/.

Chemical contamination occurs throughout the whole food chain

The scientific literature offers a goldmine of information on the adverse effects of all kinds of chemicals that clearly have no place in food and feed. This chapter does not propose to present an exhaustive list of all possible contamination problems. It does however show how large numbers of food contaminants can appear on our plates and in our mugs. We are exposed to many contaminant mixtures – to contaminant cocktails!

It is moreover vital for the purposes of food safety management to understand the nature of the contamination, its sources, and risks to the consumers, as well as the appropriate approaches to eliminate or reduce contamination levels. Sound scientific knowledge is needed to provide food products with a minimal risk of contamination. With the farm-to-fork concept in mind, Pussemier & Goeyens [in press] consider that differences between food contaminants are essentially based on their points of entry into the food chain. A first contamination source is the production environment: heavy metals, persistent organic pollutants (POP) and microorganisms present in the water, soil and air. Crop production and cattle breeding commonly make use of synthetic fertilizers, pesticides, veterinary drugs, and few additional ingredients. Harvest and post-harvest procedures, food processing and storage are other contamination routes that should not be neglected. Finally, packaging, transportation, food preparation and food consumption should be studied. A thorough evaluation of each entry route describes the food chain by considering all kinds of contaminants, whether biological or chemical in nature, naturally present in the environment or synthesised. Such a method is necessary to ensure a holistic approach, i.e. one that takes into consideration all the parameters that affect the safety and security of food products delivered to the consumers.

Agricultural land adjacent to industrial activities is vulnerable because of the risk of trace elements being accumulated into the crops. In first instance, we often think of heavy metals such as Lead (Pb), Cadmium (Cd) or Mercury (Hg). Metals such as Pb, Cd, and Hg are highly persistent in the environment due to their non-biodegradability. In addition, Cd appears to have particularly high soil-to-plant transference, making Cd exposure through the food-chain contamination an issue of concern [El-Aty et al. 2014; Satarug et al. 2017; Imseng et al. 2018]. But other metals were also found in too high concentrations. Antoniadis et al. [2019], for example, show that some soils are extremely enriched with highly toxic Thallium. Also, there were excessive concentrations of a few less expected elements, e.g. Selenium, Antimony, Molybdenum, Arsenic, Nickel as well as Chromium.

All kinds of POP are found in soils and their sources are extremely diverse: dioxins, polychlorinated biphenyls (PCB), chlorinated pesticides, but also quite a few chemicals that were recently developed such as per- and polyfluoroalkylated substances, brominated flame retardants, and synthetic musk compounds. Quite unexpectedly, it appeared that the eggs laid by privately owned hens in Belgium were significantly contaminated with dioxins, PCB and pesticides. This probably caused adverse effects on the health of consumers [Van Overmeire et al. 2009]. The fluorinated and brominated POP possibly accumulate in agricultural soils as a result of long-term regular pollutant load via sewage sludge and farmyard manure applications [Pulkrabová et al. 2019]. In spite of good intentions, there is always the possibility that farmers may have to face unexpected problems.

Pesticides – I am convinced no one knows exactly how many pesticides are used worldwide – are often characterised by strong toxicity, good stability, and biological aggregation. Their frequent and abundant use poses a huge threat to the health of humans and other organisms in the environment. Monitoring pesticide residues in foods and the environment plays an ever more important role in human health and biodiversity protection. With the continuous exploration and development of science and technology, pesticide residue detection has recently made major analytical breakthroughs [Goscinny 2017; Wang et al. 2019]. One fact should be remembered: problems are hardly ever due to one single pesticide alone but are always the result of complex mixtures of synthetic substances.

Veterinary drugs such as antimicrobials, growth promoters, non-steroidal anti-inflammatory drugs[112], tranquilizers, etc. in foods of animal origin including meat and poultry, milk and dairy products, eggs, fish and seafood, and honey [Okocha et al. 2018; Patel et al. 2018; Potes et al. 2018; von Eyken et al. 2019] have received much attention in recent years because of growing food safety and public health concerns. These drug residues may lead to immediate toxicities such as allergic reactions or longer-term health problems such as antimicrobial drug resistance, hypersensitivity reaction, carcinogenicity, mutagenicity, teratogenicity, bone marrow depression, and disruption of normal intestinal flora. Moreover, their presence in food of animal origin constitutes socioeconomic challenges for the international trade in animal and animal products. The presence of veterinary drug residues found in animal-derived foods can occur through both legal and prohibited uses. It can also occur via direct administration of the drug to the animal through the environment or in other ways with varying levels of residues depending upon animal characteristics and administration methods. The exact numbers of veterinary drugs are unknown, but in all likelihood they probably number several hundreds of different molecules.

Another extremely important and often unnoticed source of contamination is packaging materials. More than 10 years ago, Grob et al. [2006] sounded the alarm about large numbers of possibly toxic substances released from food packaging: ... *The number of substances migrating from food contact materials above the threshold of toxicological concern for genotoxic carcinogens is unknown, but might be about 100.000, i.e. the large majority has not been listed as officially approved...* So, how efficient is the European Regulation (EC) No 1935/2004 on materials and articles intended to come into contact with food? Its well-known Article 3 is very clear: *Materials and articles, including active and intelligent materials and articles, shall be manufactured in compliance with good*

---

112 Nonsteroidal anti-inflammatory drugs are more than just pain relievers; they also help reduce inflammation and lower fevers. Moreover, they prevent blood from clotting, which is good in some cases but not so in others [https://orthoinfo.aaos.org/en/treatment/what-are-nsaids/].

manufacturing practice so that, under normal or foreseeable conditions of use, they do not transfer their constituents to food in quantities which could endanger human health. This means that all possible chemicals must be identified and that their reaction products and health effects must be known. This sounds very much like a mission impossible!

The food industry sold us a line about beef

Savoury dishes, excellent wines, lovely fruit, delicious ice cream, etc. but there is more than meets the eye. What you see is not what you get because the eye cannot see the chemical contaminants. Only proper control can prevent a great deal of unpleasantness. In 1999, the naked eye did not see that a Belgian fat rendering company had contaminated tons of animal feed with dioxins. The event triggered the creation of the Federal Agency for the Control of the Food Chain. Its aim is to establish an integrated control programme to check compliance with various regulations [Maudoux et al. 2006].

The safety of our food improved both in Belgium and in Europe. There is however no such thing as zero risk. Suitable food security processes start at the farm and rules apply all the way from the farm to the dining table. They require holistic approaches: all food chain links, from the producer's farm to the consumer's table, as well as their interactions with simultaneous processes, such as waste management and recycling, must be evaluated. Sometimes, threatening contaminations or undesirable adulterations slip through the net. Unfortunately, while the food industry has made enormous progress ensuring our food is safe to eat, significantly less attention has been paid to preventing and protecting against food crime [Barnett et al. 2016].

Six years ago, the Food Safety Authority of Ireland published the news that numerous beef burgers sold by supermarkets contained horse meat. A few weeks later, beef lasagne was found to be "contaminated" with equine ingredients in 11 out of 18 products tested. "Horse gate" never posed a public health risk, but it shook confidence in the security of the food supply chain [Brooks et al. 2017] temporarily at least. Red meat sales dropped in the aftermath and for a while, retailers relied on more local suppliers. But neither of these two trends lasted. Little has changed since the scandal, because the truth is that what happened was the almost inevitable consequence of a flawed food system, not of one of its parts. The root of the problem is that farm produce is more often a commodity sold on price rather than a product bought for its distinctive value [Baggini 2018].

Sustainability is our goal

John Elkington, co-founder of the business consultancy SustainAbility introduced the term "triple bottom line" [Elkington 1994]. He referred to the business investment principle Environment, Social and Governance (ESC), which became popular in the latter part of the 20th century. ESC advocates claim that investors should target companies with a proven track record in environmental and social responsibility. Triple bottom line auditing – People, Planet and Profit, the 3P concept – was devised to measure the track record.

The People (first P) bottom line is sometimes called the social equity or human capital bottom line and is concerned with the company's stakeholders other than shareholders. The Planet (second P) bottom line or natural capital relates to the size of a company's ecological footprint and how to keep the footprint as small as possible. Conceptually, it includes lessening the environmental impact from the raw material sourcing stage to the end-of-life disposal stage. The Profit (third P) bottom line focuses on guaranteeing fair and sufficient profits to the producers.

Today, this 3P concept of sustainability is receiving increasing attention in the agricultural world [Peterson 2013]. By adopting the 3P approach, the farm tries to ensure that its current decisions will not compromise the well-being of future generations.

Fewer middlemen ensure that farmers receive a larger slice of the profit

Low-food-mile[113] systems of agricultural products restore a strong link between producers and consumers. They are opposed to both economic globalisation and standardized food production. Obviously, globalisation has profoundly changed our production methods, our transport and distribution modes as well as our purchase and consumption behaviour. In a globalised model, production is made where it is least costly and this can have a direct effect on the consumer's wallet. However, there are several risks, e.g. poor quality because of chemical contaminants and deliberate fraud, and also societal costs through the decreasing numbers of farmers and the intensive industrialisation of food production [Pussemier & Goeyens 2017].

Proximity provides consumers with a response to emerging concerns. In recent years, local markets where farmers and producers sell directly to the consumer have prospered in both rural and urban areas. The development of short food supply chains where intermediaries between farmers and consumers are removed should result in fairer remunerations for farmers and higher quality local food products, supporters say.

Consumers can easily purchase healthy products: the foods they buy are fresh and minimally processed. Since they are close to the producers, they can be assured that production methods are in line with consumer expectations of health and environmental quality. Short food supply chains also advertise the dissemination of information on the quality of the marketed foods (and drinks) and their production conditions, together with the promotion of the development of sustainable and responsible consumption [Dethier 2013]. In conclusion, by sourcing in short circuits the consumer – the first P – can take full advantage of the system, both for himself and for society in general.

---

113   An interesting concept related to carbon footprints is that of *food-miles*, the distance food travels from where it is grown to where it is ultimately purchased or consumed by the end user; the more food miles that attach to a given food, the less sustainable and the less environmentally desirable that food is – available on line at http://www.gdrc.org/uem/footprints/food-miles.html.

Additionally, short circuits contribute to the promotion of practices favourable to the environment and so are beneficial for our planet, the second P. They exert influence on the enhancement of natural heritage and landscapes, because in order to retain clients, producers will be required to maintain a welcoming and quality environment, itself an indicator of superior marketed quality products. Thus, the client-consumer can encourage the farmer to implement measures favourable to the environment, such as grassy or flowering headlands, the maintenance of a winter cover, composting biomass and manure, the reduction of input of synthetic chemicals, the development of farmland, etc. – minor interventions on the face of it, but all of them useful in reducing greenhouse gas emissions.

Finally, short supply chains enable producers to value their know-how, sell their products at fairer prices and retain customers to ensure a more stable, less fluctuating income – the third P. They offer farmers the opportunity to diversify their production and reduce their reliance on distribution chains. In many cases, it is an economic necessity and a way of ensuring the survival of the farm. Moreover, local agriculture and horticulture will contribute to significant savings of natural resources, since products are sold locally meaning fossil fuel is no longer wasted in long distance transport.

The Scottish economist Adam Smith (1723-1790) wrote more than two centuries ago: *it is the maxim of every prudent master of a family, never to attempt to make at home what it will cost him more to make than to buy.* Some believe this 250 year-old quote should still be understood as: feeding a rapidly growing world population requires long-distance trade to ensure that food is produced most efficiently at the most suitable locations.

Anyone who thinks this is clearly wrong.

However, nothing is what it seems

Thousands of individuals have now decided to reject foods that have been transported to their plates over long distances by road, air or sea. The locavores, as they are called, insist that their way is the only one to save the planet. No more environmental dangers posed by carbon-emitting imports of sugar, citrus fruits, coffee, avocados, etc. from South-America; corn, fruits, vegetables, etc. from Africa; meat and fishery products from Asia; and all those other foreign food products that now fill the shelves of our supermarkets. Is the consumption of local produce at all costs the future of ethical eating?

The concept of food-miles is not wrong; it is just too simplistic. Consider apple growing – a major fruit crop in eastern Belgium. Apples are harvested in August, September and October. Some are sold fresh and the rest is chill stored. For most of the following year, they still represent good value for fruit lovers. But by the summer of the following year, the Coxs, Braeburns etc. will have been in store for ~10 months. The amount of energy used to keep them fresh for that length of time might by then have overtaken the carbon cost of shipping them from New Zealand.

Working out carbon foot prints is extremely complicated. Food-miles alone are probably not the best way to judge whether the food we eat is sustainable. Access to uncontaminated and fraud-proof foods and beverages, guaranteeing fair prices for all stakeholders for the goods we consume, and respect for nature require efforts in many different areas. There is no one-size-fits-all solution.

Bibliography

Antoniadis et al. [2019]. Soil and maize contamination by trace elements and associated health risk assessment in the industrial area of Volos, Greece, *Environment International* 124, 79-88

Baggini [2018]. Five years on from the horsemeat scandal, our flawed food system has still not been fixed, *Prospect*, January 15, available on line at https://www.prospectmagazine.co.uk/life/five-years-on-from-the-horsemeat-scandal-our-flawed-food-system-has-still-not-been-fixed

Barnett et al. [2016]. Consumers' confidence, reflections and response strategies following the horsemeat incident, *Food Control* 59, 721-730

Brooks et al. [2017]. Four years post-horsegate: an update of measures and actions put in place following the horsemeat incident of 2013, *npj Science of Food* 1, 1, 5

Dethier [2013]. *Les circuits courts, une solution d'avenir*, Centre Permanent pour la Citoyenneté et la Participation, available on line at http://www.cpcp.be/etudes-et-prospectives/collection-au-quotidien/circuits-courts

Elkington [1994]. Towards the sustainable corporation: Win-win-win business strategies for sustainable development, *California management review* 36, 2, 90-100

El-Aty et al. [2014]. Residues and contaminants in tea and tea infusions: a review, *Food Additives & Contaminants: Part A* 31, 11, 1794-1804

Fukuda [2015]. Food safety in a globalized world, *Bulletin of the World Health Organization* 93, 212

Goscinny [2017]. *Enhanced screening methods for pesticides in food based on travelling-wave ion-mobility-high-resolution mass spectrometry*, PhD thesis, University of Liège, pp. 157

Grob et al. [2006]. Food contamination with organic materials in perspective: packaging materials as the largest and least controlled source? A view focusing on the European situation, *Critical Reviews in Food Science and Nutrition* 46, 529-536

Hanning et al. [2012]. Food Safety and Food Security, *Nature Education Knowledge* 3, 10, 9

Imseng et al. [2018]. Fate of Cd in Agricultural Soils: A Stable Isotope Approach to Anthropogenic Impact, Soil Formation, and Soil-Plant Cycling, *Environmental Science and Technology* 52, 4, 1919-1928

Maudoux et al. [2006]. Food safety surveillance through a risk based control programme: approach employed by the Belgian Federal Agency for the Safety of the Food Chain, *Veterinary Quarterly* 28, 4, 140-154

Okocha et al. [2018]. Food safety impacts of antimicrobial use and their residues in aquaculture, *Public Health Reviews* 39, 21, pp. 22

Patel et al. [2018]. Drug residues in poultry meat: A literature review of commonly used veterinary antibacterials and anthelmintics used in poultry, *Veterinary Pharmacology and Therapeutics* 41, 6, 761-789

Peterson [2013]. Sustainability: a Wicked Problem, in Kebreab (ed.) *Sustainable animal agriculture*, CAB International, Oxfordshire & Boston, 1-9

Potes et al. [2018]. Animal Health, Biosafety and Food Safety, *Archivos de Zootecnia* 68, Suplemento 1, 131-135

Pulkrabová et al. [2019]. Is the long-term application of sewage sludge turning soil into a sink for organic pollutants?: evidence from field studies in the Czech Republic, *Journal of Soils and Sediments*, 1-14

Pussemier & Goeyens [2017]. *Agricultures & Enjeux de Société*, Presses Universitaires de Liège, Agronomie Gembloux, pp. 112

Pussemier & Goeyens [in press]. *Alimentation*, Presses Universitaires de Liège, Agronomie Gembloux

Satarug et al. [2017]. Current health risk assessment practice for dietary cadmium: Data from different countries, *Food and Chemical Toxicology* 106, 430-445

Van Overmeire et al. [2009]. Assessment of the chemical contamination in home-produced eggs in Belgium: General overview of the CONTEGG study, *Science of the Total Environment* 407, 4403-4410

von Eyken et al. [2019]. Direct injection high performance liquid chromatography coupled to data independent acquisition mass spectrometry for the screening of antibiotics in honey, *Journal of Food and Drug Analysis*, in press

Wang et al. [2019]. Research progress for detection technology of pesticide residue in agricultural products and water, *Journal of Food Safety and Quality* 10, 1, 173-180

THE BETTER APPROACH CONSIDERS CHEMICAL INTERACTIONS

The fallacy of adding drug effects

... A combination of agents that is more effective than is expected from the effectiveness of its constituents is said to show synergy (other terms loosely used in the immunological literature are augmentation, potentiation, super-additivism and sometimes, quite wrongly, additivism). One less effective than expected is said to show antagonism (or depotentiation, negative interaction, negative synergy, etc.), and one no more and no less effective than expected is said to show additivism... [Berenbaum 1977].

Paracelsus' dictum heralded the modern application of the no-observed-adverse-effect level

Standard textbooks on pharmacology sometimes note that toxicology is regarded as the science of poisons. However, developing a clear definition for poison is problematic. The reason for this paradox is that, in principle, any chemical has the capacity to harm a living organism and thus to be a poison. The discovery of this conundrum is credited to the famous Renaissance physician Paracelsus (1493-1541), often referred to as the Father of Toxicology. He wrote mainly in German and a modern translation of his central dictum could be: *What is there that is not poison? All things are poison and nothing is without poison. Solely the dose determines that a thing is not a poison* [Grandjean 2016].

Paracelsus was a self-chosen academic name. He soon became known as a strong critic of old masters like Hippocrates (c. 450-c. 380 B.C.E.) and Galen of Pergamon (c. 129-c. 210) and he infuriated his academic colleagues by burning the treasured classical textbooks. In fact, he was not a particularly likeable person. Though intelligent, well-educated and deeply religious, he was also an unpredictable, stubborn, free-thinking and independent iconoclast [Grandjean 2016]. He soon aroused the anger of other physicians when he demanded that they rely on facts and not on authority alone: ... *My accusers complain that I have not entered the temple of knowledge through the right door. But which one is the truly legitimate door – Galen and Avicenna, or Nature? I have entered through the door of Nature. Her light, not the lamp of an apothecary's shop, has illuminated my way...*

The common adage in toxicology – that the dose makes the poison – is now being revisited. It implies that larger doses have greater effects than smaller ones. This makes common sense and is the core assumption underpinning regulatory testing. If the dose makes the poison, then toxicologists can safely assume that high dose tests will reveal health problems possibly caused by low dose exposures. The trouble however is that some pollutants, drugs and natural substances do not conform to this logic. Instead, they produce different effects at different levels, including violent impacts at low levels that do not occur at high doses. Sometimes the effects can even be precisely the opposite. Because regulatory testing has mostly been designed on the assumption that the dose makes the poison, it may well have missed the low dose effects.

When proceeding to identify and regulate dangerous substances government agencies usually assume that the dose makes the poison. To define exposure limits, three to five doses of a substance are tested in a laboratory. Toxicologists generally start with the highest dose chosen and lower the doses until they can identify the point where effects are no longer detectable, i.e. the dose at which the experimental animals no longer significantly differ from the controls. This safe dose is called the no-observed-adverse-effect level (NOAEL). Traditional toxicology guidance health regulations seldom advocate testing doses lower than NOAEL because of the dose makes the poison assumption.

The final acceptable level for human exposure – called the reference dose – is calculated based on the NOAEL and by adding a series of safety factors. These safety factors take into account uncertainties resulting from extrapolating animal research data to human, as well as differences in sensitivity among groups of people, such as the differences between children and adults.

Non-monotonic dose-responses go against predictable or typical dose-response patterns

In standard toxicology, as the dose increases so does the effect. Conversely, as the dose decreases so does its impact. This relationship is called a monotonic dose-response curve because effects are seen either to increase or decrease. In a monotonic curve, the effects never reverse direction. Monotonic curves can be either linear or non-linear. The key point is that the direction of the curve never changes from positive to negative or vice-versa. By contrast, non-monotonic dose-response curves (NMDRC) do change direction. Over part of the curve, response increases with dose, while over another portion it decreases as dose increases. Non-monotonic curves are often called inverted U or U curves.

For decades, investigations of endocrine disrupting chemicals (EDC) have challenged traditional concepts in toxicology, and more particularly the dose makes the poison dogma. Obviously, EDC can have effects at low doses that are not predicted by the effects at higher doses. Vandenberg et al. [2012] review two major concepts in EDC studies: low dose and non-monotonicity. Low dose effects were defined as those occurring in the range of human exposures – everybody becomes exposed to low doses over an entire lifetime, which results in higher risk in very small units [Patil et al. 2015] – or effects observed at doses below those used for traditional toxicological studies. Additionally, Vandenberg et al. [2012] provide a detailed discussion of the mechanisms responsible for generating these phenomena and illustrate that non-monotonic responses and low dose effects are remarkably common in studies of natural hormones and EDC.

The fact that low doses of EDC may influence certain human disorders is no longer a matter of conjecture, because several epidemiological studies have evidenced that environmental exposures to

EDC are associated with human diseases and disabilities. Neither can it be denied that when NMDRC occur, the effects of low doses cannot be predicted based on the effects observed at high doses. Since non-monotonicity occurs at doses or concentrations that are commonly overlooked by regulatory toxicology – for example, at doses below the toxicological NOAEL – fundamental changes in chemical testing and safety determination are now required to protect human health [Hill et al. 2018].

Vandenberg et al. [2012] encourage all scientists involved to publish data demonstrating NMDRC and low-dose effects, even if the exact mechanism of action has not yet been elucidated. This is important, because the study of EDC is a growing speciality that concerns many scientific fields. Moreover, scientists studying or regulating EDC should welcome and acknowledge the existence of NMDRC and low-dose effects, and should have access to this highly important information. They recommend expanded and generalised safety testing and surveillance to detect the potential adverse effects of this broad class of chemicals. Recent claims that crop protection products are associated with low dose effects and NMDRC raise the question whether current human exposure limits are adequate. Common sense teaches us that before new chemicals are developed, wider ranges of doses extending into the low-dose ranges should be thoroughly tested.

Total elimination may not be the best way forward

Nearly 20 years ago, Calabrese & Baldwin [2002] published a ground-breaking paper entitled *Defining Hormesis.* Since the earliest pioneering work, rapidly expanding experimental findings about the concept of hormesis have substantially contributed to a better understanding of the hormesis concept [Calabrese & Mattson 2017]. The paper by Calabrese & Baldwin [2002] provides us with a definition that addresses its historical foundations, quantitative features, and underlying evolutionary and toxicologically based mechanistic strategies. The authors argue that hormesis is an adaptive response with deviating dose-response characteristics that are induced by either direct acting or overcompensation-induced stimulatory processes at low doses.

This might for instance mean that quite a few of our ideas about toxicity may have to be modified. The term, appropriately enough, comes from the Greek word ὁρμάω, meaning rapid motion, eagerness, or excitement. According to the proponents of the hormesis theory, tiny doses of toxins in the body act in a completely different fashion from large doses and may even be beneficial. They excite the body's immune system and repair mechanisms allowing for a better response to chemical agression. Hormesis was first noted with respect to radiation. While it was clear that radiation could cause cancer, researchers also learned that extremely low doses could stimulate DNA repair and delay cancer [Sagan 1989; Wolff 1989; Feinendegen 2005]. The science is not very clear however when it comes to low dose radiation. In recent years, an increasing number of researchers – though still very much in the minority – have questioned the assumption that all radiation is bad and have begun to study whether low doses might not in fact aid in genetic repair, prevent tissue damage, etc.

Although the idea that small doses of toxins may be good for us sounds bizarre at first glance, there is actual evidence to support this assumption. Believe it or not, dioxins – perhaps the most notorious toxicants of them all – have been shown in animal experiments to have possible advantageous effects at low doses. Animals fed low doses of dioxins developed fewer liver tumours than those that had no exposure at all [Kaiser 2003]: … *Spike a rat's water with 10 parts per billion – the equivalent of 7 teaspoons of dioxin dissolved in an Olympic-sized swimming pool – and there is a 50/50 chance that the rat will die of liver cancer. Yet even tinier concentrations of dioxins fed to rats inhibit tumors...* Of course, this does not mean that we should now start thinking about taking low-dose dioxin pills. Cancer is not the only issue with dioxins and the tiny amounts that have an anti-cancer effect may still have developmental and reproductive effects. Toxins have multiple effects: EDC for example affect all hormonal systems that control the development and function of reproductive organs, regulation of metabolism, and satiety. Recent research has shown that EDC also affect physiological systems that control fat development, weight gain, and glucose levels [Thayer et al. 2012; Birnbaum 2013].

The concept *par excellence* used in toxicology to determine risk assessment and regulation is the dose-response relationship. Calabrese & Baldwin [2003] believe the dose response curve is fundamentally U-shaped, meaning it is a NMDRC. It is now clear that the toxicological community was wrong in the 1930s and 1940s when they went along with the threshold model[114]. Once it had been accepted, the model became a dogma. It provided the basis for subsequent progress and confusion, even though toxicologists, radiation biologists, pharmacologists and other scientists regularly emphasized undeniable exceptions to the so-called threshold rule, such as the effects of dioxins, numerous insecticides and herbicides, as well as pharmaceutical agents. Calabrese & Baldwin [2003] confirm that the hormetic model is not an exception to the rule: it *is* the rule.

Also, the hormetic perspective completely reshuffles the strategies and tactics used for risk communication of toxic substances for the public. Rather than expecting there may be no safe exposure level to many poisons, the risk assessment message would have to change completely. It is essential for the biomedical and clinical sciences that hormetic responses enter into the equation. Many antibiotics, antiviral and anti-tumour agents, and numerous other medicines display hormetic-like biphasic dose responses. One dose may be clinically effective, but another may be harmful. In other words, the hormetic biphasic dose-response provides not only new opportunities for clinical improvements, but also entails risks that need to be addressed. Many endogenous agonists, drugs and pollutants induce hormetic effects in humans and other animals that affect antibody production, cell migration, phagocytosis of microbes, destruction of tumour cells and other end-points. A better understanding of these phenomena would have important implications for future research and biomedical development.

---

114 Any model involving a change at some threshold value of a regressor variable, particularly models for the effects of drugs that imply zero effect below a critical level [https://stats.oecd.org/glossary/detail.asp?ID=3866].

Does this also apply to man-made xenoestrogens?

Weltje et al. [2005] discuss the similarities and differences of two types of effects that occur at low, though not at high doses of chemicals: hormesis and stimulation by oestrogenic EDC or xenoestrogens[115]. The hormetic response is a stimulatory response by an organism exposed to low doses of toxicants, while inhibition of response occurs at much higher doses. The stimulation at low doses is most probably caused by an overreaction of the organism's detoxification mechanism, which stimulates its entire metabolism. Hormesis is attributable to an array of possible working mechanisms; for many end-points it has been found to occur in a wide variety of organisms and has been documented for numerous different chemicals. It is a serious cause for concern that a huge number of chemical classes can find their way into a wide variety of food commodities. Risk factors include heavy metal contamination caused by industrial waste and pesticide accumulation due to the widespread use of chemicals in agriculture. The multitude of veterinary medicines and growth-promoting compounds used in virtually every class of livestock production can also result in animal-derived products being contaminated by drug residues. And in addition to man-made sources of contamination, chemicals derived from natural sources may also be present in food products, e.g. mycotoxins from moulds which accumulate in cereals and nuts or phycotoxins from algae found in shellfish. There are literally thousands of contaminants, and if their breakdown products, i.e. metabolites, are also taken into account, the number of contaminants increases by a factor of three or four.

Responses to natural as well as to man-made oestrogenic chemicals can be stimulated at low doses and inhibited at high doses. This is precisely what happens with hormetic agents. Oestrogenic responses

---

115 Xenoestrogens are defined as chemicals that mimic some structural parts of the physiological oestrogen compounds, therefore may act as oestrogens or could interfere with the actions of endogenous oestrogens [Słomczyńska 2008]. Environmental xenoestrogens can be divided into natural compounds (e.g. from plants or fungi), and synthetically derived agents including certain drugs, pesticides and industrial by-products [Singleton & Khan 2003].

however are induced by specific chemical substances. They exert their effects either by mimicking oestradiol (direct effects) or by interfering with the production, metabolism and transport of oestradiol and interfering with the oestrogen receptors (indirect effects). Man-made chemicals, which are classified as xenoestrogens, meet certain structural requirements that allow them to bind to the oestrogen receptors or interfere with a specific component of oestrogen biology. Weltje et al. [2005] conclude that the oestrogenic response is a specific effect – e.g. the stimulation of the female reproductive system – and one that occurs through the interaction of a chemical with the classical nuclear oestrogen receptor or via the recently discovered receptors associated with the rapid induction of second messenger systems[116]. All these chemicals mimic the natural hormone oestradiol. A typical response in female mammals is the stimulation of the uterus and other reproductive tissues at low though not at high doses. The situation in males is more complicated, with some reproductive organs being stimulated (e.g. prostate) and others inhibited (e.g. testes, epididymis and seminal vesicles).

There is definitely a difference between hormesis and responses to low doses of man-made xenoestrogens. The stimulation of performance by man-made xenoestrogens cannot be viewed as the result of defence mechanism over-reacting as in the case with hormesis. Yet, since even very low concentrations may cause responses deviating from the normal status, man-made xenoestrogens should receive special treatment in risk assessment procedures.

And let us be clear about this: man-made xenoestrogens are extremely numerous; they are omnipresent and not least in the food we eat. Every average meal is likely to contain a cocktail of pesticide and herbicide residues, additives, chemicals liberated from the packaging and food contact materials, natural toxins, etc. that might have additive or – worse still – synergistic effects.

Inconvenient as it may be, the truth is that we are exposed to complex cocktails of contaminants.

---

116 Second messengers are small intracellular molecules that mediate the effects of first messengers, i.e., neurotransmitters and hormones.

Another area of considerable concern we should pay attention to

Cocktail effects and synergistic interactions of chemicals in mixtures are an area of great concern to both the public and the regulatory authorities [Cedergreen 2014]. The main concern is whether some chemicals can enhance the effect of other chemicals and together have a much stronger effect than can be predicted by adding up the individual effects. This concern refers to two general aspects. First, there is the uncertainty as to whether we are monitoring and regulating the most harmful chemicals. But our greatest concern is whether the chemicals that are officially regulated on a single compound basis and considered safe, are in fact liable to potentiate or can be potentiated by other chemicals and so jointly have a stronger effect than predicted? The latter is called synergy and is one of the major factors that is now giving rise to substantial uncertainty regarding the proposed models for the chemical risk assessment of mixtures.

Defining synergy as two or more chemicals that together have a stronger effect than predicted implies that we can determine the joint effects of chemicals under certain assumptions. To be able to do so has been a research objective for more than a century [Fraser 1872]. Moreover, the two major concepts underlying all valid assessments of joint chemical effects were framed in the first part of the twentieth century by Loewe & Muischnek [1926] and Bliss [1939], respectively. Both these concepts assume that the chemicals do not interact chemically or affect the toxicity of each other.

But the chemicals do in fact interact – chemistry is the branch of natural science that focuses mainly on the properties of substances as well as on the changes (the chemical reactions) they undergo – and the joint effects may significantly deviate from the (additive) predictions, resulting either in synergistic or antagonistic effects. The latter are defined as those effects that are less pronounced than would be expected if the known effects of the individual substances were added together [Cedergreen et al. 2013].

Moreover, determining the experimental data is inherently subject to uncertainty (variance). For mixture studies this applies to both the toxicity data of the individual compounds used to make the model prediction as well as to the tested mixture toxicity data. As a matter of consequence, small biases or deviations from the reference models can be statistically hard to detect [Cedergreen et al. 2007]. Biologically significant and reproducible synergy can therefore be defined as a more than twofold deviation from concentration addition – a definition that was also proposed by Belden et al [2007]. In other words, the concentration predicted to yield a certain effect is more than twice the concentration actually seen to produce the proposed effect. Many of the mixtures showing ratios slightly below two most probably also include true synergists. But in order to exclude false positives and to focus on combinations where the size of the synergistic interactions might be of quantitative importance, it was suggested to set the ratio limit defining synergy at two.

Providing nutritious, abundant and safe food requires efforts

Recent foodborne illness outbreaks have highlighted food safety systems that are insufficiently effective in protecting public health. Food chain safety systems have been criticised because they only respond reactively to food safety problems and neglect their preventive functions. The complexity of the chemical contaminant cocktails in food should extend the thinking to encompass interactions between residues, additives and natural toxins when assessing food risk [Shaw 2014]. A chemical that is able to influence the way in which another chemical is absorbed, spread or eliminated in the body may result in negative effects being added so that $1 + 1 = 2$, but it can also be amplified even more so that $1 + 1 = 3$ or more.

Existing legislation concerning chemicals is generally based on our knowledge of the effects of individual substances. Only in the very small number of cases where combination effects are understood is this understanding taken into consideration when evaluating the risk of chemical substances. But we use safety factors to ensure a high level of protection (the worst-case approach) and these safety factors can to some extent provide protection against combination effects.

Recent studies introduce holistic approaches to identify the impact in terms of toxicity to humans when multiple chemical contaminants are present in the foodstuffs. Today, governmental regulatory bodies must urgently evaluate how to safeguard the population when mixtures of contaminants are found in foods. It is the duty of governments to address this outstanding critical issue [Clarke et al. 2015].

Who today can believe that we are exposed to only one contaminant at a time?

Bibliography

Belden et al [2007]. How well can we predict the toxicity of pesticide mixtures to aquatic life?, *Integrated Environmental Assessment and Management* 3, 364-372

Berenbaum [1977]. Synergy, additivism and antagonism in immunosuppression. A critical review, *Clinical and experimental immunology* 28, 1, 1-17

Birnbaum [2013]. State of the Science of Endocrine Disruptors, *Environmental Health Perspectives* 121, 4, A107

Bliss [1939]. The toxicity of poisons applied jointly, *Annals of Applied Biology* 26, 585-615

Calabrese & Baldwin [2002]. Defining hormesis, *Human & Experimental Toxicology* 21, 91-97

Calabreses & Baldwin [2003]. Toxicology rethinks its central belief, *Nature* 421, 691-692

Calabrese & Mattson [2017]. How does hormesis impact biology, toxicology, and medicine? *npj Aging and Mechanisms of Disease* 3, 13, pp. 8.

Cedergreen [2014]. Quantifying Synergy: A Systematic Review of Mixture Toxicity Studies within Environmental Toxicology, *PLOS One* 9, 5, e96580, pp. 12

Cedergreen et al. [2007]. The reproducibility of binary mixture toxicity studies. *Environmental Toxicology and Chemistry* 26, 149-156

Cedergreen et al. [2013]. Chemical Mixtures: Concepts for Predicting Toxicity, in Jorgensen (ed.) *Encyclopaedia of Environmental Management*, Taylor & Francis, New York, 2601-2610

Clarke et al. [2015]. Challenging conventional risk assessment with respect to human exposure to multiple food contaminants in food: A case study using maize, *Toxicology Letters* 238, 1, 54-64

Feinendegen [2005]. Evidence for beneficial low level radiation effects and radiation hormesis, *The British journal of radiology* 78, 925, 3-7

Fraser TR [1872]. Lecture on The Antagonism Between the Actions of Active Substances, *The British Medical Journal*, 485-487

Grandjean [2017]. Paracelsus Revisited: The Dose Concept in a Complex World, *Basic & Clinical Pharmacology & Toxicology* 119, 2, 126-132

Hill et al. [2018]. Nonmonotonic Dose–Response Curves Occur in Dose Ranges That Are Relevant to Regulatory Decision-Making, *Dose-Response* 16, 3, pp. 4

Kaiser [2003]. Sipping from a Poisoned Chalice, *Science* 302, 5644, 376-379

Loewe & Muischnek [1926]. Über kombinationswirkungen. 1. Mitteilung: Hilfsmittel der Fragestellung, *Naunyn-Schmiedebergs Archiv für Pharmakologie und experimentelle Pathologie* 114, 313-326

Patil et al. [2015]. Application environmental epidemiology to vehicular air pollution and health effects research, *Indian Journal of Occupational and Environmental Medicine* 19, 1, 8-13

Sagan [1989]. On radiation, paradigms, and hormesis, *Science* 245, 4918, 574

Shaw [2014]. Chemical residues, food additives and natural toxicants in food – the cocktail effect, *Food Science and Technology* 49, 10, 2149-2157

Singleton & Khan [2003]. Xenoestrogen exposure and mechanisms of endocrine disruption, *Frontiers in Bioscience* 8, 110-118

Słomczyńska [2008]. Xenoestrogens: mechanisms of action and some detection studies, *Polish Journal of Veterinary Sciences* 11, 3, 263-269

Thayer et al. [2012]. Role of environmental chemicals in diabetes and obesity: a National Toxicology Program workshop review, *Environmental Health Perspectives* 120, 779-789

Vandenberg et al. [2012]. Hormones and Endocrine-Disrupting Chemicals: Low-Dose Effects and Nonmonotonic Dose Responses, Endocrine Reviews, Volume 33, Issue 3, 1 June 2012, Pages 378–455

Wolff [1989]. Are radiation-induced effects hormetic?, *Science* 245, 4918, 575

Cocktail effects must be taken very seriously

Several attempts have been suggested to evaluate cumulative exposure

Europeans are consuming dozens of pesticides on a daily basis, say the Pesticide Action Network [Gore-Langton 2017]. *Toxic mixtures of pesticide residues in fruit and vegetables keep on flooding EU markets* [Pesticide Action Network 2018]. Harsh words and sentences may not be necessary, but some firmness is desirable. Quite some peer reviewed articles show there is an essential element of truth in these statements.

It is now widely accepted that humans are predominantly exposed to a wide range of chemical contaminants through their diet. A very interesting and important study [Traoré et al. 2016] studied 440 substances and identified the major mixtures to which the French adult population is exposed. Six main consumption systems and their associated contaminant mixtures were determined. The contaminant classes are heavy metals, mycotoxins, polycyclic aromatic hydrocarbons, pesticides, and xenobiotics. For example, one of the identified contaminant mixtures contains 10 pesticides, six trace elements and bisphenol A (BPA). There are 11 to 19 contaminants in each of the mixtures.

Yes, we can rightly speak of a contaminant cocktail.

In a follow-up study by Kopp et al. [2018], the genotoxic effects of the latter food contaminants were investigated using a bio-assay[117]

---

117   A bio-assay is a method for determining the concentration, purity, and/or biological

in human cell lines. Both the single molecules and the characteristic mixtures of the typical French diet were tested. Out of 49 individual organic contaminants 14 demonstrated a positive genotoxic response. Additionally, two mixtures out of six triggered significant γH2AX[118] induction after 24 hours of treatment and at concentrations for which the individual compounds did not induce any DNA damage. This suggests more than additive interactions between the chemicals. The authors conclude that two contaminant mixtures present in the French diet induce genotoxicity and mutagenicity and that the combined effects of single molecules present in the contaminant mixtures are not additive but synergistic.

The potential problems for hazard assessment related to contaminant cocktails deserve our full attention.

Mycotoxins: another class of common contaminants in food products

Mycotoxins are toxic compounds that are naturally produced by certain types of moulds[119] (fungi). Moulds that can produce mycotoxins grow on numerous foodstuffs such as cereals, dried fruits, nuts, spices, vegetables, processed flour, smoked-dried fish and dried meats [Adeyeye 2016]. Mould growth can occur either before or after harvest, during storage, on the food as well as in the food. Warm and damp conditions make the moulds proliferate. Most mycotoxins are chemically stable and food processing does not eliminate them.

Several hundreds of different mycotoxins have been identified, but the most commonly observed that constitute a health hazard for humans

---

activity of one or more substances (e.g., vitamins, hormones, plant growth factors, antibiotics, enzymes) by measuring the effect on an organism, tissue, cell, enzyme or receptor preparation and comparing it to a standard preparation.

118   γH2AX induction is widely used as a biomarker to research the fundamental biology of DNA damage and repair and to assess the risk of environmental chemicals, pollutants, radiation [Motoyama et al. 2018].

119   Moulds are multicellular fungi that form thin threadlike structures called hyphae. They are widely distributed and found wherever moisture is present; they produce secondary metabolites which are referred to as mycotoxins [Adeyeye 2016].

and livestock include aflatoxins, ochratoxin A, patulin, fumonisins, zearalenone and nivalenol/deoxynivalenol [Kabak & Dobson 2017; Kovács 2018; Gerssen et al. 2019]. Exposure to mycotoxins can happen either directly by eating infected food or indirectly through the consumption of milk and other food products from animals that were fed contaminated feed.

The effects of some food-borne mycotoxins are acute with symptoms of severe illness appearing soon after the consumption of food products contaminated with mycotoxins. Other mycotoxins occurring in food have been linked to long-term effects on health, including the induction of cancers and immune deficiency. Aflatoxins are carcinogenic to humans (Group 1); ochratoxin A is possibly carcinogenic to humans (Group 2B).

A contamination with a mycotoxin is bad enough, but the situation becomes even more disastrous when mycotoxins occur in mixtures with pesticides [Eze et al. 2018]. No one will deny that pesticide residues may also be present in our diets. Epidemiological studies have shown that we face a global decline in male fertility primarily as a result of poor sperm quality and that this is attributed to exposure to EDC in the environment, food and pharmaceutical products, including mycotoxins and pesticides. The Leydig cells[120] in the male testes are responsible for producing androgens, i.e. hormones that play major roles in male development and reproductive function. Any toxin that affects the function and morphology of the Leydig cells may therefore result in sub-fertility or infertility. The cytotoxic effects of single and binary mixtures of common mycotoxins, and of the pesticides 1,1,1-trichloro-2,2-bis(p-chlorophenyl) ethane (DDT) and 1,1-dichloro-2,2-bis(p-chlorophenyl) ethylene (DDE) on a model cell line, the MA-10 Leydig cells, were evaluated using a bio-assay after 48 h of exposure. Co-exposure with DDT or DDE enhanced the toxicity of the mycotoxins to MA-10 Leydig cells, particularly at higher concentrations.

---

120 Interstitial or Leydig cells are located in the connective tissue surrounding the seminiferous tubules. They produce testosterone, the male sex hormone responsible for the growth and maintenance of the cells of the germinal epithelium and the development of secondary sex characteristics.

Another study focused on the exceptionally adverse effects on male reproductive health following co-exposure to toxicants. These findings are particularly relevant, especially now that DDT and its degradation products such as DDE are still found in the environment as well as in our food [Van Overmeire et al. 2006 & 2009; Silva et al. 2019].

Highly profitable but illegal trade of plant protection products

Referring to the inherent dangers of pesticides does not mean that we have to ban them completely. Plant protection products – the pesticides, herbicides, and all the other "-ides" – are considered crucial tools in agriculture. They are designed to keep diseases, pests and weeds under control. The benefits that are commonly recorded include improved crop quality, reduced fungal toxins and soil disturbance, reliable production processes and less land consumption for the same amount of agricultural products [Cooper and Dobson 2007]. However, all -ides require a thorough evaluation by detailed studies before they are allowed onto the market. Since the evaluation is based on submitted data, these commercial plant production products do not come cheap. They are unique and often complex formulations that contain tens of different co-formulants – cocktails again – from different sources. The individual characteristics of a plant protection product are critical parameters that include the purity of the active substance, the identity of the solvents, emulsifiers and other co-formulants [Streloke 2018].

It is hardly surprising then that cheaper counterfeit products are becoming increasingly available. These products are unknown mixtures of chemicals that were never tested. There is almost no information concerning their formulation and consequently, nobody knows whether they are really effective or how they will react once used on crops for food and feed. Streloke [2018] calls them chemical black boxes.

The illegal trade of plant protection products is apparently a profitable business and one that generates billions of Euros worldwide. According to the European Union Intellectual Property Office (EUIPO), about 14 % of the revenue from plant protection products in the EU comes from counterfeit products (EUIPO 2017). According to a report of the United

Nations Interregional Crime and Justice Research Institute (UNICRI), other parts of the world have comparable problems, but with large disparities between different regions, some with counterfeits of up to 70 % (UNICRI 2016). The global market value of plant protection products is about 45 billion Euros. The total global revenue of illegal plant protection products can therefore be estimated at several billion Euros.

Unknown and potentially hazardous cocktails – and there is a great deal of money to be made from them – can only be regarded with a great deal of suspicion.

Food contact materials under scrupulous scrutiny

... The number of substances migrating from food contact materials above the threshold of toxicological concern for genotoxic carcinogens is unknown, but might be about 100.000, i.e. the large majority has not been listed as officially approved... [Grob et al. 2006a].

Migration from food contact materials (FCM) might be the largest source of food contamination in terms of amounts as well as of numbers of substances [Grob et al. 2006a; Grob et al. 2006b; Grob 2017]. For many years, little attention was paid to this most important issue. In the 1960s comprehensive analysis of migrants was virtually impossible because the deployment of analytical chemistry was still in an early stage. Capillary gas chromatography, high performance liquid chromatography and coupling to mass spectrometry were only available in only a small number of research laboratories. Because of the overwhelming complexity of substances migrating from FCM into foods and drinks, specific European legislation began with the raw materials used to manufacture FCM: monomers and additives. The latter were known and easily available for toxicological investigation.

It soon became abundantly clear however that checking for the major ingredients only was insufficient to protect the health of the consumers. Early European legislation was limited to the migration levels of some evaluated substances (specific migration) and, predominantly, to the gravimetrically determined overall migration. The overall migration limit (OML) was set at 60 mg per kg food – migration testing prior to the use of packaging or food contact materials is performed using food simulants – or 10 mg per square dm contact area. OML values are not molecule-specific; in other words, it is assumed that the cocktail of migrants (multiple molecules in different concentrations) should not exceed the value of 60 mg per kg food, whatever its chemical composition may be.

Because of the obvious shortcomings in the legislation, a large majority of the European Parliament voted in favour of a report that would highlight the weaknesses of what was then the current attitude towards FCM control [European Parliament 2016]. The initiative was triggered by numerous media articles about migration into packaged foods and beverages, but there would be many years of endless and often useless discussions about how to improve FCM regulation. The need for improvement was also outlined in a report ordered by the European Commission [2017].

So far the requirements, but were promising solutions generated?

Non-intentionally added substances, increasingly more unknowns

With contemporary toxicology able to detect low-dose as well as synergistic effects, and with high performance analytical chemistry fine-tuning our knowledge of the migrant substance composition, doubts arose about the capacity of OML data to sufficiently ensure packaged food safety. In the 1990s, the old approach was still being defended by arguing that the evaluation of raw materials used for manufacture would cover the other substances, since these would largely consist of reaction products, including oligomers, with structural elements corresponding or at least related to the substances used. There is however no scientific support for these arguments. And there are FCM whose migrants almost exclusively consist of reaction products, e.g. the can coatings produced from resins [Grob et al. 2010]. It is now generally accepted that reaction products do not necessarily have the same toxicological profile as starting substances for the production. Therefore, to use authorized starting substances and additives does not rule out the migration of compounds that might endanger human health. But these reaction products normally escape from controls when the safety evaluation processes merely consider the starting monomers and some additives used.

The term "non-intentionally added substances" or NIAS was introduced to magnify incomplete safety assessments. In fact, NIAS are reaction products, degradation products and impurities present in the raw materials [Aznar et al. 2012; Nerin et al. 2013]. And their numbers are huge. Let there be no doubt about this: determining the extent of NIAS will be a mammoth challenge.

The requirement laid down in Article 3 of the Framework Regulation (EC) No 1935/2004 is stricter than it seems: *Materials and articles ... do not transfer their constituents to food in quantities which could endanger human health...* This means that remediation and improvement are required whenever a problem is noted and that the possible harm by either unknown or wellknown chemicals must be ruled out on beforehand [Grob 2017]. Quite a task for the analytical chemist! To ensure the safety of a mixture migrating from the packaging materials into the foods and drinks, it must be demonstrated that none of these cocktail substances can be harmful to human health. If performed through chemical analysis, it means the detection and identification of all potentially relevant substances, including the unexpected (unknown) ones. This is called comprehensive analysis [Grob 2002; Biederman & Grob 2013]. This is hardly ever done: analyses are usually restricted to the known and potentially harmful substances selectively detected in complex mixtures of which the majority of the constituents remain unidentified and inherently uncharacterised.

Common chemical analyses are very successful in determining known substances, even at low concentrations and in complex matrices. They make use of extraction procedures adapted to these substances, selective clean-up steps, and occasional derivatisation in combination with specific chromatographic separation and detection techniques. All these steps remove sample material that does not fall within the analytical scope or render it invisible for the chromatographic separation and detection. Comprehensive analyses of largely unknown mixtures, on the other hand, are fundamentally different. They require the efficient extraction of all substances, including the unexpected ones – ranging from low to high polarity as well as from extreme acidity to strong alkalinity – minimal clean-up, chromatography covering all potential substances of interest, and detection with similar response for all substances [Biedermann & Grob 2013].

Can coatings, ingenious but harmful cocktails

Trapping can metals behind tight, ultra-thin coating screens was considered a very good idea until it turned out that molecules from the coatings were migrating into the food. Chemical migration is a simple concentration gradient-driven mass transfer and it is almost impossible to stop.

In 1996, the bisphenol A diglycidyl ether (BADGE) issue related to canned food was rocking the foundations of the established concept and caused many years of heated discussions. Not only did the migration of the starting substance BADGE into oily food exceed the legal limit by a factor of 1000 and more [Biedermann et al. 1996], the chromatograms also showed "forests of peaks" of unidentified, non-evaluated components – reaction products, degradation products, impurities? Basically, nobody was at all familiar with these unknown chemicals.

Investigations during the following years identified >100 chemical substances that were claimed to represent only a small part of the potentially health-relevant migrants [Biedermann et al. 1998; Schaefer & Simat 2004]. Evaluating only the major starting chemicals – i.e. the monomers BADGE and BPA – and blindly accepting that they "cover" all migrating reaction products and derivatives could no longer be considered a sound approach.

During the 1990s, huge migration of BADGE chlorohydrins[121] from organosol can coatings was evidenced by Biedermann et al. [1999].

---

121 Chlorohydrins are any of various organic compounds derived from diols or polyhydroxy alcohols by substitution of chlorine for part of the hydroxyl groups.

These substances caused concern because of their structural analogy to the genotoxic monochloropropanediol and other chloropropanols of relatively high biological activity. As a result, a legal limit was introduced. The Commission Regulation (EC) No 1895/2005 states that BADGE and its hydrolytic metabolites[122] are no cause for concern with regard to carcinogenicity and genotoxicity *in vivo*, and that a tolerable daily intake of 0.15 mg per kg body weight can be established for BADGE and its hydrolytic metabolites. Because of the relative dearth of data at the time on genotoxicity *in vivo* for the BADGE chlorohydrins, a specific migration limit of 1 mg per kg of food or food simulant was retained. However, Regulation (EC) No 1895/2005 points to merely five substances among the numerous reaction products migrating from can coatings. Would incorporating more substances have resulted in an unmanageable patchwork [Grob 2017]?

In 2012, enforcement requested documentation on the safety of cyclo-diBA – the cyclic product formed from BPA and BADGE during the production of epoxy resins – that is present in foods packaged in cans with internal epoxy coatings. The average concentration in canned fish amounted to 0.807 mg per kg, with a maximum of 2.64 mg per kg [Biedermann et al. 2013]. Since the industry responsible could not provide data on toxicity, toxicologists from the Swiss national authority performed an *in silico* hazard profiling. No indication of genotoxicity was found. In the EFSA guidance, a migration limit of 50 micrograms per kg food is proposed for basic ingredients. Oddly enough, a less rigorous assessment was applied for impurities such as cyclo-diBA. It was classified as Cramer Class III[123] with an exposure threshold of 90 micrograms per day and per person [EFSA 2012]. Using a conservative assumption on consumption, a migration limit of 384 micrograms per kg of canned fish was derived [Biedermann et al. 2013]. What should we think about this? Grob [2017] summarizes the situation as follows: ...

---

122   The reaction with water leads to the formation of BADGE.H_2O and BADGE.$2H_2O$.

123   The Cramer classification scheme (decision tree) is the best known approach to estimate the Threshold of Toxicological Concern (TTC) for a chemical substance based on its chemical structure. There are three Cramer classes with class III representing the most severe toxic hazard.

(1) local taxpayers financed much of the compliance work that the business operators should have done; (2) the migration limit was listed nowhere; and (3) no measures could be taken to improve the situation... This did not help at all: in 2016, the enforcement campaign by the German Chemisches und Veterinäruntersuchungsamt Münsterland-Emscher-Lippe still found the same levels of cyclo-diBA migration.

A chemical can make people sick when it is a registered FCM ingredient, but it is harmless when it is an impurity. This seems really hard to believe.

The gap between legal requirements for safety and the actual situation could not be greater. Many of the substances migrating from epoxy can coatings contained a glycidyl group, whicht was considered a genotoxic alert. The list of genotoxic carcinogens at the time included BADGE, and for these chemicals, non-detectable levels, i.e. concentrations below 10 microgram per kg, were the rule [Grob 2017].

Unfortunately, the half-baked measures that were taken at the time did not help at all. Today, some 20 years later, these coatings are still on the market with no further safety assessments. And the cocktail to which the consumer is now exposed has become somewhat larger and somewhat more dangerous.

Bibliography

Adeyeye [2016]. Fungal mycotoxins in foods: A review, *Cogent Food & Agriculture* 2, 1, pp. 11

Aznar et al. [2012]. UPLC-Q-TOF-MS analysis of non-volatile migrants from new active packaging materials, *Analytical and bio-analytical chemistry* 404, 6-7, 1945-1957

Biederman & Grob [2013]. Is comprehensive analysis of potentially relevant migrants from recycled paperboard into foods feasible?, *Journal of Chromatography A* 1272, 106-115

Biedermann et al. [1996]. Bisphenol-A-Diglycidyl Ether (BADGE) in edible-oil-containing canned foods: determination by LC-LC-fluorescence detection, *Mitteilungen aus dem Gebiete der Lebensmitteluntersuchung und Hygiene* 87, 547-558

Biedermann [1998]. Identification of migrants from coatings of food
    cans and tubes: reaction products of bisphenol-A-diglycidyl ether
    (BADGE) with phenols and solvents, *Mitteilungen aus dem Gebiete der
    Lebensmitteluntersuchung und Hygiene* 89, 529-547

Biedermann et al. [1999]. Reaction products of bisphenol-A-diglycidyl ether
    (BADGE) and bisphenol-F-diglycidyl ether (BFDGE) with hydrochloric
    acid and water in canned foods with aqueous matrix. 2. Results
    from a survey of the Swiss market, *Mitteilungen aus dem Gebiete der
    Lebensmitteluntersuchung und Hygiene* 90, 177-194

Biedermann et al. [2013]. Migration of cyclo-diBA from coatings into canned
    food: method of analysis, concentration determined in a survey and in
    silico hazard profiling, *Food and Chemical Toxicology* 58, 107–115

Cooper & Dobson [2007]. The benefits of pesticides to mankind and the
    environment, *Crop Protection* 26, 9, 1337-1348

EFSA [2012]. *Scientific opinion on exploring options for providing advice
    about possible human health risks based on the concept of Threshold of
    Toxicological Concern (TTC)*, http://www.efsa.europa.eu/en/efsajournal/
    pub/2750.htm.

EUIPO [2017]. *Die wirtschaftlichen Kosten der Verletzung von Rechten des
    geistigen Eigentums in der Pestizidindustrie*, https://euipo.europa.eu/
    tunnel-web/secure/webdav/guest/document_library/observatory/resources/
    research-and-studies/ip_infringement/study10/pesticides_sector_de.pdf

European Commission [2017]. *Mapping the industry and regulatory
    frameworks for food contact materials to support better regulation*, https://
    ec.europa.eu/jrc/en/news/mapping-industry-and-regulatory-frameworks-
    food-contact-materials-support-better-regulation

European Parliament [2016]. *Food contact materials Regulation (EC)
    1935/2004. European Implementation Assessment*, http://www.europarl.
    europa.eu/RegData/etudes/STUD/2016/581411/EPRS_STU(2016)581411_
    EN.pdf

Eze et al. [2018]. Toxicological effects of regulated mycotoxins and persistent
    organochloride pesticides: In vitro cytotoxic assessment of single and
    defined mixtures on MA-10 murine Leydig cell line, *Toxicology in Vitro* 48,
    93-103

Gerssen et al. [2019]. Food and feed safety: Cases and approaches to identify
    the responsible toxins and toxicants, *Food Control* 98, 9-18

Gore-Langton [2017]. Campaigners launch fresh attack on pesticide mixtures in EU food, *FOODnavigator.com*, https://www.foodnavigator.com/Article/2017/02/23/Campaigners-launch-fresh-attack-on-pesticide-mixtures-in-EU-food?utm_source=copyright&utm_medium=OnSite&utm_campaign=copyright

Grob [2002]. Comprehensive analysis of migrates from food-packaging materials: a challenge, *Food Additives and Contaminants* 19, 185-191

Grob [2017]. The European system for the control of the safety of food-contact materials needs restructuring: a review and outlook for discussion, *Food Additives & Contaminants Part A* 34, 9, 1643-1659

Grob et al. [2006a]. Food contamination with organic materials in perspective: packaging materials as the largest and least controlled source? A view focusing on the European situation, *Critical Reviews in Food Science and Nutrition* 46, 529-536

Grob et al. [2006b]. Food Contamination with Organic Materials in Perspective: Packaging Materials as the Largest and Least Controlled Source? A View Focusing on the European Situation, *Critical Reviews in Food Science and Nutrition* 46, 1-7

Grob et al. [2010]. Need for a better safety evaluation of food contact materials produced from resins, *Food Control* 21, 763-769

Kabak & Dobson [2017]. Mycotoxins in spices and herbs–An update, *Critical Reviews in Food Science and Nutrition* 57, 1, 18-34

Kopp et al. [2018]. Genotoxicity and mutagenicity assessment of food contaminant mixtures present in the French diet, *Environmental and Molecular Mutagenesis* 59, 8, 742-754

Kovács [2018]. Mycotoxins in the food chain, *Acta Agraria Kaposváriensis* 22, 1, 38-51

Motoyama et al. [2018]. Advantages of evaluating γH2AX induction in non-clinical drug development, *Genes and Environment* 40, 10, pp. 7

Nerin et al. [2013]. The challenge of identifying non-intentionally added substances from food packaging materials: A review, *Analytica Chimica Acta* 775, 14-24

Pesticide Action Network [2018]. Toxic mixtures of pesticide residues in fruit and vegetables keep on flooding EU markets, *Pesticide Action Network Europe*, Press Release August 1, https://www.pan-europe.info/press-releases/2018/08/toxic-mixtures-pesticide-residues-fruit-and-vegetables-keep-flooding-eu

Schaefer & Simat [2004]. Migration from can coatings: part 3. Synthesis, identification and quantification of migrating epoxy-based substances below 1000 Da, *Food Additives and Contaminants* 21, 390-405

Silva et al. [2019]. Pesticide residues in European agricultural soils – A hidden reality unfolded, *Science of the Total Environment* 653, 1532-1545

Streloke [2018]. Illegal trade of plant protection products: a highly profitable way to smuggle chemicals, *Journal of Consumer Protection and Food Safety* 13, 255-256

Traoré et al. [2016]. To which chemical mixtures is the French population exposed? Mixture identification from the second French Total Diet Study, *Food and Chemical Toxicology* 98, Part B, 179-188

UNICRI [2016]. *Illicit pesticides, organized crime and supply chain integrity*, http://www.unicri.it/in_focus/on/Illicit_Pesticides

Van Overmeire et al. [2006]. Chemical contamination of free-range eggs from Belgium, *Food Additives and Contaminants* 23, 11, 1109-1122

Van Overmeire et al. [2009]. Assessment of the chemical contamination in home-produced eggs in Belgium: General overview of the CONTEGG study, *Science of the Total Environment* 407, 4403-4410

Tackling the contaminant cocktail with a cocktail of techniques

... The chemical reactions we have studied thus far can very effectively differentiate one class of compounds from another, for example, those that can react with a base from those that do not. Full spectrometric analysis and chromatography methods provide a greater degree of discriminating power in many situations, but the lower the concentration of the analyte we wish to characterize, the greater the degree of selectivity must be. One of the remarkable aspects of the chemical reactions that occur in biological systems is their degree of selectivity, that is, the extremely limited number of compounds with which they will carry out a given reaction. This is accomplished by adding molecular shape and electron density distributions to the qualities the reactant must have in order to undergo a reaction... [Enke 2001].*

A challenge for the 21st century

Selectivity is the recommended term in analytical chemistry to express the extent to which a particular method can be used to determine specific analytes under given conditions in the presence of other components of similar behaviour. Selectivity can be graded. To avoid confusion, the use of the term specificity for the same concept is to be discouraged, since it is not correct. A method is either specific or not. Besides, very few methods are specific [Vessman et al. 2001]. Selectivity refers to the extent to which the method can be used to determine particular analytes in mixtures or matrices without interferences from other components of similar behaviour.

"Mixtures and matrices" of chemicals: never have there been so many of them!

Over the last one hundred or so years, the numbers and volumes of industrial chemicals introduced into the environment have increased exponentially. This has an irreversible anthropogenic impact on our planet Earth. Undoubtedly, chemical pollution is a serious threat [Svingen & Vinggaard 2016] and we are finding it very hard to quantify the threat because of the complexity of the problem, the large number of chemicals and living organisms involved, and the inevitable interactions (all their chemical reactions).

There is also growing evidence for the adverse health effects of many chemicals with very low concentrations, the infamous low dose effects. Moreover, adverse effects would not always be observable if the chemicals were present alone or in very small numbers. These are usually called the cocktail effects and have been demonstrated in various experimental models [Kortenkamp 2007; Relya 2009; Kerr 2017; Lukowicz et al. 2018]. Unfortunately, chemical hazards are still too often and wrongly evaluated molecule by molecule.

There are many outstanding examples in the peer reviewed scientific literature to convince us that we are exposed to cocktails of chemical contaminants. But we still favour the old risk assessment methods, based on a one-by-one approach. What we must do is look beyond the presence of one molecule or other and focus on the biological activity – the cancerogenicity, the hormonal disruption, the immunotoxic properties, the neurobehavioral disturbances, etc. – of the food and drinks we consume and of the air we breathe. The control agencies however generally highlight the only molecule whose concentration exceeds the threshold value. Yet, as explained above, it is the mixture of often very different molecules that constitutes the threat.

Sometimes, the concentration of a certain contaminant does not exceed its threshold value and yet it does make us ill because of the presence of several other chemicals. So, we should favour a control procedure that examines the cocktail effects. The time has come for a change in attitude: selectivity should no longer be our top priority.

Molecule-specific analyses are one-by-one pearls from instrumental analytical chemistry

Chromatography is a versatile separation technique that was developed in 1903 by Mikhail Semyonovich Tsvet (1872-1919), a Russian-Italian botanist. He separated plant pigments using a column of calcium carbonate. Since its discovery, chromatography has developed into a powerful laboratory tool for the separation and identification of different mixture compounds. Evidently, we are now a long way from Tsvet's first chromatographic separations. We are familiar with high performance chromatographic separation systems, sophisticated detectors such as mass spectrometers and we have significantly refined our sample preparation techniques.

A few examples will illustrate this point. The identification and quantification of the full complement of metabolites within a biological sample creates huge analytical issues with regard to metabolome[124] coverage. New liquid as well as gas chromatography techniques — e.g. higher resolution[125] instruments, novel stationary phase[126] chemistries, improved sample preparation and extraction techniques as well as new software – are rapidly emerging [Haggarty & Burgess 2017].

---

124 The metabolome is the global collection of all low molecular weight metabolites that are produced by cells during metabolism, and provides a direct functional readout of cellular activity and physiological status. It reflects the combined exogenous effects of lifestyle and environmental factors as well as the endogenous effects of genetic, developmental and pathological factors. Metabolomics is an emerging discipline that aims to profile all low molecular weight metabolites present in biological samples [Sun & Hu 2016].

125 In general, resolution is the ability to separate two signals. In terms of chromatography, this is the ability to separate two peaks (or two different molecules).

126 Chromatography is used to separate mixtures of substances into their components. All forms of chromatography work on the same principle. They all have a stationary phase (a solid or a liquid supported on a solid) and a mobile phase (a liquid or a gas). The mobile phase flows through the stationary phase and carries the components of the mixture with it. Different components travel at different rates.

Also, the detection systems are becoming increasingly efficient. Within the context of the neverending bisphenol A (BPA) saga, an improved analysis technique for BPA in water was described. Its limit of detection, usually defined as the lowest quantity or concentration of a component that can be reliably detected, amounts to 3 nanograms per litre, meaning 3 nanograms of BPA in 999.999.999.997 nanograms of water [Liu et al. 2019]. And, of course, we need extremely low detection limits since we know that very low concentrations can be hazardous.

Molecule specific analyses are very efficient and also very sophisticated. But these analyses represent a heavy burden in terms of resources and time. And by definition, they do not tell us much about the non-target analytes, molecules – sometimes very dangerous ones – whose presence is not even suspected. This is a major issue that still needs to be addressed – an issue that is and will be at the centre of research initiatives of which only a very few examples are currently available. Huysman et al. [2019] published an example of the holistic monitoring of a broad range of known and unknown plasticisers in combination with targeted quantification of alkylphenols, phthalates and primary phthalate metabolites. The hormone disruptors strike again!

Instrumental chemical analysis techniques are incredibly expensive to put into place, however, and to use them efficiently requires considerable funds and a great deal of time.

The time has come to evaluate and implement new techniques

The notorious dioxin crisis that hit Belgium in 1999 demonstrated the inadequacy of animal health and food safety provisions. Baeyens et al. [2004] summed up the situation as follows: … *Monitoring programmes, focussing on high numbers of randomly taken samples that generally show background contamination levels, appeal for fast and cheap screening methods. They are used to sift large numbers of samples for potential positives and are specifically designed to avoid false negatives (<1%) … The dioxin concentrations in samples with excessive levels need to be determined or confirmed by a confirmatory method (GC–HRMS). The latter method should provide full or complementary information, enabling* *individual dioxins and dioxin-like PCBs to be identified and quantified unequivocally at the level of interest...* This then was an unambiguous appeal for combining sophisticated and expensive physico-chemical methods – mainly chromatographic – with cheaper bio-analytical screening techniques.

In order to complement physico-chemical analyses with bio-analytical methods, biosensors and other biological approaches has been developed since the beginning of the 21th century [González-Martinez et al. 2007]. Optical biosensors for example constitute an interesting option for the analysis of many analytes since they offer numerous advantages such as high sensitivity, direct and real-time measurement in addition to multiplexing capabilities [Peltomaa et al. 2018].

Blasco & Picó [2009] emphasised the importance of applying and/ or exploring biological strategies along with deploying a chemicals-driven strategy for ecological risk assessments of pollutant mixtures. They claim that bio-assays, biosensors and effect-directed analyses to identify pollutants responsible for particular effects can no longer be neglected. They also emphasise the benefits of assessing biological monitoring in combination with chemical monitoring of priority and specific substances involved in contamination. A similar message was previously published by Denison et al. [2004]. Farré et al. [2012] review the trends in the analysis of emerging pollutants, including novel brominated flame retardants, disinfection by-products, drugs of abuse and their metabolites, hormones and endocrine disrupting chemicals (EDC), nanomaterials, organophosphate flame retardants, plasticisers, perfluorinated compounds, pharmaceuticals and personal care products, polar pesticides and their degradation and transformation products and siloxanes. The authors argue that new bio-analytical tools and the refinement of existing ones will meet most of the needs of current environmental pollution monitoring that are not or insufficiently addressed by physico-chemical methods.

Foodborne diseases, on the other hand, encompass a wide spectrum of illnesses and have become a very serious public health issue worldwide. They result from ingesting contaminated foods and drinks and range from diseases caused by a multitude of micro-organisms to those caused by chemicals. Scientists and public health agencies have developed risk assessment methods to derive safe levels of exposure for humans [Dorne et al. 2005]. An elaborate review by Dorne et al. [2009] aims at bridging the gap between chemical exposure and biological effects using analytical chemistry as a vehicle between the two. Therefore, the authors review the analytical techniques and exposure assessment applied to food contaminants together with biological and toxicological bases for setting safe exposure levels in humans. Once the food contaminants are identified and quantified, and the human exposure is determined, the biological activity (or the toxicity) of the chemicals is obtained from two basic processes, i.e. the toxicokinetics and the toxicodynamics[127]. The authors emphasise the multidisciplinarity of the approach that relies on analytical chemistry, biology, biochemistry, toxicology and quantitative modelling.

Three relatively new approaches deserve our full attention

BIO-ANALYTICAL SCREENING – The incidence of breast cancer has risen worldwide to unprecedented levels. It has now become the major form of female cancer in many parts of the world. Although several factors have been associated with the increase in breast cancer, the main identified risk factors are life exposure to hormones, including physiological variations associated with puberty, pregnancy and menopause, the use of hormonal contraceptives and/or hormone replacement therapy. Based on these facts, the exposure of the human breast to the many environmental pollutant chemicals capable of mimicking or interfering with oestrogen action is an issue that requires urgent attention. Darbre & Fernandez [2012] conclude ... *Thus, knowledge of tissue concentrations of chemicals may be inadequate because consideration must be given to their interactions, biological effects and/or potency. For these reasons, epidemiological studies on the association between environmental pollutant chemicals and breast cancer should not only identify and*

---

127 Toxicokinetics refer to what the body does to the chemical; toxicodynamics refer to what the chemical does to the body [Dorne et al. 2009].

quantify chemical residues in exposed individuals but also consider the combined effect of these compounds. The development of exposure biomarkers based on hormonal activity could provide a more accurate quantification of exposure, and the detailed analysis of samples identified by these biomarkers can reveal chemicals responsible for hormonal/ antihormonal effects...

In contrast to traditional physico-chemical analysis, bio-analytical methods provide an overall value of the sample activity, but no information about the concentrations of individual molecules. These techniques measure the biological responses, e.g. the enzymatic activity, the antigen-antibody reaction, the hormonal activity, etc. The result of this type of analysis provides information on the effect of all the molecules present (the cocktail of contaminants), without however quantifying them individually.

MULTIRESIDUE ANALYSIS – There are more than 1000 pesticides used around the world to ensure that food is not damaged or destroyed by pests[128]. Each pesticide has different properties and toxicological effects. The toxicity of a pesticide depends on its function as well as on other factors. For example, insecticides tend to be more toxic to humans than herbicides. The same chemical can have different effects at different doses; and differences can also depend on the route by which the exposure occurs, such as swallowing, inhaling, or direct contact with the skin. Risk assessments for pesticide residues in food are conducted by an independent, international expert scientific group, the Joint FAO/WHO Meeting on Pesticide Residues (JMPR). These assessments are based on all data submitted for national registrations of pesticides worldwide and on all scientific studies published in peer-reviewed journals. After assessing the risk level, the JMPR establishes limits for safe intake to ensure that the amount of pesticide residue people are exposed to through eating food over their lifetime will not result in adverse health effects. These acceptable daily intakes are used by governments and international risk managers such as the Codex

---

128 Information from https://www.who.int/news-room/fact-sheets/detail/pesticide-residues-in-food.

Alimentarius Commission (the intergovernmental standards-setting body for food) to establish maximum residue limits for pesticides in food. Codex standards are the reference for the international trade in food so that consumers everywhere can be confident that the food they buy meets the agreed standards for safety and quality, no matter where it was produced. Currently, there are Codex standards for more than 100 different pesticides.

Analyses of hundreds of different pesticides would be impossible without the most recent analytical developments. Multiresidue analyses allow us to identify and quantify several hundreds of different molecules in one single run. This could be a great victory for analytical chemistry, but one that requires a sophisticated infrastructure and specialized operators. Several recent publications [Lozowicka et al. 2016; Akutsu et al. 2018; Mebdoua 2018] and doctoral theses [Goscinny 2017] provide clear evidence for simultaneous analyses of hundreds of pesticides in a foodstuff.

That so many contaminants should still be found in human food leaves me speechless!

IN SILICO TOOLS – Finally, in silico tools or mathematical modelling methods are gaining considerable importance in toxicology, not only as a first-level screening tool, but also as a complement to in vivo and in vitro test results [Van Bossuyt et al. 2017].

Determining the toxicity of chemicals is necessary to identify their harmful effects on animals, plants, or the environment. It is also one of the main steps in drug design. Animal models have been used for a long time for toxicity testing. However, in vivo animal tests are constrained by time, ethical considerations, and cost. Computational methods for estimating the toxicity of chemicals are therefore considered useful. In silico toxicology refers to toxicity assessments that use computational methods to analyse, simulate, visualise or predict the toxicity of chemicals.

In silico toxicology aims at complementing existing toxicity tests to predict toxicity, prioritise chemicals, guide toxicity tests, and minimise late-stage failures in drugs design. The field of in silico toxicology was in continuous development through the introduction of new methods, improvement of existing ones or discarding others. Unfortunately, a method that is suited for certain types of toxicity endpoints or chemicals may not work well (or even not work at all) for others. If used correctly, in silico tools can be very effective in assessing the toxicity of chemicals.

We should not be obsessed by a single approach

Despite their undeniable usefulness, combinations of bio-analytical screening methods, multiresidue analyses and in silico techniques should not be seen as substitutes for the traditional, one-by-one approach. The identification and quantification of the great culprit, the most threatening contaminant, will always remain the first phase of successful remediation. Hence, the one-by-one approach will continue to be applied in research and development projects as well as in remediation procedures.

Obviously, the emerging new techniques offer promising new options; but considerable efforts are still needed. First and foremost, quality assurance must be guaranteed. Additionally, serious industry is eagerly awaiting the definition of standards for quality goods, i.e. the norm values, that do not harm public health (or environmental quality).

All scientific values however are subject to inherent uncertainty. Uncertainty can never be excluded, and even with the most advanced methods uncertainty will always be part of the analytical results obtained! And this must also be taken into consideration.

The inherent margin of error should never generate unethical behaviour

An analytical result is no more than the best possible compromise and 100 % certainty does simply not exist. But some industrial lobbies have constantly tried to turn this uncertainty to their advantage, to make the risk "socially acceptable". Big Tobacco industry led the way forward and many followed suit. Showing no scruples about hiding the risks associated with consuming their products, about sacrificing the health of thousands of individuals on the altar of the economic supremacy.

Several branches of the agro-chemical industry do not only corrupt the academic world; they create a new one by financing large numbers of researchers and rewarding those who arrive at "desirable" results. Doing business is about achieving success – that goes without saying. But some business concerns obstruct popular and scientific knowledge by blurring the reception of scientific signals, which constitutes an inacceptable onslaught on academic integrity. Against this show of strength, recent developments in analytical chemistry are virtually powerless.

We can only hope that international organizations such as the European Confederation of Directors' Associations will be able to agree on a code of conduct that can be shared by all businesses – a code that respects diversity and is based on principles and rules that can be applied by all [Klees 2014].

Bibliography

Akutsu et al. [2018]. Problems and solutions of polyethylene glycol co-injection method in multiresidue pesticide analysis by gas chromatography-mass spectrometry: evaluation of instability phenomenon in type II pyrethroids and its suppression by novel analyte protectants, *Analytical and bioanalytical chemistry* 410, 13, 3145-3160

Baeyens et al. [2004]. Editorial - Elucidation of sources, pathways and fate of dioxins, furans and PCBs requires performant analysis techniques, *Talanta* 63, 1095-1100

Blasco & Picó [2009]. Prospects for combining chemical and biological methods for integrated environmental assessment, *Trends in Analytical Chemistry* 28, 6, 745-757

Darbre and Fernandez [2012]. Environmental oestrogens and breast cancer: long-term low-dose effects of mixtures of various chemical combinations, *Journal of Epidemiology and Community Health* 67, 3, 203-205

Denison et al. [2004]. Recombinant cell bioassay systems for the detection and relative quantitation of halogenated dioxins and related chemicals, *Talanta* 63, 1123-1133

Dorne et al. [2005]. Human variability in xenobiotic metabolism and pathway-related uncertainty factors for chemical risk assessment: a review, *Food and Chemical Toxicology* 43, 2, 203-216

Dorne et al. [2009]. Combining analytical techniques, exposure assessment and biological effects for risk assessment of chemicals in food, *Trends in Analytical Chemistry* 28, 6, 695-707

Enke [2001]. *The Art and Science of Chemical Analysis*, John Wiley & Sons, Inc., pp. 500

Farré et al. [2012]. Achievements and future trends in the analysis of emerging organic contaminants in environmental samples by mass spectrometry and bioanalytical techniques, *Journal of Chromatography A* 1259, 86-99

González-Martinez et al. [2007]. Optical immunosensors for environmental monitoring: How far have we come?, *Analytical and Bio-analytical Chemistry* 387, 205-218

Goscinny [2017]. *Enhanced screening methods for pesticides in food based on travelling-wave ion-mobility-high-resolution mass spectrometry*, PhD, ULiège pp. 157

Haggarty & Burgess [2017]. Recent advances in liquid and gas chromatography methodology for extending coverage of the metabolome, *Current opinion in biotechnology* 43, 77-85

Huysman et al. [2019]. Targeted quantification and untargeted screening of alkylphenols, bisphenol A and phthalates in aquatic matrices using ultra-high-performance liquid chromatography coupled to hybrid Q-Orbitrap mass spectrometry, *Analytica Chimica Acta* 1049, 141-151

Kerr [2017]. A cocktail of toxins - The effects of sustained neonicotinoid exposure on bees depend on location, but are usually negative, *Science* 356, 6345, 1331-1332

Klees [2014]. *Ethique et gouvernance des entreprises*, Éditions Vanden Broele, Brugge, pp. 90

Kortenkamp [2007]. Ten Years of Mixing Cocktails: A Review of Combination Effects of Endocrine-Disrupting Chemicals, *Environmental Health Perspectives* 115 (suppl. 1), 98-105

Liu et al. [2019]. Dummy-template molecularly imprinted micro-solid-phase extraction coupled with high-performance liquid chromatography for bisphenol A determination in environmental water samples, *Microchemical Journal* 145, 337-344

Lozowicka et al. [2016]. Toxicological evaluation of multi-class pesticide residues in vegetables and associated human health risk study for adults and children, *Human and Ecological Risk Assessment: An International Journal* 22, 7, 1480-1505

Lukowicz et al. [2018]. Metabolic effects of a chronic dietary exposure to a low-dose pesticide cocktail in mice: sexual dimorphism and role of the constitutive androstane receptor, *Environmental health perspectives* 126, 6, 067007, pp. 18

Mebdoua [2018]. Pesticide Residues in Fruits and Vegetables, in Mérillon & Ramawat (eds) *Bioactive Molecules in Food*, Reference Series in Phytochemistry, Springer, Cham, pp. 39

Peltomaa et al. [2018]. Optical Biosensors for Label-Free Detection of Small Molecules, *Sensors* 18, 4126, pp. 46

Relyea [2009]. A cocktail of contaminants: how mixtures of pesticides at low concentrations affect aquatic communities, *Oecologia* 159, 2, 363-376

Sun & Hu [2016]. Chapter Three - Integrative Analysis of Multi-omics Data for Discovery and Functional Studies of Complex Human Diseases, *Advances in Genetics* 93, 147-190

Svingen & Vinggaard [2016]. The risk of chemical cocktail effects and how to deal with the issue, *Journal of Epidemiology and Community Health* 70, 322-323

Van Bossuyt et al. [2017]. Safeguarding human health using in silico tools?, *Archives of Toxicology* 91, 2705-2706

Vessman et al. [2001]. Selectivity in Analytical Chemistry (IUPAC Recommendations 2001), *Pure and Applied Chemistry* 73, 8, 1381-1386

IF WE ARE TO SEPARATE THE WHEAT FROM THE CHAFF, THEN WE NEED TO ADOPT A SOUNDER ETHICAL APPROACH

The world we live in depends on chemicals

Chemistry is everywhere

The quote *Alles ist Chemie! Nichts geht ohne Chemie* is attributed to the famous German chemist Justus von Liebig (1803-1873). Yes, everything is chemistry, and chemistry is everywhere! It even appears where we would prefer not to find it.

On September 7, 2009 when the Chemical Abstracts Service (CAS) announced the 50 millionth chemical, Professor Hideaki Chihara (1927-2013) addressed his audience with this striking but very significant comparison: ... *Achieving a milestone of 50 million small molecules registered, which I congratulate CAS for, has given us two major insights; one is that a novel substance is either isolated or synthesized every 2.6 seconds on the average during the past 12 months, day and night, seven days a week in the world, showing an almost unbelievable rate of progress in science. The other is that CAS is maintaining its reputation as the world's largest compilation of substance information that every scientist in the world relies on either directly or indirectly...* It is no longer surprising that the numbers and volumes of chemicals in the environment are increasing at an unprecedented rate.

The chemical sector is very important if not essential, but it does not always have a good image. Air, water and land pollution, ecological disasters, and diseases are obvious ills for which chemistry is directly or indirectly responsible. The anthropogenic impact on our planet has become almost irreversible: chemical pollution has now become a considerable concern and even a real threat [Svingen & Vinggaard

2016]. But let us not forget its positive role in the treatment of diseases and disabilities, in the creation of new consumer products (textiles, construction materials, packaging, toys, sporting goods, electronic devices, etc.), in the purification of air and water, in the manufacture of cosmetics, detergents and fuels, in agro-food biotechnologies, and in many more areas of human activity. Obviously, there are two sides to every coin. Although chemistry has an essential role to play in the quality of our lives, it can be a source of misfortune and disaster.

Chemistry is at the crossroads of contemporary sciences (biotechnology, nanotechnology, information technology and cognitive science). Sound chemical research is carried out in university laboratories and also in industrial companies. It increases our knowledge and yet, contrary to what we commonly think, there is another form of research! In contrast to real sound science – as intended by the French experimental biologist, science writer, and philosopher Jean Rostand (1894-1977), who once wrote in *Pensées d'un Biologiste* [Rostand 1939]: *Science, la seule façon de servir les hommes sans se rendre complice de leurs passions* (Science, the only way to serve men without being complicit with their passions) – there is a criminal science that attempts to undermine existing knowledge and whose aim is to create doubt[129]. It is the science that is meant to obscure the truth and delay the actions of regulatory authorities [Proctor 2011].

Many chemicals that ushered in the modern industrial era are pollutants

Chemical pollution has not gone unnoticed. The scientific detective story and bestseller *Our stolen future*, published by Theo Colborn (1927-2014) et al. in 1996, popularised the theory that synthetic chemicals, with properties similar to natural hormones, can affect all animals including humans. Colborn's book tells about the origin and development of the

---

129 In writing *Golden Holocaust: Origins of the Cigarette Catastrophe and the Case for Abolition,* Robert Proctor has drawn on the tobacco industry's formerly secret internal documents to describe how the industry caused the epidemic of tobacco use and the resulting massive burden of premature mortality and morbidity.

hypothesis of endocrine disrupting chemicals (EDC), and bisphenol A (BPA) has a central role herein. It was considered sufficiently important by the then Vice President of the United States Al Gore to write the preface to the book, and sufficiently disturbing for a large part of the chemical industry to severely discredit its message. Are our fertility, intelligence and survival being threatened? Today, this question has become more legitimate than ever.

Modern analytical chemistry has found traces of BPA in food crops, waste water, many everyday consumer goods, dental amalgam and even thermal paper [Geens et al. 2011]. Long regarded as safe at low exposures, several new scientific results show that even (very) low levels of BPA disrupt hormonal activity [Hirabayashia & Inoueb 2011].

Discovered at the end of the 19th century, BPA appeared around the 1930s while searching for synthetic hormones to prevent spontaneous abortion. But BPA has never been present in pharmacies because distilbene was immediately preferred as an alternative. In the 1950s, BPA reappeared when a synthetic method was developed for polycarbonate (PC) production. PC is a polymer formed by the polycondensation of BPA and phosgene. Since the 1960s, the plastics industry has been using BPA for the production of PC (~70 % of all synthesized BPA) and epoxy resins (~30 %). Global production of BPA easily exceeds 3 million tonnes per year, of which ~1 million are produced and consumed in the European Union. The presence of BPA in our immediate environment is therefore not at all surprising. The potential for human exposure to BPA is high with more than 95 % of the western populations showing traces of BPA in their urine [Calafat et al. 2005]. It is also quite alarming that the global trends are not falling. Moreover, an increasing number of publications argue that there is a correlation between environmental exposure to BPA and adverse health effects in humans [Rochester 2013].

It was not until 2016 that the European Chemicals Agency (ECHA) listed BPA as a substance of very high concern (SVHC) since its endocrine disrupting properties cause serious human health problems. So, BPA reached a level of concern equivalent to carcinogenic[130] substances,

---

130 Carcinogenic substances are capable of causing a malignant tumor.

mutagens[131] or reprotoxic[132] chemicals. However, the classification of BPA as SVHC only concerns the hazard which this substance in itself represents. It does not elaborate on the risks incurred by the population at current levels of exposure. The issue is still at the centre of a disagreement between the French Agency for Food Safety, Environment and Labour (ANSES) and the European Food Security Agency (EFSA). ANSES claims there is a risk of cancer, especially of breast cancer, while EFSA considers the risk to be non-existent for the general population. The latter agency strongly believes that exposure to BPA does not exceed the allowable daily intake of 4 µg of BPA per kg body weight, but has announced a new risk study whose general purpose will be to assess whether new scientific evidence (published after 2013 and not yet evaluated) still supports the current value.

Twenty years and more after the publication of *Our Stolen Future* we continue to almost exclusively monitor BPA even though we have been using alternative chemicals for a long time. ANSES has identified 73 alternatives to BPA [ANSES 2013]. Some are currently used in European markets, others are still in the research and development phase. Additionally, the list of 73 alternatives to BPA is not considered exhaustive and it is quite conceivable that other products have been introduced since 2013 to replace BPA. Two common alternatives, bisphenol S (BPS) and bisphenol F (BPF), are widely used. They have been detected in many consumer products, such as personal care products, paper products, and packaged or canned foods. Ideally, the alternatives to a chemical of concern should be inert or at least much less toxic than the parent compound. However, many chemical alternatives currently on the market have not been tested. Surely this is reason enough to be alarmed! Several researchers have already concluded that the hormonal activities of BPS and BPF are similar to those of BPA and that they do not constitute safe alternatives [Eladak et al. 2015; Rochester & Bolden 2015; Warner & Flaws 2018].

---

131   Mutagens are capable of changing the genome of an organism.

132   Reprotoxic substances affect the fertility and/or development of the child to born.

Quite a few companies are now advertising *BPA-free* consumer products. Indeed, manufacturers have gradually stopped using BPA as many studies have increasingly linked the substance to early puberty and increased breast and prostate cancer. Recent research however has also linked the common alternatives to BPA to these risks. So why not consider all bisphenols as a class in health assessments? In 2007, Kortenkamp wrote ... *that accumulated evidence seriously undermines continuation with the customary chemical-by-chemical approach for risk assessment of endocrine disruptors...* It is therefore strongly recommended to consider group regulation of endocrine disruptor classes [Kortenkamp 2007]. Since everyone is obviously exposed to a huge and complex cocktail of chemical contaminants, it is important to characterize co-exposure patterns and take into account exposures to BPA analogues.

Cunning and dangerous disinformation distorts the truth

As a result of subtle and deceitful propaganda by the tobacco industry smoking rates among young Singaporeans remain relatively high despite the strong and well-established tobacco control policy in force in Singapore [van der Eijk et al. 2018]. Menthol[133] tobacco products became popular among young Singaporeans in the early 1980s, largely as a result of a health-consciousness trend among young people – tobacco companies used menthol to encourage smoking among young people – and the common misperception that menthol tobacco products were safer. That was a blatant lie: *certain flavouring such as menthol together with nicotine would synergistically increase harmful effects* [Cho et al. 2018]. Still menthol tobacco products comprise ~48 % of Singapore's total tobacco market. They are the key to the tobacco industry's strategy of recruiting and retaining young smokers in Singapore.

Banning the sale of menthol tobacco products would be an important part of preventing smoking among Singapore's younger generation,

---

133 Menthol is a cyclic monoterpene alcohol possessing well-known cooling characteristics and a residual minty smell of the oil remnants from which it was obtained. Because of these attributes it is one of the most important flavouring additives [Kamatou et al. 2013].

conclude van der Eijk et al. [2018]. And anyway, there is a continuing need to protect the next generation of children in Singapore as well as anywhere else in the world from starting to smoke and from second-hand smoke exposure. Investigation into these issues remains highest priority [Edwards 2018].

Another striking case study: the recent literature review by Muneret et al. [2018] evidenced that organic farming can enhance pest control and suggested that organic farming offers a way of reducing the use of synthetic pesticides for the management of animal pests and pathogens without increasing their levels of infestation. Organic farming using no synthetic pesticides is considered to be very beneficial to biodiversity [Pussemier & Goeyens 2017]. In other words, the levels of natural processes supported by biodiversity, such as the natural regulation of pests, are higher in this context than under so-called conventional systems that are characterised by the elevated consumption of pesticides. Muneret et al. [2018] performed a meta-analysis of the scientific literature demonstrating the impact of organic practices on the stimulation of natural regulation and control of pests. They found that the natural regulation of pests was better in organic than in conventional agriculutre for all types of pests. Organic agriculture practices stimulate the natural processes responsible for pest regulation. They offer interesting perspectives to reduce the use of synthetic fungicides or insecticides without however raising the levels of pathogen or pest infestation.

... We must feed ourselves. To do that, we must have agricultural chemicals. Without them, the world population will starve... said Norman Ernest Borlaug (1914-2009), who won the Nobel Peace Prize for breeding high-yielding grains. Obviously, we should take this assumption with the proverbial grain of salt.

Can a company – let alone a multinational – consider lying to consumers?

Can a company misrepresent and conceal relevant information? Is it prepared to confirm the safety of tobacco, glyphosate, sweet foods (see also the chapter *From exceptional delicacy to addiction*), BPA-based plastics, etc.? Needless to say that in a society where everyone would be liable to do so, the very notion of promise would lose its meaning. Not only would promises become meaningless, but if everyone lied the possibility of reliable exchange of information would disappear. This is why lying is immoral.

On n'aime jamais tant la vérité que lorsque le mensonge fait loi (We never love truth so much as when lies know no law). For the eminent biologist Jean Rostand, to distance oneself from the real meaning of the truth constitutes a serious threat to humanity. Jean Rostand did not conceive truth as a dogma imposed by whatever authority; he saw truth as an effort to show perspicacity concerning the correctness of judgment and an agreement between what one thinks, says and does (or writes): *… la seule vérité à laquelle je crois en est une qui se découvre lentement, graduellement, péniblement, et qui imperceptiblement s'augmente chaque jour (the only truth I believe in is one that slowly, gradually, painfully, and imperceptibly increases each day)…* He was firmly convinced that true science, because it is aware of its own ignorance, seeks to find truth not out of a desire for power, but out of love [Rostand 1953]. It is shocking when chemical industry groups, not content with corrupting the academic world, actually create an academic world of their own by funding large numbers of researchers and rewarding those who arrive at results that best suit the interests of the industry [Proctor 2011]. No one can claim that this is done out of love for truth. Of course, businesses aim to be successful, but some are determined to obstruct popular and scientific knowledge by blurring the reception of scientific messages, which amounts to an uparalleled frontal attack on academic integrity.

Our parents and grandparents did not have to deal with the harmful effects of chemical mixtures as we do. It has only been these last 60 years that chemical cocktails have demanded our full attention. The publication in 1962 of Rachel Carson's *Silent Spring* and many other critical novels and analyses of the dark side of our society became milestones in the resistance to the rampant use of chemicals. Admittedly, the production, distribution, processing, packaging and consumption of food have changed considerably. Technological developments have altered the relationship between humans and their food products. Globalisation, urbanisation, social and political developments in commerce as well as our health and consumption patterns have greatly modified the way we use our foods. They determine the extremely complex landscape of technological and social relations relating to food as well as the ethical issues they raise.

Human food chains; successions of complex matters

Food production affects people's lives to the benefit of organisations and the well-being of the whole planet. It is not always easy to say what is right and what is wrong when it comes to food production. Many ethical questions can be raised concerning the food supply chain, including the agricultural production [Olsen & Bánáti 2014].

Climate change, animal welfare, fair trade, the health and safety of employees and consumers, fair market remuneration for employees and their social rights, economic sustainability and the use of natural resources are all important aspects of food production, processing and marketing. So there can be no doubt that food can also generate a conflict of values. In terms of food security the extent of ethics is of paramount importance. Food security exists when all people have the physical, social and economic opportunity at all times to obtain sufficient, healthy and nutritious food to meet their dietary needs and preferences for a healthy and active life [FAO 1996] – to this day a still largely unfulfilled ideal!

Some explanation of the concept of ethics may be helpful at this stage. The free dictionary defines ethics as a philosophical study of the moral value of human behaviour and the principles that should govern them[134]. And the Larousse dictionary defines it as the set of moral principles that underpin people's behaviour[135]. Morality and ethics are not synonyms, but there is a strong link between these concepts.

For Pierre Klees, morality consists of rules of conduct that ensure the smooth running of society; it brings together judgments about what is good and what is wrong. Ethics, on the other hand, is a reflection on

---

134   https://www.thefreedictionary.com/ethics

135   https://www.larousse.fr/dictionnaires/francais/%C3%A9thique/31389

the foundations of morality. It is a reasoned theory about values, moral attitudes and moral judgments [Klees 2014]. André Comte-Sponville says that morality defines absolute values (Good and Evil) and imposes commandments, whereas ethics is inspired by relative values (the good and the bad), formulates recommendations and tends towards happiness and wisdom [Bolle De Bal 2005]. Ethics are by definition individual and dynamic.

Moreover, global change, globalisation, recent technological developments, etc. confront us with several problems that are not necessarily governed by our cultural traditions and conceptions. Ethics allow us to define new standards to be morally respected. In addition, we also note the emergence of sector ethics or applied ethics [Klees 2014] such as bioethics, environmental ethics, food ethics, etc.

Olsen & Bánáti [2014] wrote: ... *Ethics is different from following the law. A good system of law incorporates many ethical standards, but law can also deviate from what is ethical ... Ethics is not the same as following culturally accepted norms either ... Ethics is not science, feelings or religions...* Although science allows us to raise cattle of the double-muscles type – the animals are not significantly heavier, but they have more muscle and less fat, which leads to an increase in yield at slaughter – we can ask ourselves whether this is indeed ethical from the point of view of animal welfare.

Since ethics is not based on feelings, religion, law, accepted social practice or science, what is then its basis? Some ethicists see ethical action as producing the greatest quantity of goods while doing the least harm possible to those concerned, i.e. the customers, the employees, the shareholders, the community and the environment. It is called the utilitarian approach and deals with the consequences by trying to increase the goods (e.g. to produce enough food to stop hunger) and reduce the damage (e.g. to avoid serious public health hazards and prevent the degradation of environmental quality).

Others suggest that ethical action is one that protects and respects the moral rights of those concerned. It is called the rights approach and is based on the belief that humans have a dignity based on their human nature or their ability to freely choose what they do with their lives. They have for example the right to consume adequate food; they have the fundamental right not to be hungry [FAO 1996].

A third approach links ethics to social responsibility and draws attention to common conditions that are important for the well-being of all: ... *The moral appeal – arguing that companies have a duty to be good citizens and "to do the right thing" – is prominent in the goal of Business for Responsibility...* [Gossner et al. 2009].

Finally, there is another and very old approach to ethics: ethical actions should be compatible with certain ideal virtues, which ensure the complete development of humanity. Olsen & Bánáti [2014] call it the approach of virtues, meaning the dispositions and habits that allow us to act according to the highest potential of our character and in the name of values, such as truth and beauty.

Each of the approaches mentioned above helps us determine which behavioural norms can be considered ethical. It is possible that different actors may disagree on the content of some of these specific approaches; that they do not all agree on the same set of human and civil rights or on what is right and wrong. Each approach provides us with important information to determine what is ethical in particular circumstances. And in any case, every human being has his or her individual ethical approach [Klees 2014].

Consumers want a wide variety of safe food choices

And at the same time, producers want to sell safe products, but preferably less regulated. These ideas are mostly incompatible. Exotic and convenience foods throughout the year, free choice of organic foods, local or imported products, value and benefit for both the producer and the consumer.

Unfortunately, food products are sometimes associated with serious health risks. The availability of safe food must take into account factors such as respect for consumer choice, the right to safety information, affordable food prices, income and working conditions for employees and workers, animal welfare, sustainability as well as commercial practices. Ethics is far from being a thoughtless and servile observation of the rules. The fundamental question of ethics is not *what should I do*, but *what kind of person should I be*. For the food industry, the question is: *what image do we want to give of ourselves and our company.*

Seen from this angle, food ethics must be based on the principles of free inquiry, the principles of action summed up in the triad *doubt, decide and convince*. This postulates the sovereignty of the search for truth and human reason.

The future of food ethics can only be in dialogue and debate, in openness and transparency, in honesty and truthful exchange of information.

Bibliography

ANSES [2013]. *Substitution du bisphénol A*, pp. 204

Bolle De Bal [2005]. *Le travail, une valeur à réhabiliter*, Éditions Labor, pp. 118

BusinessEurope [2015]. *Better Framework for Innovation - Fuelling EU policies with an Innovation Principle*, pp. 3

Calafat et al. [2005]. Urinary Concentrations of Bisphenol A and 4-Nonylphenol in a Human Reference Population, *Environmental Health Perspectives* 113, 4, 391-395

Carson [1962]. *Silent Spring*, Houghton Mifflin Harcourt, pp. 378

Cho et al. [2018]. Differential Inhalation Toxicity Induced by E-Cigarette Aerosol Flavorings in Association with Nicotine, *ISEE Conference Abstracts* 1

Colborn et al. [1996]. *Our Stolen Future: Are We Threatening Our Fertility, Intelligence, and Survival? A Scientific Detective Story*, Dutton US, pp. 306

Edwards [2018]. Lest We Forget: Harm-Reduction Research is Important and Increasing, but Other Facets of Tobacco Control Research Remain a High Priority, *Nicotine & Tobacco Research*, 145-146

Eladak et al. [2015]. A new chapter in the bisphenol A story: bisphenol S and bisphenol F are not safe alternatives to this compound, *Fertility and Sterility* 103, 1, 11-21

European Commission [2018]. *Proposal for a Regulation of the European Parliament and of the Council establishing Horizon Europe ¾ the Framework Programme for Research and Innovation, laying down its rules for participation and dissemination*, pp. 57

FAO [1996]. *Report of the World Food Summit, Rome*, http://www.fao.org/docrep/003/w3548e/w3548e00.htm

Geens et al. [2011]. Are potential sources for human exposure to bisphenol-A overlooked? *International Journal of Hygiene and Environmental Health* 214, 339-347

Gossner et al. [2009]. The Melamine Incident: Implications for International Food and Feed Safety, *Environmental Health Perspectives* 117, 12, 1803

Hirabayashia & Inoueb [2011]. The low-dose issue and stochastic responses to endocrine disruptors, *Journal of Applied Toxicology* 31, 1, 84-88 Éditions Vanden Broele, Brugge, pp. 90

Kamatou et al. [2013]. Menthol: A simple monoterpene with remarkable biological properties, *Phytochemistry* 96, 15-25

Klees [2014]. *Éthique et gouvernance des entreprises*, Éditions Vanden Broele, Brugge, pp. 90

Kortenkamp [2007]. Ten years of mixing cocktails - a review of combination effects of endocrine disrupting chemicals, *Environmental Health Perspectives* 115 (Suppl. 1), 98-105

Muneret et al. [2018]. Evidence that organic farming promotes pest control, *Nature Sustainability* 1, 361-368

Olsen & Bánáti [2014]. Ethics in Food Safety Management, in Montarjemi & Lelieveld (eds.) *Food Safety Management*, Academic Press, 1115-1125

Proctor [2011]. *Golden Holocaust: Origins of the Cigarette Catastrophe and the Case for Abolition*, University of California Press, pp. 752

Pussemier & Goeyens [2017]. *AgricultureS & Enjeux de société*, Presses Universitaires de Liège - Agronomie, Gembloux, pp. 112

Rochester [2013]. Bisphenol A and human health: A review of the literature, *Reproductive Toxicology* 42, 132-155

Rochester & Bolden [2015]. Bisphenol S and F: A Systematic Review and Comparison of the Hormonal Activity of Bisphenol A Substitutes, *Environmental Health Perspectives* 123, 7, 643

Rostand [1939]. *Pensées d'un biologiste*, Delamain et Boutelleau, pp. 93

Rostand [1953]. *Ce que je crois*, Grasset, pp. 92

Trasande [2019]. *Sicker, fatter, poorer*, Houghton Mifflin Harcourt, pp. 221

Trasande et al. [2015]. Estimating Burden and Disease Costs of Exposure to Endocrine-Disrupting Chemicals in the European Union, *Journal of Clinical Endocrinology and Metabolism* 100, 4, 1245-1255

Trasande et al. [2016]. Burden of disease and costs of exposure to endocrine disrupting chemicals in the European Union: an updated analysis, *Andrology* 4, 4, 565-572

van der Eyk et al. [2018]. How Menthol Is Key to the Tobacco Industry's Strategy of Recruiting and Retaining Young Smokers in Singapore, *Journal of Adolescent Health*, in press

Warner & Flaws [2018]. Common bisphenol A replacements are reproductive toxicants, *Nature Reviews Endocrinology* 14, 12, 691

Witteman [2018]. *Nederland hielp industrie bij potentiële ondermijning productveiligheid*, Folow the money, pp. 21

"We didn't know" is no excuse

The precautionary principle is a relatively novel concept

It is linked to the growing importance of debates on sustainable development, health and well-being risk management, evaluation of technological choices, etc. Whether it concerns the greenhouse effect, genetically modified organisms (GMO), nuclear waste, plastic soup or mad cows, the precautionary principle is increasingly invoked in political decisions that require additional, thorough investigations of long-term adverse effects because of the current void in the scientific understanding of inherent risks. The precautionary principle goes well beyond the elementary caution with which scientists must act in the interpretation of their data and which political decision-makers must show in the assessment of the consequences of their proposals and decisions. The principle proclaims that when faced with serious and irreversible risks, lack of full scientific certainty cannot be used as a reason for postponing cost-effective measures [Tallacchini 2005]. It aims to prevent risks that are still uncertain or unknown. It comes into play when there is scientific uncertainty, meaning that scientific investigation is insufficient or too controversial to demonstrate the existence of a risk.

The development of the principle appears well advanced in the field of public health[136]. It is undeniable that the precautionary principle pertains to the broader context of the risk analysis principle and includes

---

136 Regulation (EC) n° 178/2002 of the European Parliament and of the Council of 28 January 2002 lays down the general principles and requirements of food law, establishing the European Food Safety Authority, and defining procedures in matters of food safety; it enshrines the precautionary principle in relation to its application in food law.

a two-step process: risk assessment and risk management [de Sadeleer 2009]. In first instance, the occurrence probability of harm is determined using a risk assessment procedure. Experts have to examine both hazard and exposure in order to calculate an acceptable or tolerable level of contamination or exposure. However, the risk is not determined by scientific experts alone. The effect of belonging to a political, social and economic context must also be considered. When the risk assessment procedure has finally been completed, a risk management decision must be taken by responsible politicians, taking into account legislative requirements as well as the economic, political and normative dimensions of the problem. Risk management, in contrast to risk assessment, is the process that determines how safe is safe. Both risk assessment and risk management are essential. Risk assessment ensures a rigorous, scientific basis for risk management. The separation between the assessment and management phases meets a dual requirement: on the one hand, the need to base political decisions on scientific evidence and, on the other, the need to maintain political autonomy *vis-à-vis* the results of scientific assessments. This summary definition contains all ingredients of the problem: risk, uncertainty of knowledge, responsibility and legitimacy.

Problematic cases occur when there are disagreements concerning the value judgments made in the risk assessment. GMO are an example that gives rise to much debate. While GMO were strongly supported by the American science and biotechnology industry and frequently cultivated on vast agricultural land, the European citizens were fiercely opposed to GMO. Consumers were skeptical and talked about "Frankenfoods". The opponents of GMO have been relentless in their campaign to vilify genetically modified foods by describing them as unnatural and harmful Frankenfoods. Today, the European legislative framework differs from that of the United States and is predominantly in line with public perception of risk rather than with the scientific definition of risk.

The dynamic nature of the food system affects the risk assessment of food safety

The food market is becoming ever more global. As a result, not only is food but also foodborne pathogens distributed worldwide [Tauxe 2002; Koluman & Dikici 2013]. This is problematic since consumer habits and customs, often inherited from parents and grandparents, are generally not suitable for dealing with new food alerts. When foods and their pathogens change while preparation routines remain the same, then safety becomes a compelling problem. The solution to this problem raises ethical questions related to the freedom of choice, the economic prosperity of countries, the introduction of pathogens into uncontaminated areas, etc.

Moreover, food contaminations trigger ethical dilemmas. It is widely recognized that endocrine disrupting compounds (EDC) pose challenges for traditional paradigms in toxicology, since very low exposures to EDC have been shown to result in detrimental health effects. These substances – and bisphenol A (BPA) is a most notorious example – do not obey Paracelsus' poison dictum, *The right dose makes the poison*. These compounds also pose challenges for ethics and policymaking [Resnik & Elliot 2015]. When a chemical does not cause significant low-dose effects, regulators can allow it to be introduced onto the market or into the environment, provided procedures and/or rules are in place to keep exposures below an acceptable level. This option allows companies to maximise their profits by using the chemical while minimising the risks. It represents a compromise between competing values. On the other hand, if it is not possible to establish acceptable exposure levels for chemicals that pose significant health or environmental risks, the most reasonable options for risk management may be to enact a partial or complete ban on their use. These options mean that decision-makers need to make tough choices between competing values. To what extent can economic gains take precedence over environmental quality and public health?

Bisphenol A and its common alternatives: a recent story about an old culprit

The BPA case is a good example of how difficult ethical issues can be. Some governments have decided to set acceptable levels of BPA exposure through baby bottles and cups while others have decided to ban these uses of BPA [Resnik & Elliot 2015]. Making the decision to ban a particular BPA use means that government officers must compare the benefits, risks, and costs of allowing the use with those of banning it altogether. Moreover, decision-makers must consider whether there are safe and effective alternatives to BPA, since a chemical that is used instead of BPA might also pose risks to human health and environmental quality [Rosenmai et al. 2014]. In deciding whether to ban the use of BPA in manufacturing baby bottles or children's cups, regulators must ascertain whether there are alternative methods of manufacturing these items that are safer and more effective than using BPA. Recently, several teams of researchers concluded that the hormonal activities of Bisphenol S and Bisphenol F are similar to those of BPA and do not constitute safe alternatives to BPA [Viñas et al. 2013; Eladak et al. 2015; Rochester & Bolden 2015; Warner & Flaws 2018] because they also act as an EDC and have non-monotonic dose-response curves.

The decision to ban the use of BPA in baby bottles and children's cups has not posed intractable dilemmas for regulators. More challenging questions arise concerning the use of BPA in food can linings [Resnik & Elliot 2015]. Metallic cans were developed in the 19th century as a cheaper alternative to glass food recipients. The protective linings that are necessary to prevent corrosion and food spoilage are seen today as important sources of BPA contamination. Moreover, some speculate that BPA can also leach into the canned food from gloves, cutting boards and other kitchenware used in food preparation.

It is not practical to make canned food completely BPA-free. Hence, perhaps the most reasonable risk management option would be to establish standards for acceptable levels of BPA in food. However, the adverse low dose effects of BPA challenge the feasibility of this option [Resnik & Elliot 2015]. In principle, policymakers could still establish acceptable exposure levels, but such levels would not achieve the typical goal of ensuring the protection of human health. Rather, they would be the result of an effort to weigh human health protection against the social impacts of limiting the use of BPA. Policymakers will always face such difficulties. Whether to limit the use of a substance through some type of ban, establish acceptable exposure levels, or pursue a combination of both options. These are constantly recurring questions. Regulations that limit the use of BPA may help to promote human health, but have a negative impact on business. For example, if using alternatives to BPA in food can linings significantly increases the costs of canned food, this would have adverse impacts on both the food industry and the consumers. Increases in the costs of canned food could make food less affordable and would have disproportionate impacts on economically disadvantaged people, since they tend to spend a higher proportion of their income on food. It is also important to consider potential long-term costs to individuals, insurers, and society from the adverse health effects of BPA. These costs are difficult to determine at present, because the real impact of BPA on health is still insufficiently understood, but they should be factored into the assessment of BPA's social and economic impact. These and other possible consequences have to be considered in developing BPA risk management policies.

Bisphenol A is just one of many endocrine disrupting chemicals

Few scientific issues are more complex than the assessment of the effects of EDC on human health and well-being. It came as a surprise when the report of the Royal College of Obstetricians and Gynecologists (RCOG) stated that *the best approach for pregnant women is a "safety first" approach, which is to assume there is risk present even when it may be minimal or eventually unfounded* [RCOG 2013]. Many thought that the RCOG report had taken the precautionary principle too far.

An increasing number of reports have linked various EDC with human disease. However, evidence that EDC cause metabolic diseases in humans is not always very solid, and many studies cannot prove causation. The amount and type of EDC exposure varies widely across the globe and this is due to substantial differences in industrial and societal environments, and to population densities. Additionally, many low- and middle-income countries with the greatest exposure to EDC have little data on which to base governmental changes. To design a study that would provide watertight evidence for EDC harm is necessary for regulatory bodies to be able to reassess and/or introduce EDC policies. Difficult as this may be, not to do anything is not an option. The precautionary principle should perhaps be most generous towards foetuses and other populations at greatest potential risk, as suggested by van den Berg & Sly [2013].

With ~1000 EDC identified to date and the biological complexities inherent to each one of them as well as to their mixtures, to regulate will be always be complex. Regulating must also be balanced with the potential consequences for industries that rely on or make EDC-containing products. Unfortunately, the removal of all EDC from our environment will take time. The huge scientific progress in understanding the effects of EDC that has occurred in the past decade needs to continue to ensure that the acceptable threat of EDC to human health is rigorously quantified and agreed upon. This task will require the cooperation of all stakeholders. Weighing the need to protect vulnerable populations against commercial interests will be a more attainable goal if we strengthen the evidence base.

The precautionary principle: a thorn in the side of the industry

Though apparently a fairly innocent concept, the Innovation Principle has been carefully and strategically inserted into the European Union (EU) system where it could have a significant impact on the shaping of new and revised EU legislations or policies. It was produced by the European Risk Forum (ERF), a lobby platform for the chemical, tobacco and fossil fuel industries, which are invariably subject to strict health and environmental regulations. Using this principle, the ERF intends to counterbalance regulatory measures ensuring continuity of innovation while maintaining a high level of risk management. The ERF industries

– 12 CEOs of major multinational companies signed a letter in October 2013 to the Presidents of the three EU institutions proposing the adoption of the Innovation Principle – aim to ensure that whenever legislation is under consideration, its impact on innovation should be assessed and addressed[137]. Contrary to what the proponents and defenders of the principle say, the opponents claim that the biggest joint industry interest is to keep their products on the market with the least possible restrictions and regulations. Not a word about the well-being and health of the consumer in the original BusinessEurope [2015] document[138]. ERF published a cunning plea *to incorporate the Innovation Principle as an integral component of the policy-making process. Whenever EU institutions consider policy or regulatory proposals, impact on innovation should be fully assessed and addressed … Policies which simply attempt to identify and avoid technological risk maybe appear to protect health and the environment but could in the longer-term cause much greater harm by sending messages to innovators that they had better invest in other parts of the world.*

By calling it a principle, the impression is created that the concept has some kind of legal basis. In fact the so-called Innovation Principle is an industry invention and is in no way comparable to the legal principles enshrined in the EU Treaty, such as the precautionary principle. It is a lobby product formulated by a think tank and mainly promoted by the companies that finance the think tank. Did the ERF plan to use the Innovation Principle to weaken the EU's chemicals laws (REACH) concerning novel foods, pesticides, fertilisers, nanoproducts and pharmaceuticals? Did the ERF plan to undermine the legal principles of environmental protection and human health enshrined in the EU Treaty? Today the ERF's answer claims the opposite: … *The Innovation Principle is not intended to undermine or reduce the importance of the*

---

137 The ERF Innovation Principle – The overview document can be downloaded from: http://www.riskforum.eu/uploads/2/5/7/1/25710097/innovation_principle_one_pager_5_march_2015.pdf

138 The BusinessEurope document is available on http://www.riskforum.eu/uploads/2/5/7/1/25710097/businesseurope-erf-ert_innovation_principle_joint_statement.pdf

precautionary principle. In fact the two principles are complimentary. The Innovation Principle should be used alongside the Precautionary Principle, taking into account the need to protect society and the environment and also to protect Europe's ability to attract and benefit from technological innovation. The Innovation Principle aims to stimulate investment in innovation by increasing the confidence of innovators in the regulatory system... This however contradicts the earlier statement that the precautionary principle is inconsistent with scientific approaches to policy making and does not sufficiently take into account economic efficiency.

The Innovation Principle was catapulted into Competitiveness Council conclusions under the Dutch Presidency in 2016. At the initiative of the Netherlands, the criteria by which the future EU policy will be assessed were changed. The Netherlands wrote European history. At the initiative of their ministers, the EU member states decided that European laws and regulations should be subject to a new assessment, which could have a major impact on future European policy [Witteman 2018]. Continuing its rapid rise, the Innovation Principle has recently been included for the first time in an EU legal text to be voted on by the European Parliament: the draft Horizon Europe regulation and programme[139], as published by the European Commission in June 2018 Horizon Europe lays out the rules for the EU's research and innovation programme, which will succeed Horizon 2020. The adoption of the principle in Horizon Europe could mean even more EU funds may be spent on technological innovation to the detriment of civil society.

Via the ERF, the industry handed the business-friendly Innovation Principle to the EU institutions on a silver platter. The European Commission and the Council adopted it wholesale, uncritically and without too much regard for the consequences. A splendid example of corporate hijacking of how an industry that is known for its hazardous products has managed to create another instrument with which to manipulate EU laws at a very early stage, through the impact assessment

---

139 Briefing available on http://www.europarl.europa.eu/RegData/etudes/BRIE/2018/ 628254/EPRS_BRI(2018)628254_EN.pdf

phase. The European Parliament now has the opportunity to reject the innovation principle in the coming plenary session in Strasbourg. Members of the European Parliament should have been informed about the original inventors and their motivations, but this seems to have faded into the background as the EU institutions were seen to absorb the principle and even reinforce it. The stated goals of the EU cannot but raise a number of questions: ... *sustainable development based on balanced economic growth and price stability, a highly competitive market economy with full employment and social progress, and environmental protection...* Sustainability is not an idle word. Chemical substances invisible to the naked eye do not only disrupt the most important hormones in our bodies and brains; they also open up multiple paths for diseases that will impact our children and their children well into the future. This is a challenging and uncomfortable thought, especially since many of these chemicals are produced and distributed on a massive scale. Moreover, these chemicals are minimally regulated, which means they will continue to wreak havoc on our lives, generation after generation – a highly disturbing, but realistic perspective [Trasande 2019]. This represents a heavy mortgage on our future, especially for younger generations. I believe the first public disclosure that widespread use of synthetic chemicals can do harm and not just provide benefits occurred when *Silent Spring* [Carson 1962] was published. Not only is Carson's environmental science book still relevant; it serves as a reminder that we have still not yet fully resolved the issues that were raised more than half a century ago. Moreover, many synthetic chemicals are responsible for high additional disease-related costs [Trasande et al. 2015; 2016].

It is appalling that prominent public figures undermine the significance of the health and environmental issues and claim that science is wrong. Some industry representatives and their scientists also dismiss the connection between chemicals and disease. They must understand that these chemicals are real, dangerous and increasingly present in our daily lives. What is more, these chemicals will not go away if we do not actively intervene. And let us not forget that we all have a contribution to make.

Bibliography

Carson [1962]. *Silent Spring*, Houghton Mifflin Harcourt, pp. 378

de Sadeleer [2009]. The Precautionary Principle Applied to Food Safety–
Lessons from EC Courts, *European Law Journal* 12, 139-172

Eladak et al. [2015]. A new chapter in the bisphenol A story: bisphenol S and
bisphenol F are not safe alternatives to this compound, *Fertility and Sterility*
103, 1, 11-21

Koluman & Dikici [2013]. Antimicrobial resistance of emerging foodborne
pathogens: Status quo and global trends, *Critical Reviews in Microbiology*
39, 1, 57-69

RCOG [2013]. RCOG release: Mothers-to-be should be aware of unintentional
chemical exposures, say experts,

Resnik & Elliot [2015]. Bisphenol A and Risk Management Ethics, *Bioethics* 29,
3, 182-189

Rochester [2013]. Bisphenol A and human health: A review of the literature,
Reproductive Toxicology 42, 132-155

Rosenmai et al. [2014]. Are structural analogues to bisphenol a safe
alternatives?, *Toxicological sciences* 139, 1, 35-47

Tallacchini [2005]. Before and beyond the precautionary principle:
epistemology of uncertainty in science and law, *Toxicology and Applied
Pharmacology* 207, 2, Supplement, 645-651

Tauxe [2002]. Emerging foodborne pathogens, *International Journal of Food
Microbiology* 78, 1–2, 31-41

Trasande [2019]. *Sicker, fatter, poorer*, Houghton Mifflin Harcourt, pp. 221

Trasande et al. [2015]. Estimating Burden and Disease Costs of Exposure
to Endocrine-Disrupting Chemicals in the European Union, *Journal of
Clinical Endocrinology and Metabolism* 100, 4, 1245-1255

Trasande et al. [2016]. Burden of disease and costs of exposure to endocrine
disrupting chemicals in the European Union: an updated analysis,
Andrology 4, 4, 565-572

van den Berg & Sly [2013]. Protecting the human fetus against effects of
bisphenol A, *The Lancet – Diabetes & Endocrinology* 1, 2, 87

Viñas & Watson [2013]. Bisphenol S Disrupts Estradiol-Induced Nongenomic
Signaling in a Rat Pituitary Cell Line: Effects on Cell Functions,
Environmental Health Perspectives 121, 352-358

Warner & Flaws [2018]. Common bisphenol A replacements are reproductive toxicants, *Nature Reviews Endocrinology* 14, 12, 691

Witteman [2018]. Nederland hielp industrie bij potentiële ondermijning productveiligheid, *Follow the money*, https://www.ftm.nl/artikelen/productveiligheid-vs-innovatieprincipe?share=1

Mayhem caused by chemicals happens in utero

... Strong evidence now supports the notion that organophosphate pesticides damage the fetal brain and produce cognitive and behavioral dysfunction through multiple mechanisms, including thyroid disruption. A regulatory ban was proposed, but actions to end the use of one such pesticide, chlorpyrifos, in agriculture were recently stopped by the Environmental Protection Agency under false scientific pretenses... [Trasande 2017].

Organophosphates were first developed as human nerve gas agents during World War II

One can safely assume that everyone has been in contact with the insecticide chlorpyrifos [Trasande 2017] since the substance was commonly used to eradicate the annoying insects we know only too well: mosquitoes, cockroaches, and other undesirables. Dow Chemical Co. introduced chlorpyrifos in homes and farm fields in 1965. It is highly effective in deterring just about every insect. Homeowners and farmers used it as did gardeners tending golf courses and city parks. Chlorpyrifos was everywhere, and it was soon to conquer the world.

Not only are alternative methods extremely effective in reducing toxic pesticide use [Kass et al. 2009], but the ecological intensification of agro-ecosystems [Pussemier & Goeyens 2017] based on the optimisation of ecological functions such as biological pest control has also, and rather unexpectedly, turned out to be a very promising alternative to agrochemical inputs [Muneret et al. 2018]. Also, evidence documenting the adverse effects of organophosphate exposure in general and of chlorpyrifos in particular is becoming increasingly convincing. Especially the adverse effects on the foetal brain because of low-level exposure during pregnancy has raised concern [Grandjean & Landrigan 2014; Marsillach et al. 2016]. Multiple longitudinal studies have documented consistent poorer intellectual development in relationship to prenatal exposure [Bouchard et al. 2011, Zhang et al. 2014]. Prenatal exposure has been associated with magnetic resonance imaging findings in children, including frontal and parietal cortical thinning that are consistent with the neurobehavioral deficits identified in psychological testing [Rauh et al. 2012; Trasande 2017].

Thyroid hormone has long been known to be crucial for brain development. During pregnancy, subtle changes in free thyroxine within the normal range that would not prompt clinically significant increases in thyroid-stimulating hormone can induce reductions in intelligence quotient (IQ), changes in brain morphology, and even clinically apparent autism and attention deficit hyperactivity disorder [Korevaar et al. 2016].

In 2000, the Environmental Protection Agency banned chlorpyrifos in household uses but said the chemical could still be used in commercial agriculture. This ban generated interesting scientific data within an ongoing birth cohort study at Columbia University in which the research team was studying effects of pesticide exposure on the developing brain [Trasande 2017]. Data from this study provide compelling counterarguments to those who have deliberately emphasized the potential for alternative explanations.

During the last decade, several studies focused on endocrine disrupting chemicals (EDC). More particularly, the epidemiological and toxicological evidence for the role of this class of chemicals in cognitive deficits and intellectual disability was evaluated using rigorous criteria elaborated by the World Health Organization (WHO) and the Danish Environmental Protection Agency. The experts rated the probability of a causal relationship to be quite high, between 70 and 100 % [Bellanger et al. 2015]. Their calculations suggest that preventing exposure would result in substantial societal benefits.

Was there enough evidence for a total ban?

On March 29, 2017 the United States Environmental Protection Agency (USEPA) Administrator Scott Pruitt signed an order denying a petition that sought to ban chlorpyrifos, a pesticide crucial to U.S. agriculture. *We need to provide regulatory certainty to the thousands of American farms that rely on chlorpyrifos, while still protecting human health and the environment,* said EPA Administrator Pruitt. *By reversing the previous Administration's steps to ban one of the most widely used pesticides in the world, we are returning to using sound science in decision-making – rather than predetermined results*[140].

The emphasis of Administrator Pruitt on the need for sustaining the food supply by using chlorpyrifos in agriculture was abundantly commented. While concerns have been raised about the need for pesticides to "feed the world", the evidence for crop yield superiority is not as ironclad as some suggest [Trasande 2017]. As mentioned earlier, recent meta-analyses [Seufert et al. 2012; Muneret et al. 2018] show that conventional agriculture, which often uses excessive pesticide spraying, does not necessarily have better yields than organic agriculture.

Even if it is assumed that there are no good alternatives to chlorpyrifos, one still needs to consider the important trade-offs. Trasande [2017] wonders whether keeping children well fed is worth their being less smart and less able to contribute to the future of humanity. This is certainly not the first time we are faced with this kind of dilemma. Together with scientist Pete Myers and environmental journalist Dianne Dumanski, Theo Colborn (1927-2014) gives an gripping account that traces birth defects, sexual abnormalities, and reproductive failures to their source, i.e. the man-made chemicals that disrupt delicate hormone systems and derail development [Colborn et al. 1996]. In chapter 13, the dramatic consequences of an IQ drop are illustrated and brilliantly explained: ... *Consider, however, what it might mean for our society if synthetic chemicals are subtly undermining human intelligence across the entire population*

---

140 USEPA Media Relations, https://www.epa.gov/newsreleases/epa-administrator-pruitt-denies-petition-ban-widely-used-pesticide-0.

in the same manner that they have apparently undermined human male sperm count. With the current average IQ score of 100, a population of 100 million will have 2.3 million intellectually gifted people who score above 130. Though it might not sound like much, if the average were to drop just like five points to 95, it would have "staggering" implications, according to Bernard Weiss, a behavioral toxicologist at the University of Rochester who has considered the societal impact of seemingly small losses. Instead of 2.3 million, only 990,000 would score over 130, so this society would have lost over half of its high-powered minds with the capacity to become the most gifted doctors, scientists, college professors, inventors or writers... Administrator Pruitt's decision fails to consider that prenatal organophosphate exposure, and chlorpyrifos exposure especially, generates IQ shifts into the intellectual disability range and contributes to disease and dysfunction, with annual costs rising significantly [Attina et al. 2016].

There is no such thing as absolute certainty in chemical investigations

Sir Austin Bradford Hill (1897-1991) gave a landmark lecture on criteria for causation at the 1965 meeting of the Section of Occupational Medicine of the Royal Society of Medicine in London. The criteria he established in his article [Hill 1965] became known as the Bradford Hill criteria and the medical community often refers to them when determining whether or not an environmental condition causes an illness. Hill emphasises that his goal is to determine how the medical community can detect the relationship between occupational conditions and resulting disease. He warns, however, that it takes time and in-depth research, which goes beyond using his criteria, to prove that a factor can cause a disease. Hill believes his criteria will provide a relatively quick and logical way of determining whether the relationship between a factor and a disease is most likely causal. Further research remains to be carried out, however. Hill identified nine criteria [Abboud 2017] that should be considered, including consistency, exposure-response relations, biological plausibility, effect size, specificity, etc. What has all too easily been forgotten from Hill's lecture is the need for context in considering the totality of evidence.

Hill [1965] concludes his article by emphasising that ... *All scientific work is incomplete – whether it be observational or experimental. All scientific work is liable to be upset or modified by advancing knowledge. That does not confer upon us a freedom to ignore the knowledge we already have, or to postpone the action that it appears to demand at a given time...* Scientists need to emphatically declare the implications of policy failures, even if some of the scientific underpinnings remain uncertain.

There is always some uncertainty in estimating exposures from epidemiological studies, especially where there has been exposure to multiple pesticides, for example. In the case of organophosphates, there is still ample evidence to support a ban given the consistent findings among a large number of epidemiological as well as laboratory studies, which suggest a modest or perhaps minimal uncertainty of causation [Trasande 2017].

What is true for chlorpyrifos is true for other synthetic chemicals

In his inspiring book, *Sicker, Fatter, Poorer*, Trasande [2019] explains the science behind the escalating obesity, diabetes, learning disorders, autism, infertility, and food allergies which most likely result from endocrine disrupting chemicals in our food, our homes, and our personal care products: ... *The chemicals with the strongest evidence of health effects are pesticides, flame retardants, plasticizer chemicals, and bisphenols, which are used to line food and beverage cans. At first it was thought that those chemicals had to persist in the body to cause harm, like a viral or bacterial infection. Now we realize that though the chemicals themselves are often excreted within a few days, they leave lasting effects. And here is the scariest piece: the effects of this chemical contact can reverberate years later and even be passed on to the next generation. That is what I call the "hit-and-run" impact of these pernicious chemicals...* The review publication by Gore et al. [2015] speaks volumes and gives little cause for optimism about our future. It concludes that ... *Armed with this information, researchers, physicians, and other healthcare providers can guide regulators and policymakers as they make responsible decisions...*

All of this amounts to an assignment, a compelling obligation for scientists!

Scientists who raise their voices should be prepared to face criticism

A great deal of the criticism comes from those who have substantial vested interests. It is not intended to convince the scientific community, but rather to confuse the scientific data. Consequently, it promotes misinterpretation of the peer reviewed scientific reports by non-specialists, bureaucrats, politicians and other decision makers not intimately familiar with the topic of endocrine disruption and therefore liable to make incorrect generalisations based on bias and subjectivity [Bergman et al. 2015]. This is what has already been referred to as manufacturing doubt [Proctor 2011].

In general, funding sources are not stated and conflicts of interest are not declared. Who pays the piper calls the tune. The truth is not revealed; the truth is jeopardised.

Unfortunately, attacks on scientific norms are likely to continue unabated, whether they concern climate change, synthetic chemical exposures or other worrying public health and well-being issues. This day and age, when fake news is rampant, scientists and journal editors have a duty to identify knowledge gaps while documenting the need for urgent action. And this should be done vigorously and convincingly, since it has so far been very hard to make things happen. In 1962, Rachel Carson (1907-1964) published *Silent Spring*. Her "fable for tomorrow" exposed the destruction of wildlife through the widespread use of pesticides. Her passionate concern was with the future of the planet and all life on Earth. She called for humans to act responsibly, carefully, and as stewards of the living earth. She also suggested a change in how democracies and liberal societies should operate so that both individuals and groups could question which chemicals their governments allowed others to put into the environment. All too often her call has fallen on deaf ears: sixty years after her book was published [Carson 1962], the production and spraying of pesticides goes on.

Bibliography

Abboud [2017]. The Environment and Disease: Association or Causation?" (1965), by Austin Bradford Hill, *Embryo Project Encyclopedia*, ISSN: 1940-5030, http://embryo.asu.edu/handle/10776/11456, pp. 8

Attina et al. [2016]. Exposure to endocrine-disrupting chemicals in the USA: a population-based disease burden and cost analysis, *The Lancet Diabetes & Endocrinology* 4, 12, 996-1003

Bellanger et al. [2015]. Neurobehavioral Deficits, Diseases and Associated Costs of Exposure to Endocrine Disrupting Chemicals in the European Union, *The Journal of Clinical Endocrinology & Metabolism* 100, 4, 1256-1266

Bergman et al. [2015]. Manufacturing doubt about endocrine disrupter science e A rebuttal of industry-sponsored critical comments on the UNEP/WHO report "State of the Science of Endocrine Disrupting Chemicals 2012", *Regulatory Toxicology and Pharmacology* 73, 1007-1017

Bouchard et al. [2011]. Prenatal Exposure to Organophosphate Pesticides and IQ in 7-Year-Old Children, *Environmental Health Perspectives* 119, 1 189-1195

Carson [1962]. *Silent Spring*, Houghton Mifflin Harcourt, pp. 378

Colborn et al. [1996]. *Our Stolen Future: Are We Threatening Our Fertility, Intelligence, and Survival? A Scientific Detective Story*, Dutton US, pp. 306

Grandjean & Landrigan [2014]. Neurobehavioural impact of developmental toxicity, *Lancet Neurology* 13, 330-308

Gore et al. [2015]. EDC-2: The Endocrine Society's Second Scientific Statement on Endocrine-Disrupting Chemicals, *Endocrine Reviews* 36, 6, E1-E150

Hill [1965]. The Environment and Disease: Association or Causation?, *Proceedings of the Royal Society of Medicine* 58, 5, 295-300

Kass et al. [2009]. Effectiveness of an Integrated Pest Management Intervention in Controlling Cockroaches, Mice, and Allergens in New York City Public Housing, *Environmental Health Perspectives* 117, 1219-1225

Korevaar et al. [2016]. Association of maternal thyroid function during early pregnancy with offspring IQ and brain morphology in childhood:

a population-based prospective cohort study, *The Lancet Diabetes & Endocrinology* 4, 1, 35-43

Marsillach et al. [2016]. Paraoxonase-1 and Early-Life Environmental Exposures, *Annals of Global Health* 82, 1, 100-110

Muneret et al. [2018]. Evidence that organic farming promotes pest control, *Nature Sustainability* 1, 361-368

Proctor [2011]. *Golden Holocaust: Origins of the Cigarette Catastrophe and the Case for Abolition*, University of California Press, pp. 752

Pussemier & Goeyens [2017]. *AgricultureS & Enjeux de société*, Presses Universitaires de Liège - Agronomie, Gembloux, pp. 112

Rauh et al. [2012]. Brain anomalies in children exposed prenatally to a common organophosphate pesticide, *Proceedings of the National Academy of Sciences* 109, 20, 7871-7876

Seufert et al. [2012]. Comparing the yields of organic and conventional agriculture, *Nature* 485, 229-232

Trasande [2017]. When enough data are not enough to enact policy: The failure to ban chlorpyrifos, *PLoS Biology* 15, 12, e2003671, pp. 6

Trasande [2019]. *Sicker, fatter, poorer*, Houghton Mifflin Harcourt, pp. 221

Zhang et al. [2014]. Prenatal Exposure to Organophosphate Pesticides and Neurobehavioral Development of Neonates: A Birth Cohort Study in Shenyang, China, *PLoS One* 9, 2, e88491, pp. 10

Living in accordance with nature. Has anything really changed ?

... There are seven billion people. Nearly one billion are estimated to be malnourished. Several million die each year of easily preventable hunger-related conditions. Yet others are living through a culinary age: new cuisines, old cuisines brought to new places, cookbook upon cookbook, and TV shows. Food for a huge price. Food for cheap. But plenty of food for those who can afford it...

Food ethics, as an academic pursuit, is vast. It incorporates work from philosophy but also anthropology, economics, environmental sciences and other natural sciences, geography, and sociology. Scholars from these fields, including some philosophers, have been producing work for decades on the food system, and on ethical, social and policy issues connected to the food system. Yet in the last several years, there has been notable increase in philosophical on these issues – work that draws on multiple literatures within practical ethics, normative ethics, and political philosophy...
[Barnhill et al. 2018].

Several ways to critically examine food production and consumption practices

In the course of history, several events have occurred, the effects of which are still noticeable today. Hence, a comparison with the food ethics of the past will make us aware of aspects and concerns of present-day ethics. History should be explored so that the resulting account is not merely historical, but a source of inspiration for generations to come. Whereas pre-modern food ethics predominantly focused on issues relating to food consumption, modern food ethics typically develop an interest in issues relating to food production. Moreover, whereas food ethics used to be a private morality, it is the social dimension of food ethics that is now being recognized and highlighted. [Zwart 2000].

Attuning to the law of nature in ancient times

In mainstream ancient Greek and Roman ethics, the connection between nature and temperance was self-evident: *live and act in accordance with nature*[141]. Nevertheless, food products yielded by nature should be improved and refined for many and terrible were the sufferings, when men consumed crude and uncompounded foods. What is provided by nature must be actively processed by man [Zwart 2002]. To live in accordance with nature means to live in accordance with the virtues wisdom, justice, fortitude and temperance.

In the Hebrew Bible, a different moral logic is considered. It is not guided by the idea of temperance, but by the idea of a basic distinction between what is allowed and what is not allowed: *You must not eat any abominable thing ... You may eat any hoofed animal that has cloven hoofs and also chews the cud; those that only chew the cud or only have cloven hoofs you must not eat...* Leviticus and Deuteronomy both give the same general set of rules for identifying which land animals are ritually clean. Simply put, this means God's people are to differentiate between what is set apart and what is common and between what has been revealed to be clean and unclean. Many efforts have been made to explain the reason for these rules, notably in terms of health, hygiene, and other utilitarian concerns. None of them has completely succeeded in overcoming their basically arbitrary nature. The most important reason for abstaining from eating unclean food products – pork, for example – is merely the fact that the law prohibits it. This biblical approach introduces a highly

---

141 By "live according to nature" Seneca seems to be instructing to reach for the things which Nature has designed humans to desire; these things include health, safety, community, and other such things – available online at https://modernstoicism. com/what-does-living-in-accordance-with-nature-actually-mean-by-michel-daw/.

significant principle into the history of food ethics: the idea that certain food products are to be regarded as "contaminated" solely because of their origin. The contamination does in no way refer to unhealthy, tasteless, or indigestible food. It means the foods are unlawful in themselves.

The early Christian food ethics are ethics of *de-problematisation*. Be not anxious about food or drink, Jesus tells his followers: *No one is defiled by what goes into his mouth; only by what comes out of it ... Do you not see that whatever goes in by the mouth passes into the stomach and so is discharged at a certain place? But what comes out of the mouth has its origins in the heart; and that is what defiles a person* [Matthew 15: 11-17]. With this rejoinder he seems to abrogate most food restrictions. Setting all his hopes on the kingdom of heaven, Jesus simply urges his followers to lose all interest in food production and consumption.

Monastic versus "worldly" medieval life

The monastic food ethics elaborated during the Middle-Ages adhered to the Christian principle of disregard. Food in itself was seen as unimportant. In monastic regimes the focus was predominantly on the strengthening of self-discipline. The monastic nutrition approach grew into something of an obsession and abstaining from food intake became an objective in itself. Instead of functioning within the framework of a programme for moral exercise, food ethics now aimed at the mortification of the flesh and the extinction of all desire, as well as of all worldly involvement. Asceticism, in the sense of excessive abstention, became the rule and the ecclesiastical regulations had considerable impact on the food practices of the masses. Abstaining from meat was relatively widespread in the early church. It was praised when it was part of a temporary ascetic fasting regimen, but condemned if it amounted to a permanent rejection of animal foods [Zwart 2002; Frayne 2016].

Evagrius Ponticus (345-399), also called Evagrius the Solitary, was a Christian monk and ascetic. He defined and elucidated the eight kinds of evil thoughts that cause people to stumble in their race to heaven. These evil thoughts are gluttony, lust or fornication, avarice, sadness, anger, despondency or listlessness, vainglory, and pride. Later, in the west, they became the seven deadly sins. The order in which Evagrius lists the thoughts is deliberate. Gluttony and, right next to it, lust or fornication were associated from the very start of Christianity: ... *I should wonder at the Psychics, if they were enthralled to voluptuousness alone, which leads them to repeated marriages, if they were not likewise bursting with gluttony, which leads them to hate fasts...* [Lagerlund 2018].

Moreover, it was clear that the Christian tradition of the Middle-Ages followed the Stoics in their view on animals: ... *They don't have syntax, so we can eat them...* [Sorabji 1995]. They rejected the idea that animals have intrinsic moral value or even that they enter into the spheres of moral concern, since they lack reason. Many philosophers and theologians argued that humans have no obligation towards nature and can rule over it in whatever way they want [Lagerlund 2018].

But, in the sixteenth century, the monastic food ethics of mortification had become a principal target of moral criticism. Martin Luther (1483-1546) recommended the intake of food in large quantities as a remedy against temptation and melancholy. His contemporary Ignatius of Loyola (1491-1556), founder of the Jesuit order, also stressed the importance of a healthy and well-cared for body. The Renaissance rehabilitation of food intake is extremely clear in the astonishing novels of François Rabelais (1494-1553) featuring huge, healthy, vigorous giants, consuming enormous quantities of food – the very antipode of asceticism. Simultaneously, the Renaissance elite aimed at reviving the ancient Roman culinary tradition with its ravishingly abundant and exotic dishes. Very much in opposition to monastic life, the medieval worldly elite distinguished itself from the rural masses by consuming large quantities of meat. As Norbert Elias (1897-1990), the German sociologist who later became a British citizen pointed out: a civilization of food intake was to take place [Elias 1969]. It consisted of the gradual increase of delicacy and sensitivity, more particularly with regard to meat consumption.

The scientific approach: a new element in the food ethics of modernity

One of the emerging scientific practices in the 17th century was iatrophysics[142]. In 1614, the physician Sanctorio Sanctorio (1561–1636) published his famous masterpiece *Ars de Statica Medicina*. It consists of aphorisms that present the practical results of a series of weighing procedures rather than theoretical observations. Ars de Statica Medicina is the result of a large number of test series that Sanctorio carried out over ~30 years with the weighing chair he constructed himself in order to quantify the so-called *perspiratio insensibilis*, the insensible perspiration of the human body. He faithfully registered what happened – quantitatively speaking – when he was eating, drinking, sleeping, and having intercourse and by doing so he discovered, for example, that the most significant decrease of body weight occurs during sleep, while sexual intercourse is by far the most weight-consuming activity. Historical accounts of Sanctorio and his work tend to present him as a genial outsider who unexpectedly, almost out of the blue, invented a new medical science that profoundly influenced modernity [Hollerbach 2018 and references herein]. This new science is identified as either iatrophysics, iatromechanics or sometimes iatromathematics.

Modern dietetics, rather than being merely a scientific or medical endeavour also has a moral import. When Christoph Wilhelm Hufeland (1762-1836), a famous Prussian physician, published his book *Macrobiotics: The Art of Prolonging Life*, his focus was on a diet of natural and mostly vegetarian foods. The question how to extend one's own life is considered both from a medical and from a moral point of view. Hufeland understood macrobiotics as a medical philosophy that

---

142 Adherents of the first school were the Iatrophysicists, who attempted to explain fevers as the result of a defect in circulation. Iatrophysics was an attempt to view all things in nature, including animals, as though they were machines composed simply of matter in motion. Each of these moving parts, in turn, could be regarded as a smaller machine. The Iatrophysicists believed that, like all other machines, these living machines had to operate in accordance with mathematical laws. Therefore, they sought to define those laws, and, thereby, to describe precisely the mechanisms involved in life processes [Sigal 1978].

is geared towards preventing disease and prolonging life. He was not at all indoctrinated by the modern lipid hypothesis. The observation that people who live on more plant-based diets tend to have longer life spans is not some 20th century fabrication from the lipid hypothesis; it was observed at least as long ago as ancient Greece.

Dietetics was considered a moral endeavour insofar as it entails the systematic effort to subject one's sensuality to reason. So dietetics is the willingness to regulate one's life in accordance with self-ordained rules [Zwart 2000]. The influential philosopher Immanuel Kant (1724-1804) provided us with some personal dietetic experiences borrowed from daily self-observation. It is well-known, of course, that he excelled in living an extremely regular, orderly life in terms of time schedules for physical exercise and food intake. Even his mental work was accurately scheduled. In his *Metaphysik der Sitten*, Kant argued that it is morally illicit to benumb one's mind by the intake of excessive amounts of food or alcohol, thus depriving oneself of the use of one's intellectual faculties. The mere physical effects of consumption, however, in terms of well-being or health, are still regarded by him a matter of prudence rather than of practical reason.

The importance of the social dimension of food production and consumption is now recognised

According to Thomas Robert Malthus (1766-1834), there is a tendency in all animated life to increase beyond the nourishment available for it. Malthusianism is the idea that population growth is potentially exponential while the growth of the food supply is linear. In 1798, Malthus published anonymously *An essay on the principle of population as it affects the future improvement of society*. In his essay, he asked for attention to be paid to the disparity between the rate of population growth and the slower increase in the food supply. War, famine, and disease, he pointed out, were the eventual alternatives to the limitation of family size. It caused furious controversy and led him to prepare a more scholarly work. His second book, *An Essay on the Principle of Population; or, a view of its past and present effects on human happiness; with an enquiry into our prospects respecting the future removal or mitigation of the evils which it occasions*, published with acknowledged authorship in 1803, was a much larger sociological treatise deploying a mass of data in which political philosophy gave way to political economy and to the notion of moral restraint. The controversy continued. His publisher John Murray wrote: *It has been frequently remarked that no work has been so much talked of by persons who do not seem to have read it!* The book went through several editions and in 1830 he published a third work entitled *A summary view of the principle of population* [Dunn 1998].

Although his bleak view of the future actually proved incorrect, it clearly stimulated the awareness of the social dimensions of food ethics. In fact, the relationship between population increase and agriculture is still an important point of consideration [Zwart 2000].

Karl Marx (1818-1883) likewise focused on the social dimension of food. Moreover, in Marx's work attention is directed towards the production, rather than towards the consumption of food. The food products as such become the basic items of concern. They have become the incarnations of social tension and conflict. The rise of capitalism caused the destruction of the self-providing, rural communities of the past and greatly increased the distance between production and consumption. Thus, the food products generated by capitalism represent a basic experience of estrangement and alienation. In *The Jungle*, one of the best-known "muckraking" works that grew out of the Progressive Era of the early 20th century, Upton Sinclair (1878-1968) exemplifies the Marxist point of view by drawing out a dreadful picture of the Chicago meat industry in which millions of live creatures are turned into food every year.

One hundred years of literary wealth

As a result of technological and social changes in food practices, a series of critical novels and gloomy analyses of society have been published. These works raise public awareness and draw attention to ethical issues related to food production as well as food consumption They also constitute a basis for a better understanding of food ethics. The examples referred to are far from exhaustive, but they help provide a frame for the contemporary debate. The earlier mentioned Upton Sinclair revealed the terrible working conditions in the Chicago slaughterhouses run by the meat trusts. *Silent Spring*, Rachel Carson's remarkable work on the pesticide scandal published in 1962, led to the banning of DDT in the United States. This historic victory of a single individual against the lobbies of the chemical industry triggered the birth of the environmental movement in the early 1960s. Published in 1975, *Animal Liberation* by Peter Singer was to have a major impact on the emergence of animal ethics. Many readers became vegetarians or vegans and began to campaign against intensive breeding and experimenting with laboratory animals. Amartya Sen, the Indian economist who won the 1998 Nobel Prize in Economics, is well known for his book *Poverty and Famines: An Essay on Entitlements and Deprivation*, which led to the development of practical solutions to prevent or limit the effects of food shortages. Vandana Shiva examined the impact of the first green revolution on the wheat granary of India. In her convincing *The Violence of the Green Revolution - Third World Agriculture, Ecology and Politics* she showed how the promise of "quick wins" in terms of production has put aside the serious pursuit of an alternative agricultural strategy, based on respect for the environmental wisdom of peasant systems. Additionally, we are today all witnessing fierce competition in advertising and on supermarket shelves. In her fascinating *Food Politics: How the Food Industry Influences Nutrition and Health*, Marion Nestle takes a look behind the scenes to reveal how competition really works and how it affects our health [Goeyens 2019].

There are and will of course be many more other books and articles in many different languages. The selection that was made in the previous paragraph is merely my own and is therefore subjective. Books come ever faster and faster. Food ethics as a philosophical endeavour now includes work on animals and hunger. And there are several other themes: collective action, disgust, food justice and fair remuneration, food labelling, genetic modification, locavorism, obesity, diabetes, endocrine disrupting chemicals, etc.

Books help us to rediscover and never forget what is already known [Vogel 2018]. They underpin today's thinking and create the world in which posterity will live [Clifford 1876/1877].

Bibliography

Barnhill et al. [2018]. *The Oxford Handbook of Food Ethics*, Oxford University Press, pp. 802

Clifford [1876/1877]. The Ethics of Belief, *Contemporary Review* 29, 289-309

Dunn [1998]. Thomas Malthus (1766–1834): population growth and birth control, *Archives of Disease in Childhood-Fetal and Neonatal Edition* 78, 1, F76-F77

Elias [1969]. Über den Prozess der Zivilisation. Soziogenetische und Psychogenetische Untersuchungen, Francke Verlag, Bern and München, pp. 717

Frayne [2016]. On Imitating the Regimen of Immortality or Facing the Diet of Mortal Reality: A Brief History of Abstinence from Flesh-Eating in Christianity, Journal of Animal Ethics 6, 2, 188-212

Goeyens [2019]. Peur, incertitude et doute, in Susanne (ed.) *Les nouvelles Chaînes de Prométhée*, MEMOGRAMES éditions, Seneffe, 241-258

Hollerbach [2018]. The Weighing Chair of Sanctorius Sanctorius: A Replica, *NTM Zeitschrift für Geschichte der Wissenschaften, Technik und Medizin* 26, 2, 121-149

Lagerlund [2018]. Food Ethics in the Middle Ages, in Barnhill et al. (eds.) *The Oxford Handbook of Food Ethics*, Oxford University Press, pp. 802

Sigal [1978]. Fever Theory in the Seventeenth Century: Building Toward a Comprehensive Physiology, *The Yale Journal of Biology and Medicine* 51, 571-582

Sorabji [1995]. *Animal Minds and Human Morals, The Origins of the Western Debate*, Cornell University Press, Cornell Studies in Classical Philology, pp. 272

Vogel [2018]. A "rediscovered" drug against sleeping sickness gets the green light, *Science* 362, 6416, DOI: 10.1126/science.aaw0923

Zwart [2000]. A short history of food ethics, *Journal of Agricultural and Environmental Ethics* 12, 2, 113-126

Glossary

AR: antibiotic resistance
BADGE: bisphenol A diglycidyl ether
BHT: butylated hydroxytoluene
BMI: body mass index
BPA: bisphenol A
BPF: bisphenol F
BPS: bisphenol S
C: Celcius
CAP: Common Agricultural Policy
CAS: Chemical Abstracts Service
CMC: carboxymethyl cellulose
DBP: dibutyl phthalate
DEHP: bis(2-ethylhexyl) phthalate
DDE: 1,1-dichloro-2,2-bis(p-chlorophenyl) ethylene
DDT: 1,1'-(2,2,2-trichloroethane-1,1-diyl)bis(4-chlorobenzene)
DIPN: diisopropylnaphthalenes
DNA: deoxyribonucleic acid is the hereditary material in humans and almost all other organisms
ECHA: European Chemicals Agency
EDC: endocrine disrupting chemical
EFSA: European Food Safety Authority
EO: essential oil
ERF: European Risk Forum
ESC: Environment, Social and Governance
EU: European Union
EUIPO: European Union Intellectual Property Office
FAO: Food and Agriculture Organization
FCM: food contact material

FUD: fear, uncertainty and doubt
GA: gibberellins (plant hormones)
GHG: greenhouse gas
GMO: genetically modified organism
GPGP: Great Pacific garbage patch
HDL: high-density lipoprotein
IARC: International Agency for Research on Cancer
IPCC: Intergovernmental Panel on Climate Change
IQ: intelligence quotient
IRRI: International Rice Research Institute
JMPR: Joint FAO/WHO Meeting on Pesticide Residues
LDL: low-density lipoprotein
LED: light-emitting diode
LMIC: low- and middle-income countries
MOH: mineral oil hydrocarbons
MRL: maximum residue level
NHL: non-Hodgkin lymphoma
NIAS: non-intentionally added substance
NIDR: National Institute of Dental Research
NMDRC: non-monotonic dose-response curves
NOAEL: no observed adverse effect level
OML: overall migration limit
OSA: obstructive sleep apnea
OT: oxytocin
PC: polycarbonate
PCB: polychlorinated biphenyl
PET: polyethylene terephthalate
POEA: polyoxyethylene tallow amine
POP: persistent organic pollutant
PPO: polyphenol oxidase
PVAC: provitamin A carotenoids
RAS: Robotics and autonomous systems
RCOG: Royal College of Obstetricians and Gynecologists
RNA: ribonucleic acid
RNAi: RNA interference

SPI: soy protein isolate
SVHC: substance of very high concern
UN: United Nations
UNICEF: United Nations Children's Fund
UNICRI: United Nations Interregional Crime and Justice Research
   Institute
US: United States (of America)
USEPA: United States Environmental Protection Agency
USDA: US Department of Agriculture
US FDA: US Food and Drug Administration
VAD: vitamin A deficiency
VGS: Vertical Greenbox Solution
WEF: World Economic Forum
WHO: World Health Organisation

THIS BOOK IS BASED ON THE INVESTIGATIONS OF A GREAT MANY SCIENTISTS. TO QUOTE SIR ISAAC NEWTON: *"I STAND ON THE SHOULDERS OF GIANTS"*

Acknowledgments

I am very grateful to Michael Whitburn, Jean-Marie Mathot, and Pierre Klees. *Good and Bad Food Science. Separating the wheat from the chaff* would simply not have been possible without the stalwart support of these friends. Their generous encouragement and advice, their vision and creativity have contributed in various ways to making this book what it is. Michael taught English at university level for many years and has an excellent knowledge of several other languages. He proofread the manuscript and suggested changes to improve its readability. Jean-Marie is a famous artist who transforms his respect and affection for people into fascinating works of art. He managed to turn my perception and conviction into artistic illustrations. Pierre was trained as an expert in applied and management sciences and shows great interest in the philosophical and ethical trends of our modern world. Fascinated by the developments of food chemistry and food ethics, it was he who wrote the preface to this book.

I would be a serious lack of gratitude on my part if I did not express my deepest appreciation to the members of the department of Analytical and Environmental Chemistry at the *Vrije Universiteit Brussel*. I first started working there as an environmental chemist and soon realised that there is an inherent link between environmental quality and human health. *Reason and Engage* is my university's motto – a motto which I endorse unreservedly.

My heartfelt gratitude goes out to my thoughtful and passionate editor Nienke Roelants at Academic & Scientific Publishers in Brussels.

A huge thank-you also to my dear wife, Lieve. She knows what it means to live with a scientist who spends much of his time reading books or interacting with his computer. Her ability to understand and share my feelings is particularly heartwarming.

While preparing the manuscript for the book my thoughts were often with our beloved late daughter, Karen. There was hardly a day when I did not think about how much she must have suffered as she fought her losing battle against cancer. No one will ever be able to tell me precisely which chemical cocktail undermined her health. Today, it is my sincerest hope that one day we will be able to alleviate and better still, put an end to the pain that chemical cocktails can cause.

Leo Goeyens
February, 2019